Stedman's ENDOCRINOLOGY WORDS

Stedman's

ENDOCRINOLOGY WORDS

LIPPINCOTT
WILLIAMS
& WILKINS

Series Editor: Beverly J. Wolpert
Associate Managing Editor: Trista A. DiPaula
Associate Managing Editor: William A. Howard
Art Director: Jennifer Clements
Production Manager: Julie K. Stegman
Production Coordinator: Kevin Iarossi
Typesetter: Peirce Graphic Services, Inc.
Printer & Binder: Victor Graphics, Inc.

351 West Camden Street
Baltimore, MD 21201-2436

Printed in the United States of America

2001

Library of Congress Cataloging-in-Publication Data

Stedman's endocrinology words.
p. ; cm.
ISBN 0-7817-3339-1 (alk. paper)
1. Endocrinology—Terminology. I. Title: Endocrinology words. II. Stedman, Thomas Lathrop, 1853–1938.
[DNLM: 1. Endocrine Glands—Terminology—English. 2. Endocrine Diseases—Terminology—English. WK 15 S812 2001]
RC649.S74 2001
616.4'001'4—dc21

2001029224

01
1 2 3 4 5 6 7 8 9 10

Contents

Acknowledgments

An important part of our editorial process is the involvement of medical transcriptionists—as advisors, reviewers, and/or editors.

We extend special thanks to Sandy Kovacs, CMT; and Patricia White, CMT for editing the manuscript, helping resolve many difficult questions, and contributing material for the appendix sections. We also extend special thanks to our Editorial Advisory Board members, including Natasha Brown; Marty Cantu, CMT; Patty Gibson; and Nancy Hill, MT, who were instrumental to the development of this reference. They recommended sources and provided valuable judgment, insights, and perspectives.

We also extend thanks to Jeanne Bock, CSR, MT, for working on the appendix, as well as to Natasha Brown for performing the final prepublication review. Other important contributors to this edition include Ellen Atwood; Elana Bergan; Sherry G. Crawford, MT; Shemah Fletcher; Elizabeth Willard Gorsline, CMT; Deborah B. Hahn, CMT; Kathy Hess, CMT; Darcy Johnson; Robin Koza; Cheryl A. Letner, CMT; Heather Little, CMT; Kathryn C. Mason, CMT; Cheryl Miller; Cheri Sawyer, CMT; Jenifer F. Walker; MA; Sandra Wideburg, CMT; DéBorah Wiggins; Mary Chiara Zaratkiewicz; and Diane LeMieux Zook, CMT.

Barb Ferretti played an integral role in the process by reviewing the content files for format, updating the database, and providing a final quality check.

As with all our *Stedman's* word references, this resource incorporates the suggestions and expertise of our many contacts in the medical transcriptionist community. Thanks to all of our advisory board participants, reviewers, and editors; AAMT meeting attendees; and others who have written us with requests and comments—keep talking, and we'll keep listening.

Editor's Preface

Do you love new reference books? I certainly do. I am a book junkie, and when I was asked to work on an endocrinology word book, I did not hesitate to agree. After transcribing for 23 years, I am still amazed that new diseases, medications, procedures, and equipment are being discovered daily. Since I have been working for a national medical transcription service for over five years, I have become keenly aware that transcribing alone enhances the need for complete reference materials where words can be found quickly.

Unfortunately, the number of cases of type 2 diabetes mellitus in adults, as well as in children as young as 10 is growing at an alarming rate. My partner in developing this book, Patricia White, CMT, has been a great asset to me in deciding what words belong in this edition. We have included an extensive list of insulin preparations, insulin pumps, pens, monitors, and other equipment used to aid the diabetic in assessing and controlling blood sugar. As there are many systemic side effects of diabetes, terminology relating to diabetic eye disease, neuropathy, and nephropathy has been included.

Diabetes is not the only disease that is considered an endocrinology anomaly. Thyroid diseases occur in many forms, and we have included terms relating to hypothyroidism, hyperthyroidism, thyroid eye disease, Hashimoto disease, and thyroid cancers, plus pituitary abnormalities, birth defects, and gender anomalies.

You will also find an extensive list of hormones, terms relating to the male and female reproductive system, and laboratory and diagnostic studies performed for accurate diagnosis, as well as medications and treatment regimens prescribed by the treating physicians.

An often forgotten but very useful section is the appendix. There are many detailed illustrations, which will help you understand the meaning of the difficult terminology encountered when transcribing endocrinology reports. Sometimes a picture is definitely worth a thousand words!

Thanks to Lippincott Williams & Wilkins for listening to medical transcriptionists and going forth with the publication of this first edition. I also have the privilege of working with Trista DiPaula, and I appreciate her continual support and guidance in preparing this book.

I have a test that I use when assessing a new reference book. If I can find just one word in that book that I cannot find in other references, then it was definitely worth the price. I certainly hope you find the word you are looking for in this book.

Sandy Kovacs, CMT

Publisher's Preface

Stedman's Endocrinology Words offers an authoritative assurance of quality and exactness to the wordsmiths of the healthcare professions—medical transcriptionists, medical editors and copyeditors, health information management personnel, court reporters, and the many other users and producers of medical documentation.

In *Stedman's Endocrinology Words,* users will find thousands of words as they relate to the thyroid, diabetes, and hormones. Users will also find terms for protocols, diagnostic and therapeutic procedures, new techniques, and lab tests, as well as equipment names, and abbreviations with their expansions. The appendix sections provide anatomical illustrations with useful captions and labels, sample reports, and common terms by procedure, as well as normal lab values, endocrine glands and associated products, diabetes classifications, and drugs by indication.

This compilation of more than 55,000 entries, fully cross-indexed for quick access, was built from a base vocabulary of approximately 36,000 medical words, phrases, abbreviations, and acronyms. The extensive A-Z list was developed from manufacturers' literature, scientific reports, books, journals, CDs, and websites (please see list of References on page xvi).

We at Lippincott Williams & Wilkins strive to provide you with the most up-to-date and accurate word references available. Your use of this word book will prompt new editions, which we will publish as often as updates and revisions justify. We welcome your suggestions for improvements, changes, corrections, and additions—whatever will make this *Stedman's* product more useful to you. Please complete the postpaid card at the back of this book, and send your recommendations care of "Stedman's" at Lippincott Williams & Wilkins.

Explanatory Notes

Medical transcription is an art as well as a science. Both approaches are needed to correctly interpret the dictation of a physician, whose language is a product of education, training, and experience. This variety in medical language means that there are several acceptable ways to express certain terms, including jargon. *Stedman's Endocrinology Words* provides variant spellings and phrasings for many terms. These elements, in addition to complete cross-indexing, make *Stedman's Endocrinology Words* a valuable resource for determining the validity of terms as they are encountered.

Alphabetical Organization

Alphabetization of main entries is letter by letter as spelled, ignoring punctuation, spaces, prefixed numbers, or other special characters. For example:

insulin-producing cell
insulin promoter factor 1
insulin-receptor antibody

Terms beginning with Greek letters show the Greek letters spelled out and listed alphabetically. For example:

beta, β
b. blocker
b. cell replacement
follitropin b.

In subentry alphabetization, the abbreviated singular form or the spelled-out plural form of the noun main entry word is ignored.

Format and Style

All main entries are in **boldface** to expedite locating a sought-after term, to enhance distinction between main entries and subentries, and to relieve the textual density of the pages.

Irregular plurals and variant spellings are shown on the same line as the singular or preferred form of the word. For example:

canaliculus, pl. canaliculi
curette, curet

Hyphenation

As a rule of style, multiple eponyms (e.g., Mears-Rubash approach) are hyphenated. Also, hyphens have been added between a manufacturer and one or more eponyms (e.g., Vital-Metzenbaum dissecting scissors). Please note that in many cases, hyphenation is a question of style, not of accuracy, and thus is a matter of choice.

Possessives

Possessive forms have been dropped in this reference for the sake of consistency and conformance with the guidelines of the American Association for Medical Transcription (AAMT) and other groups. Please note, however, that in many cases, retaining the possessive, like hyphenating, is a question of style, not of accuracy, and thus is a matter of choice. To form the possessive of a word, simply add the apostrophe or apostrophe "s" to the end of the word.

Cross-indexing

The word list is in an index-like main entry-subentry format that contains two combined alphabetical listings:

(1) A *noun* main entry-subentry organization, which is typical of the A-Z section of medical dictionaries like *Stedman's:*

neck
- n. of pancreas
- webbed n.

fluid
- amniotic f.
- bloody f.

(2) An *adjective* main entry-subentry organization, which lists words and phrases as you hear them. The main entries are the adjectives or modifiers in a multiword term. The subentries are the nouns around which the terms are constructed and to which the adjectives or modifiers pertain:

red
- r. blood cell (RBC)
- r. bone marrow

hypoplastic
- h. gland
- h. mandible

This format provides the user with more than one way to locate and identify a multiword term. For example:

benign
b. nodular goiter

goiter
benign nodular g.

anterior
a. pituitary lobe

lobe
anterior pituitary l.

net
n. calcium absorption

absorption
net calcium a.

It also allows the user to see together all terms that contain a particular descriptor, as well as all types, kinds, or variations of a noun entity. For example:

enzyme
e. defect
e. deficiency
deiodinase e.

thyroid
t. axis.
t. biopsy
black t.

Wherever possible, abbreviations are separately defined and cross-referenced. For example:

SPA
single-photon absorptiometry

single-photon
s.-p. absorptiometry (SPA)

absorptiometry
single-photon a. (SPA)

References

In addition to the manufacturers' literature we gather at various medical meetings, scientific reports from hospitals, and the lists of our MT Editorial Advisory Board members from their daily transcription work, we used the following sources for new terms in *Stedman's Endocrinology Words:*

Books

Becker KL, Bilezikian JP, Bremner WJ, Hung W, Kahn CR, Loriaux DL, Nylen ES, Rebar RW, Robertson GL, Wartofsky L. Principles and Practice of Endocrinology and Metabolism, 3rd Edition. Baltimore: Lippincott Williams & Wilkins, 2000.

Braverman LE, Utiger RD, eds. Werner and Ingbar's, The Thyroid: A Fundamental and Clinical Text, 8th Edition. Philadelphia: Lippincott Williams & Wilkins, 2000.

Burch WM. Endocrinology, 3rd Edition. Baltimore: Lippincott Williams & Wilkins, 1994.

Bushinsky DA. Renal Osteodystrophy. Philadelphia: Lippincott-Raven Publishers, 1998.

Copeland EM, Bland KI, Deitch EA, Eberlein TJ, Howard RJ, Luce EA, Seeger JM, Souba WW, Sugarbaker DJ. Year Book of Surgery 2000. St. Louis: Mosby, 2000.

Falk SA. Thyroid Disease, 2nd Edition. Philadelphia: Lippincott-Raven Publishers, 1997.

Gass GH, Kaplan HM, eds. Handbook of Endocrinology, 2nd Edition, Volumes 1 & 2. Boca Raton: CRC Press, 1996.

Greenspan FS, Strewler GJ. Basic & Clinical Endocrinology, 5th Edition. New York: McGraw-Hill, 1997.

Guyton AC, Hall JE. Human Physiology and Mechanisms of Disease, 6th Edition. Philadelphia: Saunders, 1996.

Guyton AC, Hall JE. Textbook of Medical Physiology, 9th Edition. Philadelphia: Saunders, 1995.

Kahn CR, Weir GC, eds. Joslin's Diabetes Mellitus, 13th Edition. Philadelphia: Lea & Febiger, 1994.

Kacsoh B. Endocrine Physiology. New York: McGraw-Hill, 2000.

Kettyle WM, Arky RA. Lippincott's Pathophysiology Series: Endocrine Pathophysiology. Philadelphia: Lippincott-Raven Publishers, 1998.

Krisht A, Tindall G. Pituitary Disorders. Baltimore: Lippincott Williams & Wilkins, 1998.

Lance LL. 2000 Quick Look Drug Book. Baltimore: Lippincott Williams & Wilkins, 2000.

LeRoith D, Taylor SI, Olefsky JM. Diabetes Mellitus, 2nd Edition. Baltimore: Lippincott Williams & Wilkins, 2000.

Martin CR. Dictionary of Endocrinology and Related Biomedical Sciences. Oxford: Oxford University Press, 1995.

McDermott MT. Endocrine Secrets, 2nd Edition. Philadelphia: Hanley & Belfus, Inc., 1998.

Pyle V. Current Medical Terminology, 8th Edition. Modesto: Health Professions Institute, 2000.

Speroff K, Glass RH, Kase NG. Clinical Gynecologic Endocrinology and Infertility, 6th Edition. Philadelphia: Lippincott Williams & Wilkins, 1999.

Stedman's Medical Dictionary, 27th Edition. Baltimore: Lippincott Williams & Wilkins, 2000.

Tessier C. The AAMT Book of Style. Modesto: AAMT, 1995.

Weintraub BD. Molecular Endocrinology. New York: Raven Press, Ltd., 1994.

Wilson JD, Foster DW, Kronenberg HM, Larsen PR. Williams Textbook of Endocrinology, 9th Edition. Philadelphia: Saunders, 1998.

Journals

Current Opinion in Endocrinology and Diabetes. Philadelphia: Lippincott Williams & Wilkins, 1999–2000.

The Endocrinologist. Baltimore: Lippincott Williams & Wilkins, 1994–1999.

Endocrinology. Bethesda: The Endocrine Society, 2000.

Internal Medicine. Montvale, NJ: Medical Economics. 1996–1997.

Menopause. Baltimore: Lippincott Williams & Wilkins, 1999–2000.

Molecular Endocrinology. Bethesda: The Endocrine Society, 2000.

Pancreas. Philadelphia: Lippincott Williams & Wilkins, 1999–2000.

CDs

UpToDate Clinical Reference Library on CD, Version 8:2. Wellesley, MA: UpToDate, 2000.

Websites

http://diabetes.about.com

http://www.aace.com

http://www.diabetesnet.com

http://www.diabetes.org/professionalpublications

http://www.endo.edoc.com

http://www.endocrine.medscape.com/Medscape/features/JournalScan/public/index_JournalScan.html

http://www.eurothyroid.org

http://hpisum.com

http://www.jdf.org

http://www.mtdesk.com/newterms.shtml

http://www.niddk.nih.gov

http://www.thyroid.org

NOTES

A

α (*var. of* alpha)
α_1 (*var. of* alpha$_1$)
α_2 (*var. of* alpha$_2$)
A
alpha-preprotachykinin A
Aquasol A
beta-hydroxy-beta-methylglutaryl-coenzyme A (HMG-CoA)
beta-preprotachykinin A
botulinum toxin type A
A cell
chromogranin A
coenzyme A (CoA)
cyclosporin A
gamma-preprotachykinin A
hemoglobin A
hemophilia A
hepatitis A
hypervitaminosis A
immunoglobulin A (IgA)
inhibin A
neurokinin A
Orexin A
platelet-derived growth factor A (PDGF-A)
proenkephalin A
protein kinase A (PKA)
A-1
apoprotein A-1
A2
thromboxane A2 (TXA2, TxA2)
A9
coxsackievirus A9
A23187
Ca^{2+} ionophore A23187
A_4
leukotriene A_4 (LTA_4)
A_1
A_1 cell
vitamin A_1
A_2
A_2 cell
phospholipase A_2 (PLA_2)
vitamin A_2
A_0
hemoglobin A_0
A_{1c}
glycated hemoglobin A_{1c}
hemoglobin A_{1c} (HbA1c)
A_{1b}
hemoglobin A_{1b}
$A1_c$
spuriously elevated hemoglobin $A1_c$
(a)
lipoprotein (a)
1a
a
phosphorylase *a*
AA
arachidonic acid
platelet-derived growth factor AA
A_1a
hemoglobin A_1a
AA-NAT
arylalkylamine *N*-acetyltransferase
AASH
adrenal androgen-stimulating hormone
AAV
adeno-associated virus
Ab
antibody
anti-IL-2R Ab
antiinterleukin-2 antibody
TPO Ab
thyroperoxidase antibody
A_1b
hemoglobin A_1b
ABA
abscisic acid
AB amyloidosis
abarelix
Abbott AxSYM assay
ABCD
avidin-biotin complex assay
abciximab
abdominal
a. obesity
a. paracentesis
a. stria
abdominoperineal resection
abducent nerve
aberrant
a. behavior
a. expression
a. mediastinal thyroid tissue
a. motility
a. ribonucleic acid
abetalipoproteinemia
recessive a.
abiotic
a. environmental factor
ablation
alcohol a.
cell-specific a.
ovarian a.
thyroidal a.
abluminal compartment
abnormal
a. ocular movement
a. parathyroid gland

abnormal *(continued)*
a. regulation of calcium-dependent parathyroid hormone secretion
a. set point
abnormality
congenital a.
craniofacial a.
endocrine a.
gastric myoelectric a.
multiple endocrine a.'s (MEA)
primary immunoregulatory a.
pupillary a.
receptor-binding a.
set point a.
skeletal a.
thyroid-stimulating hormone a.
abortion
spontaneous a. (SAB)
ABP
androgen-binding protein
abscess
amebic brain a.
gas-containing a.
parathyroidal a.
peritonsillar a.
abscisic acid (ABA)
abscissa
absence of nocturnal TSH surge
Absidia
absolute
a. leptin deficiency
a. leptin resistance
a. thyroidal uptake rate
absorbable gelatin film roll
absorptiometry
dual-energy x-ray a. (DEXA, DXA)
dual-photon a.
dual-x-ray a.
single-photon a. (SPA)
absorption
calcium a.
enhanced proximal tubular salt a.
enteral aluminum a.
gastrointestinal calcium a.
insulin a.
net calcium a.
salt a.
absorptive
a. endocytosis
a. hypercalciuria
abzyme
AC
Pepcid AC
Robafen AC
acalculous cholecystitis
acanthosis
a. nigricans (AN)
acarbose
ACAT
acyl-coenzyme A cholesterol acyltransferase
ACC
acinar cell carcinoma
ACC_β
acetyl-CoA carboxylase
accelerated
a. catabolism
a. thyrotoxicosis
Accelerator
Triax Metabolic A.
accessory
a. adrenocortical rest
a. molecule
a. olfactory bulb (AOB)
Access Ostase blood test
acclimation
acclimatization
accommodative target
accretion
bone mass a.
bone mineral a.
Accu-Chek
A.-C. Advantage glucose meter
A.-C. Advantage glucose meter system
A.-C. Advantage non-wipe blood glucose monitoring system
A.-C. Complete blood glucose monitoring system
A.-C. Complete glucose meter system
A.-C. II Freedom
A.-C. II Freedom system
A.-C. III
A.-C. Instant glucose meter
A.-C. Instant glucose meter system
A.-C. InstantPlus
A.-C. InstantPlus system
A.-C. Simplicity blood glucose monitoring system
A.-C. SoftClix lancet device
accuDEXA bone mineral assessment device
Acculink Modem
accumulation
aluminum a.
osteoid a.
visceral fat a.
accurate pacemaker
Accutane
Accutility Software
ACE
angiotensin-converting enzyme
acebutolol
acellular desquamated keratin

Acephen
acervulus, pl. **acervuli**
acervuli cerebri
Acesulfame K
Aceta
acetaminophen
a. and codeine
oxycodone and a.
a. and phenyltoloxamine
propoxyphene and a.
acetaminophen, aspirin, and caffeine
acetate
buserelin a.
calcium a.
cortisone a.
Cortone A.
[13C]-a. test
cyproterone a.
depot medroxyprogesterone a. (DMPA)
desmopressin a.
estradiol/norethindrone a.
Florinef A.
leuprolide a.
medroxyprogesterone a. (MPA)
megestrol a. (MA)
nomegestrole a.
norethindrone a.
paramethasone a.
pexiganan a.
pramlintide a.
sermorelin a.
sodium a.
acetazolamide
Acetest
acetoacetate
acetoacetic acid
acetoacetyl-CoA
a.-C. thiolase
acetohexamide
acetylate
acetylation
histone a.
acetylcholine (ACh)
a. receptor (AChR)
acetyl-CoA
a.-CoA carboxylase (ACC_β)
a.-CoA deficiency
acetyl-coenzyme A
acetylcysteine
acetylglucosamine
acetylsalicylic acid
acetyltransferase
bacterial chloramphenicol a.
choline a. (ChAT)
histone a. (HAT)
***N*-acetyltransferase**
arylalkylamine *N*-a. (AA-NAT)
ACh
acetylcholine
ACh receptor-inducing activity (ARIA)
achalasia
Aches-N-Pain
achillean xanthoma
Achilles reflex
achlorhydria
gastric a.
syndrome of watery diarrhea, hypokalemia, and a.
watery diarrhea, hypokalemia, a. (WDHA)
achondrogenesis type II
achondroplasia
AChR
acetylcholine receptor
acid
aberrant ribonucleic a.
abscisic a. (ABA)
acetoacetic a.
acetylsalicylic a.
3′,5′ adenylic a.
alanine amino a.
alpha-amino-3-hydroxy-5methyl-4-isoxazole propionic a.
amino a.
aminoisobutyric a. (AIB)
antidouble-stranded deoxyribonucleic a.
arachidonic a. (AA)
ascorbic a.
a. ash diet
aspartic a.
azaprostanoic a.
bile a.
branched-chain amino a.
calcitroic a.
carbonic a.
a. cholesteryl ester hydrolase deficiency
9-*cis* retinoic a. (RXR)
13-*cis* retinoic a.
citric a.

NOTES

acid *(continued)*
complementary deoxyribonucleic a. (cDNA)
deoxyribonucleic a. (DNA)
dicarboxylic a.
dihomo-gamma-linoleic a.
2′4-dihydroxybenzoic a.
dihydroxymandelic a. (DOMA)
dihydroxyphenylacetic a. (DOPAC)
4,4′-di-isothiocyanatostilbene-2,2′-disulfonic a. (DIDS)
dimercaptosuccinic a. (DMSA, DMSA-V-Tc99-m)
docosahexaenoic a. (DHA)
edetic a.
eicosapentaenoic a. (EPA)
ergogenic a.
essential fatty a. (EFA)
ethacrynic a.
ethylenediaminetetraacetic a. (EDTA)
excitatory amino a.
fatty a.
ferrous salt and ascorbic a.
ferrous sulfate, ascorbic acid, vitamin B complex, and folic a.
fibric a.
flufenemic a.
folic a.
gamma-aminobutyric a. (GABA)
gamma-carboxyglutamic a. (GLA, Gla)
gamma-carboxylated glutamic a.
gamma-linolenic a. (GLA)
glucuronic a.
glutamic a.
glycyrrhetinic a.
glycyrrhizinic a.
homogentisic a.
homovanillic a. (HVA)
hyaluronic a.
5-hydroperoxyeicosatetraenoic a. (5-HPETE)
12-hydroperoxyeicosatetraenoic a. (12-HPETE)
hydrophobic amino a.
hydroxyeicosatetraenoic a. (HETE)
5-hydroxyeicosatetraenoic a.
12-hydroxyeicosatetraenoic a. (12-HETE)
15-hydroxyeicosatetraenoic a.
2-hydroxyglutaric a.
5-hydroxyindoleacetic a. (5-HIAA)
hydroxyisovaleric a.
13-hydroxyoctadecadienoic a. (13-HODE)
iodoamino a.
iopanoic a.
isobutyric a.
isovaleric a.
lactic a.
L-alpha-aminomethyl-encyclopropylproprionic a.
linoleic a.
mefenamic a.
messenger ribonucleic a. (mRNA)
5-methoxyindoleacetic a.
2-methylbutyric a.
methylmalonic a.
mitochondrial deoxyribonucleic a. (mDNA, mtDNA)
monosaturated fatty a.
nalidixic a.
nicotinic a.
N-methyl D-aspartic a.
nondissociated a.
nonesterified fatty a. (NEFA)
okadaic a.
oleic a.
omega-3 polyunsaturated fatty a.
orotic a.
palmitic a.
palmitoleic a.
pantothenic a.
paraaminobenzoic a.
paraaminosalicylic a.
peracetic a.
a. phosphatase deficiency
phosphatidic a.
potassium citrate and citric a.
pyroglutamic a.
pyrophosphoric a.
a. resistant/coated preparation
resorcyclic a.
retinoic a.
ribonucleic a. (RNA)
sialic a.
small nuclear ribonucleic a. (snRNA)
a. solochrome azurin
stearic a.
sulfhydryl amino a.
technetium-99m dimercaptosuccinic a. (^{99m}Tc-DMSA)
tetraiodoacetic a.
tetraiodothyroacetic a.
thyroacetic a.
tiglic a.
tranexamine a.
transfer ribonucleic a. (tRNA)
trans-retinoic a. (RAR)
tricarboxylic a. (TCA)
triiodoacetic a.
triiodothyroacetic a.
3,5,3′-triiodothyroacetic a. (TRIAC)

A

unesterified arachidonic a.
unsaturated fatty a.
uric a.
ursodeoxycholic a. (UDCA)
valproic a.
vanillylmandelic a. (VMA)
vitamin B complex with vitamin C and folic a.

acid-base balance

acidemia
glutaric a. type II
isovaleric a.
methylmalonic a.
propionic a.

acidic fibroblast growth factor (aFGF)

acidification

acid-labile subunit (ALS)

acidophil
mammotrope a.
somatotroph a.

acidophilic
a. adenoma
a. cell
a. tumor

acidophilus
lactobacillus a.

acidosis
aldosterone-deficient hyperkalemic a.
anion-gap a.
chronic metabolic a.
hyperchloremic metabolic a. (HCMA)
lactic a.
metabolic a.
nonketotic hypoglycemic a.
renal tubular a. (RTA)
respiratory a.
type 4 renal tubular a.
uncompensated metabolic a.
uremic metabolic a.

acidotic coma

acid-Schiff
periodic a.-S. (PAS)
a.-S. reaction
a.-S. stain

acid-Schiff-positive
periodic a.-S.-p.

acid-stable protein

aciduria
argininosuccinic a.
methylmalonic a.
propionic a.
pyroglutamic a.

acinar
a. cell carcinoma (ACC)
a. gland

acinus, pl. **acini**
glandular acini

Aciphex

acipimox

ackee tree

ACL
acromegaly, cutis verticis, leukoma
ACL syndrome

acne
cystic a.
steroid a.

acneiform eruption

acquired
a. diabetes insipidus
a. end-organ resistance
a. hypogonadotropic hypogonadism
a. immune deficiency
a. immune deficiency syndrome (AIDS)
a. immunity
a. immunodeficiency syndrome (AIDS)
a. immunodeficiency syndrome-related complex
a. organification defect
a. perforating dermatosis (APD)
a. von Willebrand disease (AvWD)

acral
a. enlargement
a. overgrowth

acrodermatitis

acrodynia

acrodysostosis

acromegalic
a. feature
a. patient
a. rosary
a. symptom

acromegaloidism

acromegaly
a., cutis verticis, leukoma (ACL)
a., cutis verticis, leukoma syndrome
ectopic a.
hypothalamic a.
pituitary tumor-related a.

acromelic shortening

acroosteolysis

NOTES

acropachy
thyroid a.
acrophase
acrosin
acrosomal
a. cap
a. enzyme
a. reaction
a. vesicle
acrosome
a. phase
a. reaction
Act
Medicare Bone Mass Measurement Standardization A.
Actagen-C
ACTH
adrenocorticotrophin hormone
adrenocorticotropic hormone
ACTH hypersecretion
ACTH resistance
Acthar
ACTH-dependent Cushing syndrome
ACTH-independent
A.-i. bilateral macronodular hyperplasia (AIBH)
A.-i. Cushing syndrome
ACTH-producing thymoma
Acthrel
actin
a. fibril
a. filament
a. scavenger system
actin-binding protein
actin-myosin complex
Actinobacillus actinomycetemcomitans
Actinomyces
A. naeslundii
actinomyces
actinomycetemcomitans
Actinobacillus a.
actinomycin-D
actinomycosis
action
altered androgen a.
antigonadotropic a.
antinociceptive a.
antipsoriatic a.
autocrine a.
extracellular cathepsin a.
glucocorticoid a.
hemocrine a.
hypotriglyceridemic a.
insulin a.
intracrine a.
nongenomic a.
paracrine a.
phosphaturic a.
pituitary resistance to thyroid hormone a.
a. potential
thyroid hormone a.
thyromimetic a.
Action-II
Actiprofen
Actiq
A. Oral Transmucosal
activated
a. Hageman factor
a. protein C resistance
activating
a. cytokine
a. factor
activation
adrenergic receptor a.
B-cell a.
ectopic intrapancreatic protease a.
a. energy
gonadotropin-releasing hormone a.
G protein a.
neutrophil a.
purinergic a.
steroid hormone receptor a.
activational hormone
activator
allosteric a.
kallikrein a.
plasminogen a.
a. protein-1 (AP-1)
a. protein-1 element
tissue plasminogen a. (TPA)
tissue-type plasminogen a.
urokinase plasminogen a.
urokinase-type plasminogen a.
active
a. immunity
a. renin
a. salt transport
a. variceal hemorrhage
a. vitamin D_3
Activelle
activin
a. cell-surface receptor type I
a. cell-surface receptor type II
a. receptor (ActR)
a. receptor I (ActRI)
a. receptor IB (ActRIB)
a. receptor II (ActRII)
a. receptor IIB (ActRIIB)
a. signaling
activinlike receptor kinase
activin-nonresponsive pituitary tumor
activity
ACh receptor-inducing a. (ARIA)
adenylate cyclase a.
adenylyl cyclase a.

adrenomedullary a.
1-alpha-hydroxylase a.
5-alpha-reductase a. (5α-RA)
anticonvulsive a.
antidiuretic a.
antirachitic a.
bactericidal a.
baroreflex a.
calorigenic a.
carbonic anhydrase a.
differentiation-inhibiting a.
epileptiform a.
fibrinolytic a.
hCG-modulated thyroid a.
human chorionic gonadotropin-modulated thyroid activity
hepatic fibrogenic a.
hepatic lipase a.
high-impact a.
histone deacetylase a.
human chorionic gonadotropin-modulated thyroid a. (hCG-modulated thyroid activity)
increased adenyl cyclase a.
insulinlike a. (ILA)
melanoma growth stimulatory a. (MGSA)
monodeiodinase a.
5′-monodeiodinase a.
monodeiodination a.
neutrophil respiratory burst a. (NRBA)
nonsuppressible insulinlike a. (NSILA)
osteoclast a.
osteoclastic a.
phagocytic a.
phosphatase a.
plasma aldosterone concentration/plasma renin a. (PAC/PRA)
plasma renin a. (PRA)
plasmin renin a. (PRA)
platelet a.
postreceptor pyruvate dehydrogenase a.
protein-dimerizing a.
proteolytic a.
receptor tyrosine kinase a.
a. rhythm
serum vasopressinase a.
stromal osteoclast-forming a. (SOFA)
suppressed plasma renin a.
thyroid peroxidase a.
thyroid trapping a.
transmembrane Ser/Total hip replacement kinase a.
tyrosine kinase a.
uterine contractile a.

Actonel

Actos

ActR
activin receptor

ActRI
activin receptor I

ActRIB
activin receptor IB

ActRII
activin receptor II

ActRIIB
activin receptor IIB

Actron

acuity
visual a.

Acular Ophthalmic

Acusyst-Xcell monoclonal antibody culturing system

acute
a. addisonian crisis
a. arterial occlusion
a. fatty liver of pregnancy
a. gouty arthritis
a. hemorrhagic pancreatitis (AHP)
a. infectious hepatitis
a. insulin response (AIR)
a. insulin response testing
a. lymphoblastic leukemia
a. lymphocytic leukemia (ALL)
a. lymphocytic thyroiditis
a. myelogenous leukemia
a. necrotizing pancreatitis
a. phase reactant
a. phase response (APR)
a. phase response syndrome
A. Physiology and Chronic Health Evaluation (APACHE, APACHE II)
a. primary hyperparathyroidism
a. recurrent pancreatitis (ARP)
a. streptococcal gangrene
a. suppurative thyroiditis
a. uric acid nephropathy

NOTES

acute *(continued)*
a. water intoxication
a. Wolff-Chaikoff effect
Acutrim
A. 16 Hour
A. II, Maximum Strength
A. Late Day
acyclovir
acylcarnitine
fatty a.
acyl-CoA
long chain fatty a.-C. (LCFA-CoA)
acyl-coenzyme A cholesterol acyltransferase (ACAT)
acyltransferase
acyl-coenzyme A cholesterol a. (ACAT)
alpha-glycerophosphate a.
lecithin-cholesterol a. (LCAT)
AD
androstenedione
AD-36 adenovirus
ADA
adenosine deaminase
American Diabetes Association
Adagen
adamantinomatous
a. craniopharyngioma
adaptation
hypothermic cold a.
adaptational response
adaptor protein
ADCC
antibody-dependent cell cytotoxicity
antibody-dependent cellular cytotoxicity
ADD1
adipocyte determination and differentiation factor-1
add-back regimen
Adderall
Addison disease
addisonian crisis
adduct
ketamine a.
Adeflor
ADEKs pediatric drops
adenine
a. nucleotide translocase
a. phosphoribosyltransferase
a. phosphoribosyltransferase deficiency
adeno-associated virus (AAV)
adenocarcinoma
mucin-producing a.
pancreatic a. (PAC)
adenocyst
adenohypophysial, adenohypophyseal
a. capillary
a. corticotroph cell
a. gangliocytoma
a. hormone
a. neuronal choristoma
a. system
adenohypophysial-thyroid axis
adenohypophysis
adenoid
a. appearance
a. facies
adenoma
acidophilic a.
adrenal a.
adrenocortical a.
adrenocorticotropic hormone cell a.
aldosterone-producing a. (APA)
aldosterone-secreting a.
alpha subunit-secreting pituitary a.
basophilic a.
C cell a.
chromophobe a.
chromophobic a.
clinically nonfunctioning pituitary a. (CNFA)
colloid a.
corticotroph a.
corticotropin-secreting a.
cortisol-producing cortical a.
cortisol-secreting a.
dense staining of a.
ectopic adrenal a.
ectopic pituitary a.
embryonal a.
endocrine-inactive pituitary a.
fetal a.
follicular a.
gangliocytoma-pituitary a.
GH cell a.
growth hormone cell adenoma
GH-secreting pituitary a.
growth hormone-secreting pituitary adenoma
giant invasive pituitary a.
glycoprotein-producing a.
gonadotrope a.
gonadotroph cell a.
gonadotroph pituitary a.
gonadotropic a.
gonadotropin-producing pituitary a.
gonadotropin-secreting a.
growth hormone cell a. (GH cell adenoma)
growth hormone-producing giant invasive a.
growth hormone-prolactin cell a.
growth hormone-secreting pituitary a. (GH-secreting pituitary adenoma)

Hürthle cell a.
hyalinizing trabecular a.
intraductal pancreatic a.
intrapituitary a.
intrasellar a.
invasive hormonally active pituitary a.
invasive hormonally inactive pituitary a.
islet cell a.
lactotroph a.
left anterior mediastinal a.
macrofollicular a.
mammosomatotroph cell a.
mediastinal parathyroid a.
mixed GH cell-prolactin cell a.
mixed GH-PRL cell a.
mixed GH- and prolactin-secreting a.
mixed growth hormone cell-prolactin cell a.
mixed growth hormone-prolactin cell a.
mixed growth hormone- and prolactin-secreting a.
multicentric islet cell a.
nonfamilial parathyroid a.
nonfunctional pituitary a.
nonfunctioning pituitary a. (NFPA)
nonsecreting pituitary a.
nonsecretory a.
nonsecretory adrenal a.
nontoxic thyroid a.
null-cell a.
oncocytic a.
oxyphilic a.
papillary a.
parathyroid a.
pituitary a.
plurihormonal a.
PRL-cell a.
PRL-secreting a.
prolactin cell a.
prolactin-producing pituitary a.
prolactin-secreting a.
recurrent a.
residual a.
secreting pituitary a.
silent ACTH a.
silent corticotrope a. subtypes I, II, III
silent corticotroph cell a.
silent gonadotroph cell a.
silent somatotroph a.
solitary a.
somatotroph cell a.
thyroid gland a.
thyrotrope a.
thyrotroph cell a.
thyrotroph-derived a.
thyrotropin-secreting pituitary a.
toxic a.
trabecular a.
TSH-secreting pituitary a. (TSH-oma)
unilateral aldosterone-producing a.

adenoma-carcinoma sequence

adenoma-gangliocytoma
mixed pituitary a.-g.

adenomatosis
islet cell a.
multiple endocrine a.

adenomatous
a. adrenal gland
a. goiter
a. hyperplasia
a. polyposis
a. tumor

adenomectomy
surgical a.
transrhinosphenoidal a.
transsphenoidal microsurgical a.
transsphenoidal pituitary a.
transsphenoidal selective a.

adenomyomatosis

adenopathies
multiple endocrine a. (MEA)

adenosine
a. cyclic monophosphate
a. deaminase (ADA)
a. deaminase deaminate
a. deaminase locus
a. 5′ diphosphate (ADP)
a. diphosphate ribosylation
a. 5′ monophosphate (AMP)
a. monophosphate deaminase 1 (AMPD1)
a. monophosphate deaminase deficiency
a. triphosphatase (ATPase)
a. 5′ triphosphate (ATP)

adenosis
sclerosing a.

adenosyltransferase
methionine a.

NOTES

adenovirus
AD-36 a.
a. E1A protein
recombinant a.
adenylate
a. cyclase
a. cyclase activity
a. cyclase desensitization
a. cyclase moiety
a. cyclase stimulator
a. cyclase system
adenylation
adenyl cyclase
3′,5′ adenylic acid
adenylosuccinate lyase deficiency
adenylyl
a. cyclase
a. cyclase activity
a. cyclase agonist forskolin
a. cyclase cascade
a. cyclase pathway
ADH
antidiuretic hormone
adherens
cumulus a.
a. junction
zonula a.
adhesion
a. molecule
a. molecule-like from the X-chromosome (ADMLX)
periovarian a.
adhesiveness
platelet a.
ADICOL
advanced insulin infusion with a control loop
ADICOL system
Adione
Adipex-P
adipocyte
a. determination and differentiation factor-1 (ADD1)
adipogenesis
adipokinetic hormone
adipoleptin growth hormone axis
adipose
a. tissue
a. tissue regulation
a. tissue-uncoupling protein
adiposity
intraabdominal a.
truncal a.
adiposogenital
a. dystrophy
a. syndrome
adipostat
adipsia
type A a.
type B a.
type C a.
adipsic disorder
adipsin
adjuvant
a. arthritis
a. chemotherapy
complete Freund a. (CFA)
ad libitum
Adlone Injection
ADM
atypical diabetes mellitus
administration
glycerol a.
intensive insulin a.
mannitol a.
pharmacologic estrogen a.
pulsed a.
ADMLX
adhesion molecule-like from the X-chromosome
adnexa
cutaneous a.
adolescence
constitutional delay in growth and a. (CDGA)
ADP
adenosine 5′ diphosphate
adrenal
a. adenoma
a. androgen
a. androgen deficiency
a. androgenesis
a. androgen excess
a. androgen-stimulating hormone (AASH)
a. cancer
a. capsular distention
a. carcinoma
a. cortex
a. cortex cell
a. corticosteroid (mineralocorticoid)
a. cortisol
a. crisis
a. diabetes
a. dysfunction
a. gland
a. gland limb
a. gland margin
a. hemorrhage
a. hypoplasia congenita (AHC)
hypothalamopituitary a. (HPA)
a. incidentaloma
a. insufficiency
a. medulla
a. medullary disease

a. medullary hormone
a. medullary hyperplasia
a. medullary paraganglioma
a. necrosis
a. pheochromocytoma
a. pseudotumor
a. remodeling
a. reserve
a. rest
a. rest tissue
a. scintigraphy
a. steroidogenesis
a. steroidogenic cascade
a. steroid precursor
a. tuberculosis
a. vein
a. vein aldosterone ratio
a. vein sampling
a. vein thrombosis
a. venous sampling (AVS)
a. zona fasciculata
a. zona glomerulosa

adrenalectomize

adrenalectomy (ADX)
laparoscopic a. (LA)
open a. (OA)
unilateral a.

adrenalectomy/oophorectomy

Adrenalin Chloride

adrenaline

adrenalitis
autoimmune a.
infectious a.

adrenarche
precocious a.
premature a.

adrenergic
a. agent
a. receptor
a. receptor activation

α-adrenergic (*var. of* alpha-adrenergic)

β-adrenergic (*var. of* beta-adrenergic)

adrenocortical
a. adenoma
a. atrophy
a. carcinoma
a. cell
a. hormone
a. regeneration
a. tumorigenesis

adrenocorticotrophic
a. hormone hypersecretion

adrenocorticotrophin
a. hormone (ACTH)
a. stimulation test

adrenocorticotropic
a. hormone (ACTH)
a. hormone cell adenoma
a. hormone-dependent Cushing syndrome
a. hormone-dependent Cushing syndrome
a. hormone hypersecretion

adrenocorticotropic-adrenal axis

adrenocorticotropin

adrenodoxin
a. reductase

adrenogenital syndrome

adrenoleukodystrophy
familial a.
neonatal a.
recessive a.
sex-linked a.
X-linked recessive a.

adrenomedullary
a. activity
a. cell
a. hormonal system
a. hyperplasia

adrenomedullin (AM)
a. hormone

adrenomyeloneuropathy

adrenopause

Adriamycin

adult
a. adrenal cortex
a. cystinosis
growth hormone-deficient a.
hypopituitary a.
a. Leydig cell failure
a. polycystic kidney disease
a. respiratory distress syndrome
a. rickets
a. T-cell leukemia (ATL)
a. zone

adult-onset
a.-o. diabetes
a.-o. diabetes mellitus

adults
latent autoimmune diabetes of a. (LADA)

advanced
a. glycation end product

NOTES

advanced *(continued)*
a. glycosylation end product (AGEP)
a. insulin infusion with a control loop (ADICOL)
adventitia
perithyroidal a.
ADX
adrenalectomy
adynamia
adynamic
a. bone
a. bone disease
a. bone disorder
a. bone lesion
AEIOU TIPS
alcohol, epilepsy, insulin, overdose, uremia, trauma, infection, psychiatric, stroke
Aerobacter
Aerodiol
aeruginosa
Pseudomonas a.
AERx
A. diabetes management system
AF-1
antifertility factor-1
affective illness
afferent
a. arteriole
a. arteriole hyalinization
a. axon
beta-endorphinergic a.
histaminergic a.
noradrenergic a.
a. pathway
a. signal
a. system
vagal a.
affinity
a. attenuated total reflectance spectroscopy
a. chromatography
a. evanescent wave spectroscopy
a. fluorescence spectroscopy
insulin binding a.
a. surface plasmon spectroscopy
aFGF
acidic fibroblast growth factor
AFP
alpha-fetoprotein
African trypanosomiasis
AFTN
autonomously functioning thyroid nodule
agammaglobulinemia
AGD
antigonadotropic decapeptide
age
delayed bone a.
large for gestational a. (LGA)
a., metastases, extent and size (AMES)
a., metastases, extent and size risk criteria
a. pigment
small for gestational a. (SGA)
Agency
International Atomic Energy A. (IAEA)
agenesis
Leydig cell a.
müllerian a.
pituitary a.
unilateral renal a.
agent
adrenergic a.
alkylating a.
alpha-adrenergic a.
antidiabetic a.
antimycotic a.
antiresorptive a.
antiserotonergic a.
beta-adrenergic a.
biguanide oral antihyperglycemic a.
bipyridine inotropic a.
bone formation-stimulating a.
bone-resorbing a.
bone resorption-inhibiting a.'s
calcimimetic a.
class 1B cardiac antiarrhythmic a.
dopamine a.
first-generation a.
formation-stimulating a.
formation-stimulation a.
gastric prokinetic a.
goitrogenic a.
hypolipidemic a.
inactive a.
lipid-lowering a.
nonsteroidal antiinflammatory a.
oral antidiabetic a.
oral hypoglycemic a.
orexigenic a.
paracrine a.
phosphate-binding a.
rheologic a.
second-generation a.
serotonergic a.
thiazide diuretic a.
tocolytic a.
uricosuric a.
AGEP
advanced glycosylation end product
age-related osteoporosis

agglutination
labial fusion a.
agglutinin
fluorescein-labeled pea a.
fluorescein-labeled peanut a.
aggregated human IgG (AHuG)
aggregation
arachidonate-induced platelet a.
platelet a.
aggressive
a. hypothalamic lymphoma
a. xanthomatosis
aging
programmed theory of a.
stochastic theory of a.
agoiterous autoimmune thyroiditis
agonist
beta a.
beta-adrenergic a.
beta-receptor a.
calcium receptor a.
D_2 a.
dopamine receptor a.
dopaminergic a.
E_2 a.
GnRH a.
gonadotropin-releasing hormone agonist
gonadotropin-releasing hormone a. (GnRH agonist, GnRHa)
mineralocorticoid a.
partial a.
purinergic a. (PIA)
agonist-antagonist
mixed a.-a.
agonist-receptor interaction
***agouti* protein**
***agouti*-related**
a.-r. peptide
a.-r. transcript
AGP
$alpha_1$ acid glycoprotein
agranulocytosis
infantile a.
AHA
autoimmune hemolytic anemia
AHC
adrenal hypoplasia congenita
AHG
antihemophilic globulin
AHO
Albright hereditary osteodystrophy
AHP
acute hemorrhagic pancreatitis
AhR
arylhydrocarbon receptor
AhR nuclear translocator (ARNT)
Ah receptor
AHuG
aggregated human IgG
A-hydroCort Injection
AIB
aminoisobutyric acid
AIB1
A. coactivator
AIBH
ACTH-independent bilateral macronodular hyperplasia
AICAR
aminoimidazole carboximide riboside
AIDS
acquired immune deficiency syndrome
acquired immunodeficiency syndrome
AIDS-related complex (ARC)
AIGF
androgen-induced growth factor
AILD
angioimmunoblastic lymphadenopathy with dysproteinemia
AIR
acute insulin response
air
alveolar a.
AIRE
autoimmune regulator
AIRE gene
Airet
AIS
androgen insensitivity syndrome
AITD
autoimmune thyroid disease
autoimmune thyroid disorder
AKR
aldo-keto reductase
AKR gene
alacrima
alanine
a. amino acid
a. aminotransferase
a. cycle
a. transaminase
alar-like extension
alar plate

NOTES

ALB
albumin
alba
Albers-Schönberg disease
Albert Glyburide
albicans
Candida a.
corpus a.
albinism
ocular a.
oculocutaneous a. (OCA)
oculocutaneous a. type I
Albright
A. hereditary osteodystrophy (AHO)
A. hereditary osteodystrophy syndrome
albumin (ALB)
antibovine serum a. (anti-BSA)
bovine serum a. (BSA)
serum a.
a. solution
albumin-bound
a.-b. calcium
a.-b. testosterone level
albuminoid protein
albuminuria
albuterol
ipratropium and a.
Alcian
A. blue
A. blue stain
alcohol
a. ablation
a. dehydrogenase
a., epilepsy, insulin, overdose, uremia, trauma, infection, psychiatric, stroke (AEIOU TIPS, AEIOU TIPS)
a. intolerance
sugar a.
alcoholic ketoacidosis
alcohol-induced birth defect
alcoholism
pseudo-Cushing syndrome of a.
alcohol-related chronic pancreatitis (ARCP)
Aldactone
aldehyde
a. dehydrogenase
a. fuchsin
a. thionin
a. thionin staining technique
aldehyde-thionin-positive vesicle
Aldo
aldosterone
aldo-keto reductase (AKR)
a.-k. r. g. gene
aldolase level
aldose
a. reductase
a. reductase inhibitor (ARI)
aldosterone (Aldo)
a. escape
a. escape phenomenon
a. excretion
plasma a.
a. receptor
recumbent a.
a. resistance
a. secretory rate
serum a.
a. synthase deficiency
a. synthesis
urine a.
aldosterone-deficient hyperkalemic acidosis
aldosterone-18-glucuronide
aldosterone-producing adenoma (APA)
aldosterone-secreting adenoma
aldosterone-stimulating hormone (ASH)
aldosterone-to-renin ratio
aldosteronism
glucocorticoid-remediable a. (GRA)
glucocorticoid-suppressible a.
idiopathic a.
primary a.
aldosteronoma
Aldurazyme
alendronate (ALN)
a. sodium
Alesse
Aleve
alfa
dornase a.
epoetin a.
thyrotropin a.
alfacalcidol
Alfenta
alfentanil
alglucerase
algodystrophy
algogenic
alimentary
a. form
a. hypoglycemia
aliquot
alkali
alkaline
a. phosphatase
a. phosphatase antialkaline phosphatase (APAAP)
a. phosphatase antialkaline phosphatase antibody test
alkaloid
ergot a.

A

opium a.
semisynthetic ergot a.
alkalosis
hypokalemic metabolic a.
metabolic a.
respiratory a.
Alka-Mints
alkaptonuria
Alkphase-B serum bone turnover assay
alkylated androgenic steroid
alkylating agent
ALL
acute lymphocytic leukemia
Allbee With C
allele
DQ a.
DR a.
DR4 a.
HLA a.
human leukocyte antigen allele
human leukocyte antigen a. (HLA allele)
mutant a.
5T a.
allele-specific
a.-s. oligonucleotide (ASO)
a.-s. oligonucleotide hybridization
Allen test
Allerfrin w/Codeine
allergy
insulin a.
AllerMax Oral
Allescheria boydii
Allgrove syndrome
allograft
fetal a.
freeze-dried a.
alloimmunity
allosteric
a. activator
a. effect
a. effector
a. inhibitor
a. stimulator
allowance
recommended daily a. (RDA)
recommended dietary a. (RDA)
alloxan
ALN
alendronate
alone
pancreas transplantation a. (PTA)
alopecia
a. androgenica
a. areata
total a.
Alor 5/500
Alora
A. transdermal
alpha, α
a. antagonist
a. cell
ER a.
estrogen receptor a.
follitropin a.
3-a.-hydroxysteroid dehydrogenase (3-alpha-HSD)
a. subunit-secreting pituitary adenoma
a. subunit-secreting tumor
thyrotropin a.
transforming growth factor a. (TGF-A, TGFα)
$alpha_1$, α_1
$a._1$ acid glycoprotein (AGP)
thymosin $a._1$ ($T\alpha_1$)
$alpha_2$, α_2
$alpha_2$ antagonist
$alpha_2$ receptor
alpha-1 antitrypsin deficiency
alpha-adrenergic, α-adrenergic
a.-a. agent
a.-a. blocker
a.-a. effect
a.-a. receptor
$alpha_2$-adrenergic
$alpha_2$-a. catecholamine
$alpha_2$-a. receptor
$alpha_1$-adrenergic receptor
alpha-amidation
alpha-amino-3-hydroxy-5methyl-4-isoxazole propionic acid
5-alpha-androstane-3-alpha,17-beta-diol
5-alpha-a.-d. glucuronide
alpha-antitrypsin deficiency
Alphabetic multivitamin supplement
alpha-cell
islet a.-c.
5-alpha-dihydrotestosterone
3-alpha-diol
3-alpha-diol-G
alpha-fetoprotein (AFP)
9alpha-fludrocortisone
9alpha-fluorocortisol

NOTES

alpha-glucosidase
alpha-glucosidase inhibitor
alpha-glutamyl
alpha-glycerol phosphate
alpha-glycerophosphate
a.-g. acyltransferase
a.-g. acyltransferase
a.-g. dehydrogenase
alpha-hCG
alpha-human chorionic gonadotropin
3-alpha-HSD
3-alpha-hydroxysteroid dehydrogenase
alpha$_2$-HS-glycoprotein
alpha-human chorionic gonadotropin (alpha-hCG)
16-alpha-hydroxyestrone
1-alpha-hydroxylase
1α-h. activity
25-hydroxy-vitamin D 1α-h. (1-alpha-OHase)
17-alpha-hydroxylase
17-alpha-h. deficiency
20-alpha-hydroxylase
17-alpha-hydroxylase/17,20-lyase
17-alpha-h.-l. deficiency
17-alpha-h.-l. (p450c17) deficiency
1-alpha-hydroxylation
1-alpha-hydroxyvitamin D$_3$
alpha-lactalbumin
alpha$_2$-macroglobulin
alpha-mannosidosis
alpha-melanocyte-stimulating (alpha-MSH)
alpha-melanocyte-stimulating hormone
alpha-melanocyte-stimulating hormone
alpha-methyldopa
alpha-methyldopamine
alpha-methylnorepinephrine
7-alpha-methyl-19-nortestosterone (MENT)
alpha-methyl-tyrosine
alpha-MSH
alpha-melanocyte-stimulating
alpha-MSH hormone
1-alpha-OHase
25-hydroxy-vitamin D 1α-hydroxylase
1-alpha-OH-cholecalciferol
alpha-preprotachykinin A
5-alpha-reductase
5-alpha-r. activity (5α-RA)
5-alpha-r. type II
5-alpha-reductase activity (5α-RA)
5-alpha-reductase type I
alpha v beta 3
alpha v beta 3 vitronectin receptor integrin
alprenolol
alprostadil
intraurethral a.
Alredase
alrestatin
ALS
acid-labile subunit
amyotrophic lateral sclerosis
antilymphocytic serum
Alstrom syndrome
Altea
A. MicroPor
A. MicroPor laser
alteration
gain-of-function a.
altered
a. androgen action
a. degradation of parathyroid hormone
a. set point
ALternaGEL
alternate cover test
Alu-Cap
Aludrox
aluminum
a. accumulation
a. bone disease
a. bone level
a. burden
a. carbonate
a. deposit
a. effect
a. gel
a. hydroxide
a. hydroxide and magnesium carbonate
a. hydroxide, magnesium hydroxide, and simethicone
a. hydroxide and magnesium trisilicate
a. intoxication
a. loading
Maloney stain for a.
a. overload
a. retention
a. salt
tissue a.
a. toxicity
aluminum-associated osteomalacia
aluminum-containing
a.-c. medication
a.-c. phosphate binder
aluminum-contaminated
a.-c. casein hydrolysate
a.-c. dialysate
aluminum-induced osteomalacia
aluminum-related
a.-r. bone disease
a.-r. osteomalacia

Alu-Tab
alveolar
a. air
a. bone
a. type II cell
ALZA
Alzheimer disease
AM
adrenomedullin
Amadori product
Amadori-type rearrangement
Amaryl
A. glimepiride tablet
amastia
ambient temperature
ambiguous genitalia
ambisexual development
Amcort Injection
AME
apparent mineralocorticoid excess
amebic brain abscess
ameloblast
amelogenesis imperfecta
Amen Oral
amenorrhea
exercise-related a.
functional hypothalamic a. (FHA)
hypothalamic a.
lactational a.
postpill a.
primary a.
psychogenic a.
secondary a.
amenorrhea-galactorrhea
a.-g. syndrome
American
A. Association of Clinical Endocrinologists
A. Diabetes Association (ADA)
A. Diabetes Association guidelines
A. Joint Commission on Cancer
A. Thyroid Association
A. Urologic Association (AUA)
A. Urologic Association symptom score
Amerlite MAB free T4 assay
AMES
age, metastases, extent and size
AMES risk criteria
Ames
A. dwarf mice
A-methaPred Injection
AMF
autocrine motility factor
AMH
anti-müllerian hormone
amidating enzyme
amidation
amide
tripeptide a.
amikacin
amiloride
amine
a. precursor uptake and decarboxylation (APUD)
a. precursor uptake and decarboxylation cell
a. precursor uptake and decarboxylation series
sympathomimetic a.
amino
a. acid
a. acid delivery
a. acid-peptide hormone
a. acid sequence
a. acid sequence analysis
a. acid substitution
5-a. group
a. terminal domain
a. terminus
aminoaciduria
dibasic a.
aminoacyl-tRNA complex
Amino-Cerv Vaginal Cream
aminoglutethimide
a. therapy
aminoglycoside
aminoguanide
aminoguanidine
aminoimidazole carboximide riboside (AICAR)
aminoisobutyric acid (AIB)
Amino-Opti-E
aminopeptidase
a. A
a. B
cysteine a.
aminophylline
aminoterminal leader
aminotransferase
alanine a.
aspartate a.
serum alanine a.
tyrosine a.

NOTES

aminotriazole
amiodarone
a. thyrotoxicosis
amiodarone-associated thyrotoxicosis
amiodarone-induced
a.-i. destructive thyrotoxicosis
a.-i. hypothyroidism
Amipaque
Amitone
amitriptyline
ammonium chloride
amnesia
retrograde a.
amnioblast
amniocentesis
amnionic cavity
amniotic fluid
amorphous
a. calcium
a. calcium phosphate
a. urate
amoxicillin
Amoxil
AMP
adenosine 5′ monophosphate
cyclic AMP (cAMP)
AMP-activated protein kinase (AMPK)
AMPD1
adenosine monophosphate deaminase 1
amperometric
a. glucosensor
a. glucose oxidase electrode
amphenone
amphetamine
dextroamphetamine and a.
amphetamine-related transcript system
amphiregulin
Amphojel
amphotericin B
amphoteric molecule
ampicillin
AMPK
AMP-activated protein kinase
amplification
a. factor
germline a.
a. refractory mutation system (ARMS)
somatic a.
amplified in breast-1 coactivator
amplitude
cycle a.
prolactin pulse a.
pulse a.
ampulla
a. of the vas deferens
ampullary stone
amrinone
Amsterdam-type biliary stent
AMV
avian myeloblastosis virus
amygdala
amylacea
corpora a.
amylase
amylin
amyloid
a. deposit
a. fibril
a. goiter
immune a.
a. peptide
pituitary a.
amyloidogenesis
amyloidogenicity
amyloidosis
AB a.
beta$_2$-microglobulin a.
dialysis-associated a.
dialysis-related a. (DRA)
familial oculoleptomeningea a.
senile systemic a.
amyotrophic lateral sclerosis (ALS)
amyotrophy
diabetic a.
AN
acanthosis nigricans
ANA
antinuclear antibody
anabolic
a. steroid
a. therapy
anabolic-androgenic
a.-a. steroid
a.-a. steroid binding
Anabolin
anabolism
Anadrol
anagen
analbuminemia
analog, analogue
bromoaurone a.
gastrin a.
GnRH a.
gonadotropin-releasing hormone a.
insulin a.
narcotine a.
noncalcemic a.
somatostatin a.
steroid a.
thromboxane a.
vitamin D a.
analysis
amino acid sequence a.
computer-aided sperm a. (CASA)
computer-assisted semen a. (CASA)

crystallographic stone a.
energy-dispersive x-ray a. (EDAX)
flow cytometric a.
immunocytochemical a.
immunohistochemical a.
isobologram a.
Kyte-Doolittle hydropathy a.
mass isotopomer distribution a. (MIDA)
Northern blot a.
pedigree a.
phenotype-genotype a.
Pulsar a.
semen a.
single-stranded conformation polymorphism a.
Southern blot a.
a. of variance (ANOVA)
Western blot a.

analyte

analytical sensitivity

analyzer
pulse-height a.

anamnestic
a. antibody response
a. element

anandamide

anaphylaxis

anaplastic
a. astrocytoma
a. thyroid cancer
a. thyroid carcinoma

Anaprox

Anaspaz

anastomosis
jejunocolic a.

anastomotic blood supply

anastrozole

Anatuss

Anavar

ancephaly

Andractim

Andro

androblastoma

Androcur
A. Depot

Androderm
A. testosterone transdermal patch
A. Transdermal System

Andro/Fem

Androgel

androgen
adrenal a.
estrogen/a. therapy
a. excess
a. insensitivity syndrome (AIS)
a. milieu
a. receptor (AR)
a. receptor gene
a. receptor gene mutation
a. replacement therapy (ART)
a. resistance
a. resistance syndrome
a. sensitivity

androgen-binding protein (ABP)

androgenesis
adrenal a.

androgenica
alopecia a.

androgenic follicle

androgen-induced growth factor (AIGF)

androgen-lowering therapy

androgen-producing tumor

androgen-secreting neoplasm

androgen-type hirsutism

androgynous

android
a. fat distribution
a. obesity

Andro-L.A. Injection

Androlone-D

Andropatch

andropause
surgical a.

Andropository Injection

Androsorb

androstane
a. derivative

androstanediol glucuronide

androstenedione (AD, D4-A)

androsterone
a. glucuronide (AoG)

anechoic
a. foci

anemia
autoimmune hemolytic a. (AHA)
Cooley a.
a. of end-stage renal disease
Fanconi a.
hemolytic a.
hypoproliferative a.
leukoerythroblastic a.
megaloblastic a.

NOTES

anemia *(continued)*
microcytic a.
myelophthisic a.
normocytic normochromic a.
pernicious a.
sickle cell a.
sideroblastic a.
unexplained microcytic a.
anencephaly
anephric
anergy
clonal a.
anestrina
anestrous condition
aneuploid
aneuploidia
aneuploidy
sex chromosome a.
aneurysm
carotid a.
giant carotid a.
pituitary a.
Anexsia
ANF
atrial natriuretic factor
ANG
angiogenin
angiotensin II
Angel Hypoglycemic capsule
Angelman syndrome
Anger gamma camera
anhydrase
carbonic a. II (CA II)
angiitis
Angio-Conray
angioedema
angiofibroma
angiogenesis
angiogenin (ANG)
angiography
digital subtraction a. (DSA)
nonselective arterial digital a.
nuclear a.
postmortem pancreatic a.
venous digital a.
angioimmunoblastic lymphadenopathy with dysproteinemia (AILD)
angioinvasion
angioma
retinal capillary a.
angiomyelolipoma
angiosarcoma
angiostatin
angiotensin
a. I (AT-I)
a. II (ANG, AT-II)
a. II antidiuretic hormone
a. III (AT-III)
a. I and II assay
angiotensin-converting
a.-c. enzyme (ACE)
a.-c. enzyme inhibitor
angiotensinergic fiber
angiotensinogen
angstrom
angular cheilitis
ANH
atrial natriuretic hormone
anhedonia
anhidrosis
distal a.
anicteric cholestasis
animal protein diet
Animas
A. R-1000 insulin pump
A. R-1000 sensor
anion
bicarbonate a.
a. gap
a. of the Hofmeister series
peroxynitrite a.
anion-gap acidosis
anisocoria with ipsilateral mydriasis
anisotropine
ankle
a. pressure
a. reflex time
ankyrin deficiency
anlage
cartilaginous a.
lateral a.
lateral thyroid a.
medial a.
median a.
anlagen
annexin
a. I
a. II
a. V
annual cycle
annular
a. array
a. pancreas
annulare
granuloma a.
annulus
Zinn a.
Anodynos-DHC
anomalous pancreaticobiliary union
anomaly
congenital forebrain a.
conotruncal a.
ectodermal a.
endocrine a.
anophthalmos

A

anorchia
bilateral a.
congenital a.
anorectal atresia
anorectic
anorectin
anorexia
a. nervosa
anosmia
anosmin
ANOVA
analysis of variance
anovulation
chronic hyperandrogenic a.
chronic hypoandrogenic a.
eugonadotrophic a.
hyperandrogenic a.
hypothalamic a.
anovulatory
a. cycle
a. infertility
Anovulin
anoxia
ANP
atrial natriuretic peptide
ansa
a. cervicalis nerve
a. hypoglossal nerve
Antagon
antagonism
insulin a.
antagonist
alpha a.
$alpha_2$ a.
dihydropyridine a.
histamine (H_2) a.
$5HT_2$ receptor a.
5-hydroxytryptamine subtype 2 receptor a.
inotropic glutamate receptor a.
insulin a.
interleukin-1 receptor a. (IL-1RA)
nonpeptide a.
partial agonist-partial a.
selective aldosterone a.
selective $5HT_2$ receptor a.
antegrade instrumentation
antenatal Bartter syndrome
antenatal-hypercalciuric variant
anterior
a. choroidal artery
a. clinoid process
a. commissure
a. communicating artery
a. incisural space
a. pituitary
a. pituitary function
a. pituitary gland
a. pituitary lobe
a. pole
a. scalene muscle
anterograde flow
anteroventral 3rd ventricle (AV3V)
anthracycline
anthropometry
anthropozoonosis
anti-37K antibody
antiadrenal antibody
antiandrogen
antibiotic resistance gene
antibody (Ab)
antiadrenal a.
antibovine serum albumin a.
anti-BrDU a.
anti-bromodeoxyuridine a.
anti-BSA a.
anticarcinoembryonic antigen monoclonal a.
anticardiolipin immunoglobulin M a.
anti-CEA monoclonal a.
antiidiotype a.
antiidiotypic a.
antiinsulin a.
antiinterleukin-2 a. (anti-IL-2R Ab)
antiislet cell a.
anti-37K a.
anti-La a.
antimicrosomal a.
antineutrophil cytoplasmic a.
antinuclear a. (ANA)
antipituitary a.
anti-Ro a.
antisomatostatin a.
anti-Tg a.
antithyroglobulin a. (ATA)
antithyroid peroxidase a.
antithyroid-stimulating hormone a.
anti-TPO a.
anti-TSH a.
complement-fixing thyroid a.
cytoplasmic islet-cell a.
DuPan-2 a.
a. epitope

NOTES

antibody *(continued)*
growth-blocking a.
growth-stimulating a.
heterophilic a.
insulin receptor a.
islet cell surface a. (ICSA)
a. Ki
maternal a.
MIB-1 a.
microsomal a.
monoclonal a. (MAb, Mab)
pituitary cell-surface a.
polyclonal anti-T-cell a.
primary a.
a. response
secondary a.
serum antiinsulin a.
serum microsomal a.
thyroglobulin a.
thyroid microsomal a.
thyroid peroxidase a.
thyroid-stimulating a. (TSAb)
thyroid-stimulating-blocking a. (TSBAb)
thyroid-stimulating hormone-binding inhibitor a. (TBIAb)
thyroid-stimulating hormone receptor a. (TSH-RAb)
thyroid stimulation-blocking a. (TSBAb)
thyroperoxidase a. (TPO Ab)
thyrotropin receptor a.
thyrotropin receptor-stimulating a. (TSH-RAb)
a. titer
transplacental a.
TSH-binding inhibitory a.
TSH-R a.
TSH receptor-blocking a.
TSH receptor-stimulating a.
TSH stimulation blocking a. (TSBAb)

antibody-dependent
a.-d. cell cytotoxicity (ADCC)
a.-d. cell-mediated cytotoxicity
a.-d. cellular cytotoxicity (ADCC)
a.-d. cytotoxicity test

antibovine serum albumin (anti-BSA)

antibovine serum albumin antibody

anti-BrDU
anti-bromodeoxyuridine
anti-BrDU antibody

anti-bromodeoxyuridine (anti-BrDU)
a.-b. antibody

anti-BSA
antibovine serum albumin
anti-BSA antibody

anticarcinoembryonic
a. antigen (anti-CEA)
a. antigen monoclonal antibody

anticardiolipin immunoglobulin M antibody

anti-CEA
anticarcinoembryonic antigen
anti-CEA monoclonal antibody

anticholinergic
a. side effect

anticipatory control

anticonvulsive activity

Anticort

anticus
scalenus a.

antidepressant
tricyclic a. (TCA)

antidiabetic
a. agent
a. medication

antidiuresis

antidiuretic
a. activity
a. hormone (ADH)

antidouble-stranded
a.-s. deoxyribonucleic acid
a.-s. DNA

antiestrogen
a. drug

antifertility factor-1 (AF-1)

anti-GAD
antiglutamic acid decarboxylase
anti-GAD autoantibody

antigalactic

antigen
anticarcinoembryonic a. (anti-CEA)
autoimmune thyroid-related a.-1 (ATRA1)
B8 a.
B-cell a.
breast cancer a. (BRCA)
carcinoembryonic a. (CEA)
CD1 a.
cell-surface a.
cognate a.
cryptococcal a.
factor VIII-related a.
factor VIII ristocetin cofactor a.
histocompatibility locus a. (HLA)
HLA-A a.
HLA-B a.
HLA-B8 a.
HLA-C a.
HLA-D a.
HLA-DP a.
HLA-DQ a.
HLA-DR a.
HLA-DR3 a.

HLA-DR4 a.
HLA-DR5 a.
HLA-Dw3 a.
HNK-1 a.
homologous thyroid a.
human leukocyte a. (HLA)
H-Y a.
immune response a.
islet cell a. (ICA)
leu-7 a.
leukocyte common a.
microsomal a.
proliferating cell nuclear a. (PCNA)
prostate-specific a. (PSA)
prostate-specific membrane a. (PSMA)
Rh blood group a.
Rhesus factor blood group antigen
Rhesus factor blood group a. (Rh blood group antigen)
SV40 large T a.
T-cell a.
testis-determining a. (TDA)
thyroglobulin a.
thyroid peroxidase a.
tumor-specific a. (TSA)

antigen-1
fertilization a. (FA-1)
lymphocyte function-associated a. (LFA-1)

antigen-4
cytotoxic lymphocyte a. (CTLA-4)

antigenic property

antigen-presenting cell (APC)

antigen-specific
a.-s. preventive therapy
a.-s. suppressor T cell

antiglucocorticoid

antiglutamic
a. acid decarboxylase (anti-GAD)
a. acid decarboxylase autoantibody

antigonadotropic
a. action
a. decapeptide (AGD)

antigonadotropin
pineal a. (PAG)

antihemophilic globulin (AHG)

antihormone
estrogen receptor a.
steroid hormone receptor a.

antihyperglycemic
biguanide oral a.

antiidiotype
a. antibody

antiidiotypic antibody

anti-IL-2R Ab

antiinsulin
a. antibody
a. autoantibody
B-cell a.

antiinterleukin-2 antibody (anti-IL-2R Ab)

antiislet cell antibody

antiknock mix

anti-La antibody

antilipolytic effect

antilymphocytic serum (ALS)

antimetabolite

antimicrobial therapy

antimicrosomal antibody

antimitotic effect

antimongoloid

anti-müllerian
a.-m. hormone (AMH)
a.-m. hormone deficiency

antimycotic agent

antineutrophil cytoplasmic antibody

antinociceptive action

antinuclear antibody (ANA)

antiovulatory

antioxidant
probucol a.

antiperistaltic

antiphospholipid (APL)

antipituitary antibody

antiporter

antiprogestin

antipsoriatic action

antipyretics

antipyrine

antirachitic
a. activity
a. effect
a. property

antirachitogenic effect

antiresorptive
a. agent
a. therapy

antiretroviral therapy

anti-Ro antibody

antisense nucleotide

antisera

NOTES

antiserotonergic agent
antiserotoninergic effect
antiserum
antisomatostatin antibody
antistress effect
anti-Tg
antithyroglobulin
anti-Tg antibody
antithrombin III level
antithymocyte globulin
antithyroglobulin (anti-Tg)
a. antibody (ATA)
antithyroid
a. antibody titer
a. drug (ATD)
a. medication
a. peroxidase
a. peroxidase antibody
antithyroid-stimulating
a.-s. hormone (anti-TSH)
a.-s. hormone antibody
antithyroperoxidase (anti-TPO)
a. level
anti-TPO
antithyroperoxidase
anti-TPO antibody
anti-TSH
antithyroid-stimulating hormone
anti-TSH antibody
antral follicle
antrum
antrum-sparing modified Whipple procedure
Anxanil Oral
AOB
accessory olfactory bulb
AoG
androsterone glucuronide
aortic
a. allograft conduit
a. arch
a. root dilatation
AP
area postrema
AP-1
activator protein-1
AP-1 element
APA
aldosterone-producing adenoma
unilateral APA
APAAP
alkaline phosphatase antialkaline phosphatase
Apacet
APACHE
Acute Physiology and Chronic Health Evaluation
APACHE II
APACHE II score
Apatate
apathetic
a. hyperthyroidism
a. thyrotoxicosis
apatite
a. crystal
APC
antigen-presenting cell
APD
acquired perforating dermatosis
APECED
autoimmune polyendocrinopathy-candidiasis-ectodermal dystrophy
ApEn
approximate entropy
Apert syndrome
aphagia
aphrodisiac drug
Aphrodyne
apical
a. iodide channel
a. membrane
a. membrane of proximal convoluted tubule cell
apituitarism
APL
antiphospholipid
aplasia
congenital bilateral a.
congenital thymic a.
a. cutis
germinal cell a.
Leydig cell a.
pituitary a.
renal a.
aplastic
a. bone disease
a. bone disorder
a. bone lesion
a. uremic osteodystrophy
apnea
sleep a.
Apo
A. Bromocriptine
apo
apolipoprotein
apo A-I concentration
apo E genotype
apo B
apolipoprotein B
apo B mRNA-editing catalytic polypeptide-1 (apobec-1)
apobec-1
apo B mRNA-editing catalytic polypeptide-1
Apo-Chlorpropamide

A

apocrine
a. body odor
a. secretion
a. sweat gland
Apo-Gain
Apo-Glyburide
Apo-Ibuprofen
Apo-Indomethacin
apolipoprotein (apo)
a. A-I
a. A-II
a. A-IV
a. B (apo B)
a. B gene
C a.
D a.
a. deficiency A-I
a. deficiency B
a. deficiency E
E a.
a. E
a. type 3
apomorphine
aponeurosis
levator a.
apophyseal joint
apoplectic hemorrhage
apoplexy
pituitary tumor a.
Apo-Prednisone
Apo-Propranolol
apoprotein
a. A-1
apoptosis
osteoclast a.
a. pathway
aporeceptor
apoT3R-mediated repression
Apo-Tolbutamide
apparatus
distal Golgi a.
Golgi a.
juxtaglomerular a. (JGA)
proximal Golgi a.
Warburg a.
apparent mineralocorticoid excess (AME)
appearance
adenoid a.
cotton-wool a.
dripping-candle-wax a.
signet-ring a.
sucked-candy a.
appendiceal carcinoid
appendicular skeleton
appetite
salt a.
a. suppressant
apple-green birefringence
appositional
a. crystal proliferation
a. growth
Appraise
A. diabetes monitoring system
approach
bayesian a.
candidate gene a.
pterional a.
sublabial transseptal a.
transcallosal-transforaminal a.
translateral retroperitoneal a.
transnasal-transseptal a.
transsphenoidal a.
approximate entropy (ApEn)
APR
acute phase response
APRIL
A proliferation-inducing ligand
Aprodine w/C
aprotinin
high-dose intraperitoneal a.
APUD
amine precursor uptake and decarboxylation
APUD cell
APUD series
apudoma
AQ
Nutropin AQ
AQ2
aquaporin-2
AQ2 water channel
AQP
aquaporin
Aquacare Topical
AquaMEPHYTON Injection
Aquaphyllin
aquaporin (AQP)
aquaporin-2 (AQ2)
a. water channel
Aquasol
A. A
A. E

NOTES

Aquatensen
aqueduct
nonsyndromic familial enlarged vestibular a.
a. of Sylvius
aqueous
a. humor
a. solution
Aquest
AR
androgen receptor
Axid AR
arabinoside
cytosine a.
arachidonate
arachidonate-induced platelet aggregation
arachidonic
a. acid (AA)
a. acid cascade
arachnoid
a. cyst
a. membrane
arachnoidal sheet
arachnoiditis
chiasmal a.
arborization
arbovirus
ARC
AIDS-related complex
arcuate nucleus of the hypothalamus
arch
aortic a.
arci (*pl. of* arcus)
arcing spring
ARCP
alcohol-related chronic pancreatitis
arcuata
pars a.
arcuate
a. nucleus
a. nucleus of the hypothalamus (ARC)
arcus, pl. **arci**
corneal a.
a. senilis
area
extrasplanchnic a.
hypophysiotropic a. (HTA)
lateral retrochiasmatic a.
osteoid a. (OA)
parapituitary a.
periaqueductal gray a.
posterior hypothalamic a. (PHA)
a. postrema (AP)
retrochiasmatic a.
rostral a.
sacral autonomic a.
areata
alopecia a.
Aredia
areflexia
arenacea
corpora a.
Arg
A. mutation
argentaffin
a. cell
a. reaction
a. stain
argentaffinoma
Argesic-SA
arginase
arginine
a. infusion test
a. tolerance test (ATT)
a. vasopressin (AVP)
a. vasopressor precursor
a. vasotocin (AVT)
argininosuccinate lyase
argininosuccinic aciduria
argon laser
argyrophil cell
argyrophilic stain
ARI
aldose reductase inhibitor
ARIA
ACh receptor-inducing activity
ariboflavinosis
Arimidex
A-ring
aromatic A-ring
Aristocort
A. Forte Injection
A. Intralesional Injection
A. Oral
Aristospan
A. Intraarticular Injection
A. Intralesional Injection
Arm-a-Med
A.-a.-M. isoetharine
A.-a.-M. isoproterenol
A.-a.-M. metaproterenol
Armour Thyroid
ARMS
amplification refractory mutation system
Arnold-Healy-Gordon syndrome
ARNT
AhR nuclear translocator
arom
P450 a.
aromatase
cytochrome P450 a.
a. deficiency
a. enzyme complex
a. gene

a. inhibition
a. inhibitor
a. inhibitor testolactone
a. P450

aromatic
A. Ammonia Aspirols
a. ammonia spirit
a. A-ring
a. L-amino acid decarboxylase

aromatization

aromatize

ARP
acute recurrent pancreatitis

array
annular a.

arrest
follicular a.
germinal a.

arrested follicular cyst

Arrestin

arrhenoblastoma

arrhythmia
atrial a.
cardiac a.
junctional a.
ventricular a.

arrhythmogenesis
nocturnal a.

arsenite

ART
androgen replacement therapy
assisted reproductive technology

arterial
a. bruit
a. stimulation and venous sampling (ASVS)

arteriogram
left internal mammary a.

arteriography
celiac axis a.

arteriole
afferent a.
efferent a.
juxtaglomerular afferent a.

arteriosclerosis obliterans

arteriosum
ligamentum a.

arteriosus
patent ductus a.
truncus a.

arteriovenous
a. difference
a. malformation (AVM)

arteritis
giant-cell a.
secondary a.

artery
anterior choroidal a.
anterior communicating a.
carotid a.
celiac a.
cerebral a.
choroid a.
communicating a.
coronary a.
dorsal pancreatic a.
feeding a.
gastroduodenal a.
helicine a.
hepatic a.
hypophysial a.
iliac a.
inferior pancreaticoduodenal a.
inferior parathyroid a.
inferior phrenic a.
inferior thyroid a.
mesenteric a.
ophthalmic a.
posterior cerebral a.
posterior communicating a.
profunda penis a.
renal a.
splenic a.
superior hypophyseal a.
superior mesenteric a.
superior pancreaticoduodenal a.
superior parathyroid a.
thyroid ima a.
uterine arcuate a.

Artha-G

arthralgia

arthritis
acute gouty a.
adjuvant a.
psoriasiform a.
psoriatic a.
rheumatoid a.

arthrogryposis multiplex congenita

Arthropan

arthropathy
Charcot a.
destructive a.

NOTES

arthropathy *(continued)*
diabetic neuropathic a.
neuropathic a.
pyrophosphate a.
Arthus phenomenon
articular
a. cartilage
a. overgrowth
articulation
vomerosphenoidal a.
artifact
starburst a.
artifactual hypoglycemia
artificial insemination with donor sperm
ARVDD-1
type 1 autosomal recessive vitamin D dependency
arylalkylamine *N*-acetyltransferase (AA-NAT)
arylhydrocarbon receptor (AhR)
arylmethyl group
arylsulfatase C
arytenoid
oblique a.
transverse a.
ASA
Lortab ASA
ascending pyelonephritis
Aschoff body
ascites
tense a.
ascitic fluid test
ascorbate
sodium a.
ascorbic acid
Ascorbicap
Ascriptin
aseptate hypha
aseptic necrosis
ASH
aldosterone-stimulating hormone
Asherman syndrome
Ashkenazi Jew
asialo-galacto-Tg
asialo-galacto-thyroglobulin
asialo-galacto-thyroglobulin (asialo-galacto-Tg)
asialoglycoprotein receptor
asialo-hCG
asialo-human chorionic gonadotropin
asialo-human chorionic gonadotropin (asialo-hCG)
asialyloglycoprotein
Askanazy cell
Asmalix
ASO
allele-specific oligonucleotide
asparaginase
asparagine
asparagine-linked glycosylation moiety
aspartamine
aspartate
a. aminotransferase
aspartic
a. acid
a. acid/glutamic acid-tyrosine (Asp/Glu-Tyr)
a. endopeptidase cathepsin D
aspart insulin
aspartyl endoprotease
aspartylglycosaminuria
A-Spas S/L
aspergillosis
Aspergillus
A. flavus
A. fumigatus
A. thyroiditis
Aspergum
aspermia
Asp/Glu-Tyr
aspartic acid/glutamic acid-tyrosine
aspiration
CT-guided fine-needle a.
cyst a.
fine-needle a. (FNA)
pulmonary a.
aspirin
a. and codeine
oxycodone and a.
propoxyphene and a.
aspirin-sensitive asthma syndrome
Aspirols
Aromatic Ammonia A.
assay
Abbott AxSYM a.
Alkphase-B serum bone turnover a.
Amerlite MAB free T4 a.
angiotensin I and II a.
avidin-biotin complex a. (ABCD)
binding a.
blood spot a.
chemiluminescence a.
chemiluminescent a.
Chiron ACS:180 a.
colorimetric a.
combination a.
competitive zona binding a.
cortisol a.
enzyme-linked immunosorbent a. (ELISA)
hemizona a.
immunochemiluminescence a. (ICMA)
immunochemiluminescent a. (ICMA)
immunochemiluminometric a. (ICMA)

immunometric a. (IMA)
immunoprecipitation a.
immunoradiometric a. (IRMA)
lithostathine a.
mutation-enriched restriction fragment length polymorphism a.
nuclear runoff a.
Optiquant a.
parathyroid hormone a.
pigeon crop sac-stimulation a.
proliferation a.
Pyrilinks-D deoxypyridinoline crosslinks urine a.
radioreceptor a. (RRA)
reverse hemolytic plaque a.
TBII a.
third-generation a.
thyroglobulin a.
thyroxine radioisotope a. (T_4RIA)
TSI a.
in vitro collagen invasion a.
Xenopus oocyte expression a.

assessment
histomorphometric a.
visual field a.
in vivo a.
volume a.

assisted
a. reproduction technique
a. reproductive technology (ART)

association
American Diabetes A. (ADA)
American Thyroid A.
American Urologic A. (AUA)
British Diabetes A.
cell a.
HLA DR antigen a.
human leukocyte antigen DR antigen a.

Assure blood glucose monitoring system

asteroides
Nocardia a.

asthenia

asthenospermia

AsthmaNefrin

Astramorph PF Injection

astressin

astrocytoma
anaplastic a.
juvenile pilocytic a.
low-grade a.

ASVS
arterial stimulation and venous sampling

asymptomatic
a. hyponatremia
a. pheochromocytoma
a. synechia

ATA
antithyroglobulin antibody

Atarax Oral

ataxia
familial cerebral a.
Friedreich a.
gait a.
hereditary a.
limb a.
myxedema a.
a. telangiectasia
a. telangiectasia mutated (ATM)
a. telangiectasia mutated gene

ATD
antithyroid drug

atenolol

Atgam

athelia

atherogenesis

atherogenicity

atherosclerosis

athetoid movement

athymia

athyreosis

athyreotic
a. cretin

athyrotic

AT-I
angiotensin I

AT-II
angiotensin II

AT-III
angiotensin III

ATL
adult T-cell leukemia

AtLast blood glucose monitoring system

ATM
ataxia telangiectasia mutated
ATM gene

atmospheric pressure

Atolone Oral

atom
orthoiodine a.
orthotyrosyl iodine a.
phenolic orthohydrogen a.

atomic absorption spectrophotometry

NOTES

atomization
atony
gastric a.
uterine a.
atorvastatin
a. calcium
Atozine Oral
ATP
adenosine 5′ triphosphate
ATPase
adenosine triphosphatase
ouabain-sensitive Na^+-K^+ ATPase
sarcoplasmic/endoplasmic reticulum calcium ATPase (SERCA)
ATRA1
autoimmune thyroid-related antigen-1
atresia
anorectal a.
biliary a.
follicular a.
atretic
a. follicular cyst
atrial
a. arrhythmia
a. myxoma
a. natriuretic factor (ANF)
a. natriuretic hormone (ANH)
a. natriuretic peptide (ANP)
a. tachyarrhythmia
atriopeptidergic fiber
atriopeptin
atrophic
a. chronic autoimmune thyroiditis
a. gastritis
a. Hashimoto thyroiditis
atrophy
adrenocortical a.
band a.
bow-tie a.
bull's-eye type macular a.
cortical a.
dentatorubral-pallidoluysian a. (DRPLA)
disuse a.
exhaustion a.
fiber a.
fibrous a.
genital a.
gyrate a.
interosseous a.
multiple system a.
neurogenic a.
olivopontocerebellar a.
postinflammatory testicular a.
postpubertal testicular a.
spinal muscular a. types I, II, III
spinobulbar muscular a.
Sudeck a.
testicular a.
type II muscle fiber a.
atropine
Atrovent
ATT
arginine tolerance test
AtT20 pituitary cell line
Attache food scale
attention-deficit hyperactivity disorder
attenuate
attenuation
attractin
atypia
cytologic a.
nuclear a.
atypical
a. diabetes
a. diabetes mellitus (ADM)
a. mycobacterium
a. teratoma
AUA
American Urologic Association
AUA symptom score
AUG codon
Aurbach pseudohypoparathyroidism
aureus
Staphylococcus a.
aurintricarboxylic acid stain
aurone
autacoid
autoantibodies against insulin
autoantibody
anti-GAD a.
antiglutamic acid decarboxylase a.
antiinsulin a.
competitive insulin a.
heat shock protein a.
insulin a. (IAA)
insulin-receptor a.
plasmic islet cell a.
a. production
receptor a.
sperm a.
thyroglobulin a.
thyroid peroxidase a.
thyroid-stimulating hormone receptor a. (TSH-RAb)
thyrotropin receptor a. (TRAb)
TSH receptor a.
autoantigen
extrathyroid a.
islet a.
Autoclix fingerstick device
autocrine
a. action
a. cell
a. motility factor (AMF)
a. secretion

a. suppressor
a. system
autograft bone
autoimmune
a. adrenalitis
a. diabetes
a. diabetes mellitus
a. endocrine disease
a. hemolytic anemia (AHA)
a. hyperthyroidism
a. hypoparathyroidism
a. hypophysitis
a. neuromuscular junction disorder
a. oophoritis
a. polyendocrinopathy-candidiasis-ectodermal dystrophy (APECED)
a. polyglandular endocrinopathy
a. polyglandular failure
a. polyglandular hypofunction
a. regulator (AIRE)
a. regulator gene
a. signal
a. thyroid disease (AITD)
a. thyroid disorder (AITD)
a. thyroid hyperfunction
a. thyroiditis
a. thyroid-related antigen-1 (ATRA1)
a. thyrotoxicosis
autoimmunity
islet a.
polyglandular a.
autoinfarction
complete a.
Autolet fingerstick device
automated perimetry
autonomic
a. cooling mechanism
a. dysfunction
a. nervous system
a. neuropathy
a. polyneuropathy
a. postganglionic nerve terminal
autonomous
a. adrenal hyperplasia
a. hyperfunction
a. nodular hyperplastic gland
a. nodule
a. parathyroid chief cell proliferation
a. toxic nodule
autonomously functioning thyroid nodule (AFTN)
autonomy
masked thyroid a.
nodular a.
thyroid gland a.
autophosphorylation
insulin-stimulated a.
autoproteolysis
autoradiography
receptor a.
thyamidine a.
thymidine a.
autoregulation
autosomal
DAZ-like a. (DAZLA)
deleted in azoospermia-like a. (DAZLA)
a. dominant condition
a. dominant diabetes mellitus
a. dominant disorder
a. dominant hypocalcemia
a. dominant hypoparathyroidism
a. dominant osteosclerosis
a. dominant toxic thyroid hyperplasia
a. karyotypic disorder
a. recessive disease
a. recessive disorder
a. recessive hypophosphatemic rickets
autosome
X chromosome to a. (X:A)
autosympathectomy
autotransplantation
parathyroid a.
Avandia
aversion
a. center
aversive stimulus
avian-intracellulare
Mycobacterium a.-i.
avian myeloblastosis virus (AMV)
avidin
avidin-biotin complex assay (ABCD)
avidity
Avitene
avium-intracellulare
Mycobacterium a.-i.

NOTES

AVM
arteriovenous malformation
AVP
arginine vasopressin
AVS
adrenal venous sampling
AVT
arginine vasotocin
AV3V
anteroventral 3rd ventricle
AvWD
acquired von Willebrand disease
axial
a. osteomalacia
a. QCT
a. quantified computed tomography
a. skeleton
Axid AR
axillary hair
axis
adenohypophysial-thyroid a.
adipoleptin growth hormone a.
adrenocorticotropic-adrenal a.
brain-gut a.
endocrine a.
enteroinsular a. (EIA)
fetal-hypothalamic-pituitary-adrenal a.
GHRH-GH-IGF a.
gonadal a.
growth hormone a.
growth hormone/insulin-like growth factor a.
growth hormone-releasing hormone-growth hormone-insulin-like growth hormone a.
HPA a.
HPG a.
HPT a.
hyperparathyroidism a.
hypothalamic-pituitary a.
hypothalamic-pituitary-adrenal a.
hypothalamic-pituitary-gonadal a.
hypothalamic-pituitary-ovarian a.
hypothalamic-pituitary-thyroid a.
hypothalamopituitary-adrenocortical a.
pituitary-gonadal a.
pituitary-thyroid a.
pituitary-thyroidal a.
putative neural a.
renin-aldosterone a.
renin-angiotensin-aldosterone a.
serotonergic a.
somatotropic a.
thyroid a.
axon
afferent a.
a. response of Lewis
sympathetic preganglionic a.
axonemal
a. complex
a. structure
axoneme
Ayala disease
Aygestin
azaprostanoic acid
azathioprine
AZF
azoospermia factor
azide
sodium a.
azidothymidine (AZT)
azithromycin
azoospermia
deleted in a. (DAZ)
deleted in a.-homologue (DAZH)
a. factor (AZF)
azotemia
prerenal a.
AZT
azidothymidine
azurin
acid solochrome a.

β (*var. of* beta)
B
amphotericin B
apolipoprotein B (apo B)
cathepsin B
B cell
compound B
coxsackievirus B
hepatitis B
inhibin B
liposomal amphotericin B
B lymphocyte
neurokinin B
B oncogene
Orexin B
procarboxypeptidase B (PCPB)
proenkephalin B
protein kinase B (PKB)
B vitamin therapy
2B
protein phosphatase 2B
B2
thromboxane B2 (TXB2, TxB2)
B6
vitamin B6
B100
familial defective apolipoprotein B100
17B
17B estradiol
Vagifem 17B
B19
parvovirus B19
B_4
leukotriene B_4 (LBA_4)
B_2
prostaglandin B_2
B_c
vitamin B_c
B_x
vitamin B_x
1b
b_4
b
phosphorylase *b*
B8 antigen
Babcock clamp
bacillus, pl. **bacilli**
b. Calmette-Guérin (BCG)
b. Calmette-Guérin vaccine
Döderlein b.
tubercle b.
bacteremia
bacterial
b. chloramphenicol acetyltransferase
b. overgrowth (BO)
b. thyroiditis
b. translocation
bactericidal
b. activity
b. killing
bacteriophage
b. lambda repressor
bacteriuria
Bacteroides
B. dermatitidis
B. fragilis
baculovirus vector
bafilomycin A
B/Akt
protein kinase B/Akt
balance
acid-base b.
calcium b.
glomerulotubular b.
nitrogen b.
phosphate b.
phosphorus b.
water b.
balanced electrolyte solution (BES)
balding
frontotemporal b.
temporal b.
baldness
male pattern b.
ballismus
balloon
b. dilation of the pancreatic duct sphincter
intragastric b.
Bancap HC
band
b. atrophy
Broca diagonal b.
C b.
floating beta b.
G b.
hypoechoic b. (halo)
b. keratopathy
Q b.
banding
gastric b.
Bannayan-Ruvalcaba-Riley (BRR)
Bannayan-Ruvalcaba-Riley syndrome
Bannayan-Zonana syndrome
Banophen Oral
Banthine
bar
Greenberg b.
ZNP B.

Barbidonna
barbiturate
Bardet-Biedl syndrome
bare lymphocyte syndrome
barium
b. contrast esophagography
b. swallow
βARK
beta-adrenergic receptor kinase
baroreceptor
carotid sinus b.
high-pressure b.
low-pressure b.
baroreflex
b. activity
baroregulation
barostat
electronic b.
Barr body
barrel deformity
barrier
blood-brain b. (BBB)
blood-cerebrospinal fluid b.
blood-testis b.
perivitelline b.
Bartholin gland
Bartter syndrome
basal
b. aluminum level
b. body temperature (BBT)
b. catecholamine secretion
b. cell nevus syndrome
b. compartment
b. encephalocele
b. ganglia
b. ganglion calcification
b. glycemia
b. 24-hour UFC excretion
b. 24-hour urine free cortisol excretion
b. insulin secretion
b. insulin therapy
b. lamina
b. level
b. metabolic rate (BMR)
b. metabolism
b. plasma cortisol
b. plasma GH level
b. plasma growth hormone level
b. plate
b. promoter element (BPE)
b. serum prolactin level
b. sphincter pressure
b. surface
b. telencephalon
b. thyroxine
basal body temperature (BBT)
basale
stratum b.
basal ganglia
basalis
decidua b.
Basaljel
base
Schiff b.
skull b.
Basedow
B. disease
B. paraplegia
baseline
b. aldosterone/plasma renin activity ratio
b. BMI
b. body mass index
base-substitution effect
basic
b. fibroblast growth factor (bFGF)
b. helix-loop-helix (bHLH)
b. helix-loop-helix transcription factor
b. multicellular unit (BMU)
One Touch B.
B. Rest-Activity Cycle (BRAC)
basilar
b. cistern
b. meningitis
b. sinus
basis pedunculi
basisphenoid
basolateral plasma membrane
basophil
basophilic
b. adenoma
b. cell
b. cell invasion
Bassen-Kornzweig syndrome
BAT
brown adipose tissue
battered baby syndrome
bayesian approach
Bayes rule
bayoneted Jannetta microdissector
#11 bayonet-handled scalpel
BB
platelet-derived growth factor BB
BBB
blood-brain barrier
4-1BBL
4-1BB ligand
4-1BB ligand (4-1BBL)
BBM
brush-border membrane
BBS
BES buffered saline

BBT
basal body temperature
B-cell
B-c. activation
B-c. antigen
B-c. antigen receptor (BCR)
B-c. antiinsulin
B-c. autoimmune thyroid disease
B-c. function
B-c. growth factor (BCGF)
B-c. ontogeny
B-c. repertoire
BCG
bacillus Calmette-Guérin
BCG vaccine
bCgA
bovine chromogranin A
synthetic bCgA
BCGF
B-cell growth factor
B-complex
ferrous sulfate, ascorbic acid, and vitamin B.-c.
BCR
B-cell antigen receptor
BCX-34
BD
bile duct
BDGF
bone-derived growth factor
B-D Glucose
BDNF
brain-derived neurotropic factor
beaked nose
becaplermin
Beckwith-Wiedemann syndrome
Becotin Pulvules
bed
splanchnic b.
bedtime
b. insulin
b. insulin, daytime sulfonylurea (BIDS)
bedwetting
beef insulin
Beepen-VK
beer potomania
behavior
aberrant b.
hyperoral b.
b. modification
oscillatory b.
behavioral rhythm
Belix Oral
belladonna
b. and opium
b., phenobarbital, and ergotamine tartrate
Bellatal
Bellergal
Bellergal-S
Bel-Phen-Ergot S
Benadryl
B. Oral
Ben-Allergin-50 Injection
bendroflumethiazide
Benecol
Benedict test
benfluorex
benign
b. cystic lesion
b. cystic teratoma
b. cystinosis
b. familial hypercalciuria
b. hypocalciuric hypercalcemia
b. intracranial hypertension
b. nodular disease
b. nodular goiter
b. optic glioma
b. pituitary cyst
b. prostatic fibroadenoma
b. prostatic hypertrophy
b. sporadic adrenal pheochromocytoma
Benylin
benzene
benzoate
benzodiazepine (BZD)
gamma-aminobutyric acid/b. (GABA/BZD)
benzonatate
benzothiophene
benzoyl peroxide
benzphetamine
Berardinelli-Seip syndrome
Bercu
B. patient
B. patient of Kindred S
B. syndrome
beriberi
Berocca
Berry ligament
Berubigen
berylliosis

NOTES

beryllium
BES
balanced electrolyte solution
BES buffered saline (BBS)
Besnier prurigo
Beta-2
beta, β
b. agonist
b. blocker
b. cell
b. cell destruction
b. cell dysmaturation syndrome
b. cell hyperplasia
b. cell polypeptide
b. cell replacement
b. cell secretory granule
b. cell transplant
ER b.
estrogen receptor b.
follitropin b.
integrin alpha v b. 3
retinoic acid X receptor b.
thymosin $b._4$ (Tb_4)
transforming growth factor b. (TGF-B, TGFβ)
beta-adrenergic, β-adrenergic
b.-a. agent
b.-a. agonist
b.-a. blocker
b.-a. effect
b.-a. receptor
b.-a. receptor kinase (βARK)
b.-a. vasodilation
$beta_2$-adrenergic
b.-a. catecholamine
b.-a. receptor
$beta_1$-adrenergic receptor
beta-alanine
b.-a. transaminase
beta-aminobutyrate
beta-aminoisobutyrate
beta-arrestin protein
beta-carotene
beta-cell
b.-c. impairment
islet b.-c.
beta-cellulin
Betachron
Betadine
beta-END
beta-endorphin
beta-endorphin (beta-END)
plasma b.-e.
beta-endorphinergic afferent
beta-estradiol
17-beta-estradiol
17-b.-e. valerate
beta-galactosidase
beta-gamma complex
beta-glucuronidase
17-beta-glucuronide
betaglycan
beta-granin
beta-granin
3-beta-HSD
3-beta-hydroxysteroid dehydrogenase
11-beta-HSD
11-beta-hydroxysteroid dehydrogenase
11-beta-HSD1
11-beta-hydroxysteroid dehydrogenase type 1
11-beta-HSD2
11-beta-hydroxysteroid dehydrogenase type 2
17-beta-HSD
17-beta-hydroxysteroid dehydrogenase
17-beta-HSD1
17-beta-hydroxysteroid dehydrogenase type 1
17-beta-HSD2
17-beta-hydroxysteroid dehydrogenase type 2
17-beta-HSD3
17-beta-hydroxysteroid dehydrogenase type 3
17-beta-HSD4
17-beta-hydroxysteroid dehydrogenase type 4
17-beta-HSD5
17-beta-hydroxysteroid dehydrogenase type 5
beta-human chorionic gonadotropin (β-hCG)
17-beta-hydroxyandrogen
beta-hydroxy-beta-methylglutaryl-coenzyme A (HMG-CoA)
beta-hydroxybutyrate
beta-hydroxybutyrate
beta-hydroxylase
dopamine b.-h. (DBH)
11-beta-hydroxylase (CYP11B1)
11-b.-h. deficiency
21-beta-hydroxylase (CYP21B1)
beta-hydroxysteroid
3-beta-hydroxysteroid
3-b.-h. dehydrogenase (3-beta-HSD)
3-b.-h. dehydrogenase deficiency
11-beta-hydroxysteroid
11-b.-h. dehydrogenase (11-beta-HSD)
11-b.-h. dehydrogenase type 1 (11-beta-HSD1)
11-b.-h. dehydrogenase type 2 (11-beta-HSD2)

17-beta-hydroxysteroid
17-b.-h. dehydrogenase (17-beta-HSD)
17-b.-h. dehydrogenase type 1 (17-beta-HSD1)
17-b.-h. dehydrogenase type 2 (17-beta-HSD2)
17-b.-h. dehydrogenase type 3 (17-beta-HSD3)
17-b.-h. dehydrogenase type 4 (17-beta-HSD4)
17-b.-h. dehydrogenase type 5 (17-beta-HSD5)
betaine
beta-lactamase
BetalinS
beta-lipoprotein (beta-LPH)
beta-lipotropin
beta-LPH
beta-lipoprotein
beta-mannosidosis
beta-melanocyte-stimulating hormone
betamethasone
beta$_2$-microglobulin
b.-m. amyloid deposition
b.-m. amyloidosis
beta$_2$-microglobulinemia
beta-MSH,
beta-nerve growth factor
11-beta-OHD
beta-ol-dehydrogenase deficiency
beta-preprotachykinin A
beta-receptor
b.-r. agonist
pinealocyte b.-r.
beta-secretase
beta-sitosterol
beta-thalassemia
beta-thyroid-stimulating
b.-t.-s. hormone (beta-TSH)
b.-t.-s. hormone gene
beta-TSH
beta-thyroid-stimulating hormone
beta-TSH gene
bethanechol
bexarotene
Bexophene
bFGF
basic fibroblast growth factor
BFR
bone formation rate
bG
blood glucose
Chemstrip bG
BGP
bone G1a protein
BGP protein
bHLH
basic helix-loop-helix
bHLH transcription factor
biallelic
b. expression
biantennary
bicalutamide
bicarbonate
b. anion
serum b.
sodium b.
Bicitra
bicolored irides
bicuspid aortic valve
BIDS
bedtime insulin, daytime sulfonylurea
BIDS therapy
bifid
b. scrotum
bifidus
lactobacillus b.
bifrontal craniotomy
biglycan
b. bone sialoprotein
biguanide
b. oral antihyperglycemic
b. oral antihyperglycemic agent
bihormonal effector
bilateral
b. adrenal disease
b. adrenal vein catheterization
b. anorchia
b. hemianopsia
b. idiopathic hyperaldosternism
b. IHA
b. macronodular hyperplasia
b. pes cavus deformity
b. salpingo-oophorectomy (BSO)
bile
b. acid
b. acid resin
b. acid sequestrant
b. duct (BD)
b. sequestrant
bile-binding resin
bile-salt malabsorption

NOTES

biliary
b. atresia
b. colic
b. fistula
b. sludge
b. worm
biliointestinal bypass
biliopancreatic bypass
bilirubin
conjugated b.
bilirubinemia
biliverdin
Billroth II operation
bimanual synkinesis
bimodal pattern
binder
aluminum-containing phosphate b.
phosphate b.
binding
anabolic-androgenic steroid b.
b. assay
calcium b.
b. capacity
fragment antigen b. (Fab)
^{3}H-imipramine b.
insulin b.
nonspecific b. (NSB)
phosphate b.
phosphorus b.
protein b.
receptor ligand b.
total androgen b.
bioactivation
bioactive
b. mediator
b. parathyroid hormone
bioamine neurotransmitter
bioartificial pancreas
bioassay
cytochemical b. (CBA)
endogenous estrogen b.
in vitro b.
in vivo b.
bioavailable
b. fluoride
b. testosterone level
Biocef
biochanin A
biochemical
b. gate
b. hypothyroidism
b. marker
b. remission
biochemically euthyroid
bioeffect
bioelectrical impedance
bioequivalence
bioflavanoid
bioinactive
bioinactivity
gonadotropin b.
bioincompatibility
hemodialysis membrane b.
bioineffective
biologic
b. catalyst
b. half-life
bioluminescence detection
biopsy
bone b.
fine-needle aspiration b. (FNAB)
FNA b.
iliac crest bone b.
large-needle aspiration b. (LNAB)
percutaneous b.
thyroid b.
transrectal b.
transurethral ultrasound-guided b.
TRUS-guided b.
biorhythm
pseudoperiodic b.
true periodic b.
biorhythmicity
biosensor
implantable b.
Biostator
biosynthesis
catecholamine b.
cortisol b.
hormone b.
prolactin b.
steroid b.
biosynthetic human insulin
biotechnology
biotic
biotin cofactor deficiency
biotinylated-nucleotide protocol
Biozyme-C
biphasic
biphenyl
polybrominated b. (PBB)
polychlorinated b. (PCB)
biphosphonate
bipolar cautery unit
bipyridine
inotropic b.
b. inotropic agent
Birbeck granule
bird-like facies
birefringence
apple-green b.
birefringent
b. collagen fibril
b. pattern
bisalbuminemia

BISF-W
Brief Index of Sexual Functioning for Women
Bismatrol
bismuth subsalicylate
4,5-bisphosphate
phosphatidylinositol -b. (PIP_2)
bisphosphonate
bitemporal
b. defect
b. hemianopia
b. hemianopsia
bitolterol
black
b. pus
b. thyroid
Blackfan-Diamond syndrome
blade-of-grass lesion
blastocoele
blastocyst
blastogenesis
blastolemmase
blastomere
Blastomyces dermatitidis
blastomycetica
erosio interdigitalis b.
blastomycosis
North America b.
bleach method
bleomycin
blepharitis
blepharophimosis, ptosis, epicanthus inversus syndrome
blepharoptosis
recurrent b.
blind hemihypophysectomy
blind-loop syndrome
blindness
chiasmatic postfixational b.
red-green color b.
blockade
Evaluation of PTCA to Improve Long-Term Outcome by C7E3 GpIIb/IIIa Receptor B. (EPILOG)
blocker
alpha-adrenergic b.
beta b.
beta-adrenergic b.
calcium-channel b.
dopaminergic b.
glycoprotein IIb and IIIb b.
noradrenergic b.
block-replace regimen
Blomstrand lethal chondrodysplasia
blood
circulating b.
citrated b.
b. clotting cascade
b. free thyroxine
b. glucose (bG)
b. glucose buffer system
b. glucose concentration
b. glucose monitoring
b. glucose testing
petrosal sinus b.
b. pressure (BP)
b. pressure dysregulation
b. purification therapy
b. sampling
b. spot assay
b. urea nitrogen (BUN)
b. volume
b. volume change
blood-borne pathogen
blood-brain barrier (BBB)
blood-cerebrospinal fluid barrier
blood-testis barrier
bloody fluid
Bloom syndrome
blot
Northern b.
Southern b.
Western b.
blue
Alcian b.
b.-diaper syndrome
methylene b.
b. patch
b. tinge sclera
b.-toe syndrome
Urolen b.
blueberry lesion
blues
postpartum b.
blunt estrogenic stimulation
blunting
b. of nocturnal thyroid-stimulating hormone surge
b. of nocturnal TSH surge
BMAL1
brain/muscle ARNT-like protein 1
BMAL1 protein
BMD
bone mineral density

NOTES

BMI
body mass index
baseline BMI

BMP
bone morphogenetic protein
bone morphogenic protein

BMR
basal metabolic rate

BMU
basic multicellular unit

BNP
brain natriuretic peptide

BO
bacterial overgrowth

body
Aschoff b.
Barr b.
Call-Exner b.
carotid b.
b. cell mass
b. composition
b. densitometry
Doehle b.
F b.
b. fluid osmolality
Herring b.
hyaline b.
ketone b.
lysosomal dense b.
mammillary b.
b. mass index (BMI)
oxytocinergic cell b.
polar b.
psammoma b.
Schumann b.
ultimobranchial b. (UB)
b. water
b. water osmolality
b. weight
X b.
Y b.
yellow b.

BodyGem metabolism monitor

bombesin
b. infusion
b.-like peptide
mammalian b.

bond
noncovalent b.
selenosulfide b.

bone
adynamic b.
b. alkaline phosphatase
alveolar b.
autograft b.
b. biopsy
cancellous b.
b. carbonate
b. cell
b. cell receptor
compact b.
b. consolidation
cortical b.
b. crisis
b. deficiency
b. densitometry
b. effect
b. embedding
fibrous dysplasia of b.
b. fluid
b. formation rate (BFR)
b. formation-stimulating agent
b. G1a protein (BGP)
b. growth
b. histology
b. hunger
hungry b.
hyoid b.
intramembranous b.
lamellar b.
long b.
b. marrow
b. marrow-derived myogenic progenitor
b. marrow-derived stromal cell
b. marrow element
b. marrow function
b. marrow stroma
b. marrow transplantation
b. mass
b. mass accretion
b. mass density
b. mass maintenance
membranous b.
b. mineral
b. mineral accretion
b. mineral density (BMD)
b. mineral metabolism
b. morphogenetic protein (BMP)
b. morphogenetic protein-2
b. morphogenetic protein-4
b. morphogenetic protein-7
b. morphogenic protein (BMP)
b. mucormycosis
osteoclastic b.
Paget disease of b.
pagetic b.
b. pain
b. quantum
rachitic b.
b. reconstruction
b. remodeling
b. resorption
b. resorption-inhibiting agent
sarcomatous b.
b. scan

b. sialoprotein (BSP)
sphenoid b.
spongy b.
spotted b.
b. structural unit
trabecular b.
b. turnover
undercalcified b.
von Recklinghausen disease of b.
wormian b.
woven b.

bone-age radiography

bone-derived growth factor (BDGF)

bone-forming
b.-f. cell
b.-f. cell transplantation

bone-related protein

bone-resorbing
b.-r. agent
b.-r. cytokine
b.-r. osteoclast

bone-specific
b.-s. alkaline phosphatase
b.-s. cathepsin
b.-s. protein

bone-within-bone

Bontril
B. PDM
B. Slow-Release

bony
b. exostosis
b. reservoir

boot
hyperbaric b.

borborygmus

border
ruffled b.

Borrelia

bossing
frontal b.

B&O Supprettes

botulinum
b. A toxin
b. toxin
b. toxin type A

bound
b. hormone
total b. (TB)

bovine
b. chromogranin A (bCgA)
b. insulin
b. parathyroid hormone (bPTH)
pegademase b.
b. serum albumin (BSA)
b. viral diarrhea mucosal disease (BVD-MD)
b. viral diarrhea mucosal disease virus

bow
Cupid b.
b. leg

bowel-associated dermatosis-arthritis syndrome

Bowman
B. capsule
B. gland

bow-tie atrophy

box
CAAT b.
consensus TATA b.
Goldberg-Hogness b.
high mobility group b.
HMG b.
TATA b.
toe b.

boydii
Allescheria b.

BP
blood pressure

BPE
basal promoter element

B2036-PEG

bPTH
bovine parathyroid hormone

BR
Velosulin BR

BRAC
Basic Rest-Activity Cycle

brachial
b. plexus
b. pressure

brachial-to-penile Doppler blood pressure ratio

brachydactyly

bradycardia

bradykinesia

bradykinin
desArg b.

Bragg peak proton irradiation therapy

brain
b. development
gliotic b.
b. hormone
b. isoenzyme

NOTES

brain *(continued)*
b. monoamine
b. natriuretic peptide (BNP)
b. necrosis
b. tumor
brain-derived neurotropic factor (BDNF)
brain-gut
b.-g. axis
b.-g. peptide
brain/muscle
b./m. Ahr nuclear translocator-like protein 1
b./m. ARNT-like protein 1 (BMAL1)
brainstem
b. reticular formation
branch
b. chain 2-ketoacid decarboxylase
b. chain ketoaciduria
choroidal b.
b. retinal vein occlusion
thymic b.
branched-chain amino acid
branchial
b. pouch
b. pouch dysembryogenesis
brandenberg
Salmonella b.
Bra Pocket pump holder
brawny edema
Braxton-Hicks contraction
BRCA
breast cancer antigen
BRCA gene
BRCA 1 mutation
BRCA 2 mutation
BRCA1 gene
BRCA2 gene
BrDU
bromodeoxyuridine
breast
b. cancer
b. cancer antigen (BRCA)
b. cancer antigen 1 mutation
b. cancer antigen 2 mutation
b. cancer cell
b. cancer gene
b. development
fibroadenomatous hyperplasia of b.
b. lobule
b. milk
b. parenchyma
pigeon b.
b. silicone implant
b. stimulation
b. tumor
breastfeeding
breast/ovarian cancer syndrome
Brenner tumor
Breonesin
2-Br-alpha-ergocryptine mesylate
Brethaire
Brethine
Brevicon
Bricanyl
bridge
cytoplasmic b.
disulfide b.
intermolecular dityrosine b.
bridged sella turcica
Brief Index of Sexual Functioning for Women (BISF-W)
British Diabetes Association
brittle-bone disease
brittle diabetes
broad
b. beta disease
b. ligament
Broca diagonal band
Bromanate DC
bromide
butylscopolamine b.
cyanogen b.
bromoaurone analog
bromocriptine
Apo B.
b. therapy
bromodeoxyuridine (BrDU)
b. uptake
bromodiphenhydramine and codeine
bromoflavone
bromophenolic ring
brompheniramine, phenylpropanolamine, and codeine
Bromsulphalein (BSP)
bronchial
b. carcinoid variant syndrome
b. lavage
b. microcarcinoid
bronchial asthma
bronchiectasis
bronchocentric granulomatosis
bronchoconstriction
bronchopneumonia
Bronkometer
Bronkosol
Brontex Tablet
bronze
b. diabetes
b. disease
brown
b. adipose tissue (BAT)
b. fat
b. tumor
Brown-Schilder disease

BRR
Bannayan-Ruvalcaba-Riley
BRR syndrome
brucei
Trypanosoma b.
Brucella
B. melitensis
brucellosis
Bruchner reflex
bruit
arterial b.
Brunner gland
brush-border
b.-b. alpha-glucosidase enzyme
b.-b. membrane (BBM)
brush cytology
brushite
Bruton
B. disease
B. tyrosine kinase (BTK)
B. tyrosine kinase gene
BSA
bovine serum albumin
BSO
bilateral salpingo-oophorectomy
BSP
bone sialoprotein
Bromsulphalein
BTK
Bruton tyrosine kinase
BTK gene
bubble boy disease
buccal
b. smear
b. testosterone
buciclate
testosterone b.
buffalo hump
buffer
b. nerve
proton b.
buffered citrate
Bufferin
buffering
hydrogen ion b.
buildup
callus b.
bulb
accessory olfactory b. (AOB)
jugular b.
olfactory b.
bulbospongiosus
b. muscle
bulbourethral
b. gland
b. gland of Cowper
bulbus
b. penis
b. vestibuli
bulging
chondrocostal junction b.
bulimia nervosa
bullosa
epidermolysis b.
bullosis diabeticorum
bullous
b. diabeticorum
b. pemphigoid
bull's-eye type macular atrophy
bulsulfan
bumetanide
b.-sensitive sodium-postassium-2 chloride cotransporter
Bumex
bumpy lips
BUN
blood urea nitrogen
bundle
medial forebrain b.
myelinated fiber b.
nigrostriatal b.
ventral adrenergic b.
Buprenex
buprenorphine
burden
aluminum b.
Burkitt lymphoma
Buschke-Ollendorff syndrome
buserelin
b. acetate
busulfan
butalbital compound and codeine
butanol-extractable iodine
butanone
butorphanol
button infuser
butylscopolamine bromide
B-variant
estrogen receptor B.-v.
BVD-MD
bovine viral diarrhea mucosal disease
BVD-MD virus

NOTES

bypass
- biliointestinal b.
- biliopancreatic b.
- gastric b.
- intestinal b.
- jejunoileal b.

bystander stimulation

BZD
- benzodiazepine

C

C apolipoprotein
C band
C cell
C cell adenoma
C cell hyperplasia
hemoglobin C
hepatitis C
mitomycin C
C peptide
phospholipase C (PLC)
protein kinase C (PKC)
very low density lipoprotein C (VLDL-C)

C-19

C. progestin
C. steroid

C-21

C. progestin
C. steroid

C_4

leukotriene C_4 (LTC_4)

C-18 steroid

CA

CA125

Ca^{2+}

cytoplasmic Ca^{2+}
free Ca^{2+}
Ca^{2+} ionophore A23187
Ca^{2+} ionophore drug
Ca^{2+} pump
total Ca^{2+}

CAAT box

Ca^{2+}-ATPase

calmodulin-dependent C.-A.

cabergoline

cachectin

cachexia

cancer c.
diencephalic c.
exophthalmic c.
neuropathic c.

cadaveric

c. pancreas transplantation

cadaver pancreas

cadherin

cadmium telluride detector

café au lait

c. a. l. lesion
c. a. l. macule
c. a. l. pigmentation
c. a. l. spot

cafeteria diet

caffeine

acetaminophen, aspirin, and c.
orphenadrine, aspirin, and c.

Caffey syndrome

CAH

congenital adrenal hyperplasia

CA II

carbonic anhydrase II
CA II deficiency
CA II gene

Calan

calbindin

c. D_{28K}
c. D_{9K}
c.-D9k
c. 9-kDA

Cal Carb-HD

calcemic

c. effect
c. response

Calci-Chew

Calciday-667

calcifediol

calciferol

c. metabolite

calcification

basal ganglion c.
dystrophic c.
ectopic c.
extracellular c.
extraskeletal c.
laminated c.
metastatic extraosseal c.
ocular c.
pathologic c.
popcorn c.
provisional c.
soft-tissue c.
tumor-like c.
vascular c.
visceral c.
zone of provisional c.

calcified

c. desquamated debris
c. malignant insulinoma

Calcijex

Calcimar

calcimimetic

c. agent
c. compound
c. drug

Calci-Mix

calcineurin

c. inhibitor

calcinosis
c. circumscripta
toxic c.
tumoral c.
c. universalis
calciopenic
c. rickets
calciotropic peptide hormone
calcipenia
calciphylaxis
calcipotriol
calcitonin (CT)
c. gene
c. gene expression
c. gene-related hormone (CGRH)
c. gene-related peptide (CGRP)
human c.
c. monomer
c. receptor
salmon c.
calcitonin-induced phosphaturia
calcitriol
c. deficiency
c. therapy
calcitriol-mediated hypercalcemia
calcitroic acid
calcitrol
calcitropic hormone
calcium
c. absorption
c. acetate
albumin-bound c.
amorphous c.
atorvastatin c.
c. balance
c. bilirubinate granule
c. binding
c. carbonate
c. carbonate and magnesium carbonate
c. carbonate oxyphil cell
c. carbonate and simethicone
circulating c.
c. citrate
c. complex
complexed c.
cytoplasmic c.
cytosolic free c.
c. deficiency
c. degradation
c. deposition
c. efflux
endogenous fecal c.
c. flux
c. glubionate
c. glucoheptonate
c. gluconate
c. gradient
c. homeostasis
c. homeostatic factor
c. hydrogen phosphate
immunoradiometric assay of circulating c.
intracellular c.
c. ion
c. ion concentration
ionic c.
c. ionophore
c. ionophore challenge
c. lactate
c. loading
c. malabsorption
c. oxalate
c. oxalate dihydrate crystal
c. oxalate monohydrate crystal
c. oxalate renal stone
c. phosphate compound
c. phosphate crystal
c. phosphorus metabolism
physiologically active c.
c. pump
c. pyrophosphate
c. receptor agonist
c. release
c. resorption
c. salt
c. sensor
serum ionized c.
c. stimulation test
c. times phosphorus product
total intestinal c.
c. transport
urinary c.
calcium-binding
c.-b. protein
c.-b. protein synthesis
calcium-channel blocker
calcium/creatinine
c. ratio
calcium-dependent protein kinase
calcium-lowering hormone
calcium-regulating hormone
calcium-sensing receptor (CaR)
calcium-to-creatinine ratio
calculation
Friedewald c.
calculus, pl. **calculi**
intrapancreatic c.
renal c.
Calderol
caldesmon
calendar
PRISM c.
California Diabetes and Pregnancy Sweet Success Guidelines

californica
Torpedo c.
calipers
Prader c.
Call-Exner body
callosum
corpus c.
dysgenesis of corpus c.
callus
c. buildup
Calmette-Guérin
bacillus C.-G. (BCG)
calmodulin
c. protein
calmodulin-dependent
c.-d. Ca^{2+}-ATPase
c.-d. protein kinase (CaM-kinase)
Calm-X Oral
calnexin
caloric intake
calorigenic activity
calorimetry
calpactin
Cal-Plus
Caltrate
C. 600
C. Jr.
calvarial
c. osteomalacia
c. thickening
CAM
cell-cell adhesion molecule
camera
Anger gamma c.
gamma c.
Planar gamma c.
scintillation c.
CaM-kinase
calmodulin-dependent protein kinase
cAMP
cyclic adenosine monophosphate
cyclic 3′,5′-adenosine monophosphate
cyclic AMP
cyclic arginine monophosphate
dibutyryl cAMP
nephrogenous cAMP
cAMP response element-binding (CREB)
cAMP-response
c.-r. element (CRE)
c.-r. element modulator (CREM)
camptodactyly
camptomelic
c. dwarfism
c. dysplasia
camsylate
trimethaphan c.
Camurati-Engelmann disease
Canadian-Dutch Mennonite kindreds
canal
craniopharyngeal c.
Dorello c.
haversian c.
optic c.
Volkmann c.
canalicular testis
canaliculus, pl. **canaliculi**
Canavan disease
cancellous bone
cancer
adrenal c.
American Joint Commission on C.
anaplastic thyroid c.
breast c.
c. cachexia
endometrial c.
estrogen receptor-positive breast c.
European Organization for Research and Treatment of C. (EORTC)
familial colorectal c.
familial gastric c.
familial medullary thyroid c. (FMTC)
familial ovarian c.
follicular thyroid c.
hereditary nonpolyposis colon c. (HNPCC)
hormone-resistant breast c.
liver c.
medullary thyroid c. (MTC)
pancreas c.
papillary thyroid c.
Union Internationale Contre le C. (UICC)
Candida
C. albicans
candidal vaginitis
candidate gene approach
candidiasis
c. endocrinopathy syndrome
hypoparathyroidism, adrenal insufficiency, mucocutaneous c. (HAM)

C

NOTES

candidiasis *(continued)*
mucocutaneous c.
vaginal c.
candiduria
canine
c. distemper
c. distemper virus
cannula
#7 French suction c.
Jarcho c.
cantharides
canthomeatal line
Cantil
CAP
catabolite activator protein
chronic alcoholic pancreatitis
contraction-associated protein
cap
acrosomal c.
c. phase
19S c. complex
capacitation of the spermatozoa
capacity
binding c.
reduced exercise c.
reserve c.
CAPD
chronic ambulatory peritoneal dialysis
continuous ambulatory peritoneal dialysis
capillary
adenohypophysial c.
c. basement membrane width (CBMW)
c. blood glucose monitoring
c. blood sugar (CBS)
c. endothelium
c. filtrate collector (CFC)
c. leak syndrome
Capital and codeine
capitalis
plexus pancreaticus c.
Capoten
caproate
hydroxyprogesterone c.
capsaicin
Capsin
capsularis
decidua c.
capsulatum
Histoplasma c.
capsule
Angel Hypoglycemic c.
Bowman c.
Diabetes Hypoglucose c.
internal c.
c. of islet
Pearl Hypoglycemic c.
tense tumor c.
Tongyi Tang Diabetes c.
Zhen Qi c.
captopril
c. test
caput
c. epididymis
Capzasin-P
CaR
calcium-sensing receptor
Carafate
carbamazepine
carbamide drug
carbamoyl
c. phosphate synthase
c. phosphate synthetase I deficiency
carbamoyltransferase
ornithine c.
carbamylcholine
muscarinic agonist c.
carbenoxolone
carbetapentane
Carb-HD
Cal C.-H.
carbidopa
levodopa and c.
carbimazole
carbodiimide modified heteroduplex screening method
carbohydrate
complex c.
c. intolerance
c. malabsorption
c. moiety
carbohydrate-deficient
c.-d. glycoprotein (CDG)
c.-d. glycoprotein syndrome
carbohydrate-induced hypertriglyceridemia
carbonate (CO_3^{2-})
aluminum c.
aluminum hydroxide and magnesium c.
bone c.
calcium c.
calcium carbonate and magnesium c.
dihydroxyaluminum sodium c.
c. ion
lithium c.
magnesium c.
carbon disulfide
carbonic
c. acid
c. anhydrase activity
c. anhydrase enzyme
c. anhydrase II (CA II)
c. anhydrase II deficiency

c. anhydrase II gene
c. anhydrase II isoenzyme
c. anhydrase inhibitor
carboplatin
carboxamide-Dome
dimethyl triazeno imidazole c.-D. (DTIC-Dome)
carboxyesterase
carboxykinase
carboxylase
acetyl-CoA c. (ACC_β)
hydroxymethylglutaryl-coenzyme A c.
3-methylcrotonyl c.
propionyl-coenzyme A c.
pyruvate c.
carboxyl kinase
carboxyl-terminal region
carboxyl-terminus
carboxymethylation
carboxypeptidase
dipeptidyl c.
c. E
c. H
carboxyterminal cross-linked telopeptide of type I collagen (ICTP)
carboxytermini
carbuncle
carcinoembryonic antigen (CEA)
carcinogenesis
radioactive iodine-induced c.
RAI-induced c.
carcinogenic
carcinoid
appendiceal c.
c. crisis
primary ovarian c.
sporadic c.
c. syndrome
thymic c.
c. tumor
type 1, 2, and 3 gastric c.
carcinoid-like tumor
carcinoma
acinar cell c. (ACC)
adrenal c.
adrenocortical c.
anaplastic thyroid c.
colon c.
differentiated thyroid c.
embryonal c.
encapsulated angioinvasive c.
epithelial thyroid c.
familial medullary thyroid c. (FMTC)
follicular thyroid c.
giant cell c.
infantile embryonic c.
infiltrating ductal c.
infiltrating lobular c.
insular c.
invasive ductal c. (IDC)
islet cell c.
lipid-laden homogeneous adrenocortical c.
medullary thyroid c. (MTC)
Merkel cell c.
mucoepidermoid c.
nevoid basal cell c.
nonpapillary thyrogenic c.
nonsmall cell c.
occult c.
pancreatic duct cell c. (PDC)
papillary renal c.
papillary thyroid c. (PTC)
parathyroid c.
pituitary c.
pleomorphic c.
radiation-associated papillary thyroid c.
c. of Sakamoto
small cell c.
spindle cell c.
thyrogenic c.
thyroglossal duct c.
thyroid gland c.
thyroid papillary c.
thyrotroph c.
Warthin-like papillary c.
c. with thymus-like differentiation (CASTLE)
c. with thymus-like differentiation tumor
carcinomatosa
peritonitis c.
cardiac
c. arrhythmia
c. endocrine aldosterone system
c. fibrosis
c. gene expression
c. index
c. mucormycosis
c. output (CO)
c. steroidogenic system

C

NOTES

cardiofaciocutaneous syndrome
cardiomyocyte
cardiomyopathy
diabetic c.
hypertrophic c.
cardiotropin-1 (CT-1)
cardiovascular
c. disorder
c. dysmetabolic syndrome
c. effect
Cardura
CARE
Cholesterol and Recurrent Events
CARE study
Caribbean fruit
carinatum
carinii
Pneumocystis c.
C-arm
fluoroscopic C.-a.
carmoisin
Carmol Topical
Carney
C. complex
C. syndrome
C. triad
triad of C.
carnitine
c. acylcarnitine translocase deficiency
c. palmitoyltransferase deficiency
c. palmitoyltransferase I (CPTI)
c. palmitoyltransferase I deficiency
c. palmitoyltransferase II (CPTII)
c. palmitoyltransferase II deficiency
c. shuttle
Carnitor
carnosinase
carnosine
carotenoderma
carotid
c. aneurysm
c. artery
c. body
c. body tumor
c. sinus
c. sinus baroreceptor
carpal tunnel syndrome
carpopedal spasm
carpotarsal osteolysis
carrier
c. detection
dolichol phosphate c.
c. protein
CART
cocaine and amphetamine regulated transcript
cartilage
articular c.
c. calcification failure
cricoid c.
hyaline c.
Meckel c.
preosseous c.
thyroid c.
cartilaginous anlage
cartridge
Genotropin two-chamber c.
Novolin 85/15 PenFill c.
sorbent dialysis c.
CASA
computer-aided sperm analysis
computer-assisted semen analysis
cascade
adenylyl cyclase c.
adrenal steroidogenic c.
arachidonic acid c.
blood clotting c.
insulin phosphorylation c.
MAPK c.
mitogen-activated protein kinase c.
protein kinase C c.
protein kinase/phosphatase c.
caseating granuloma
casein
c. hydrolysate
c. kinase I
c. kinase II
CASH
cortical androgen-stimulating hormone
Casodex
cassava
CASTLE
carcinoma with thymus-like differentiation
CASTLE tumor
Castleman disease
castration
c. cell
chemical c.
CAT
chloramphenicol acetyl transferase
catabolic stress
catabolism
accelerated c.
fat c.
muscle c.
statin c.
catabolite
c. activator protein (CAP)
c. regulatory protein
Cataflam Oral
catagen
catalysis

catalyst
biologic c.
catalytic homodimer
catamenial epilepsy
cataplexy
Catapres
cataract
subcapsular c.
catch trial
catecholamine
$alpha_2$-adrenergic c.
$beta_2$-adrenergic c.
c. biosynthesis
fetal c.
fractionated urinary c.
c. receptor gene
c. response
c. surge
catecholaminergic
c. system
catecholamine-secreting cell
catechol compound
catecholestrogen
catechol-*O*-methyltransferase (COMT)
cathepsin
c. B
c. B enzyme
bone-specific c.
c. D
c. H
c. K
c. K gene
c. L
c. O
c. S
catheter
lumbar cerebrospinal fluid c.
radiopaque silastic c.
Soehendra dilating c.
Tracker c.
catheterization
bilateral adrenal vein c.
cationic trypsinogen gene
Caucus
Congressional Diabetes C.
caveola
cavernosum
corpus c.
cavernous
c. hemangioma
c. sinus
c. sinus sampling (CSS)
c. sinus syndrome
c. sinus thrombophlebitis
cavity
amnionic c.
endometrial c.
intrasellar c.
medullary c.
nasal c.
CBA
cytochemical bioassay
CBAVD
congenital bilateral absence of the vas deferens
CBC
complete blood count
CBD
common bile duct
CBF
cerebral blood flow
CBG
corticosteroid-binding globulin
cortisol-binding globulin
CBMW
capillary basement membrane width
CBP
CREB-binding protein
CBS
capillary blood sugar
c/c
Snp5 c/c
CCAAT/enhancer binding protein (C/EBP)
CCCT
clomiphene citrate challenge test
CCD
cortical collecting duct
C cell
C-cell complex
ccHRT
continuous-combined hormone replacement therapy
CCK
cholecystokinin
CCK-A and CCK-B
cholecystokinin A and cholecystokinin B
CCK-A and CCK-B receptor
CCK-8-S
CCPT
chronic calcific pancreatitis of the tropics
C-Crystals
CD
C. 27 ligand (CD 27L)

NOTES

CD *(continued)*
C. 30 ligand (CD 30L)
C. 40 ligand (CD 40L)
CD1 antigen
CD4 helper lymphocyte
CD4+ T cell
CD8+
C. phenotype
C. T cell
CD8 suppressor lymphocyte
CDE
Certified Diabetes Educator
CDG
carbohydrate-deficient glycoprotein
CDGA
constitutional delay in growth and adolescence
CDI
central diabetes insipidus
CDK
cyclin-dependent kinase
Cdk
cyclin-dependent kinase
CD 27L
CD 27 ligand
CD 30L
CD 30 ligand
CD 40L
CD 40 ligand
cDNA
complementary deoxyribonucleic acid
complementary DNA
CDR3
third complementarity determining region
CDU
color Doppler ultrasonography
CEA
carcinoembryonic antigen
Cebid
C/EBP
CCAAT/enhancer binding protein
C/EBP transcription factor
cecocentral
c. defect
c. scotoma
Cecon
cecum
foramen c.
CEE
conjugated equine estrogen
CEEP
conjugated equine estrogen plus norgestrel
cefadroxil
Cefanex
cefdinir
Cefol Filmtabs
ceftazidime
Celebrex
celecoxib
Celestone
C. Oral
C. Phosphate Injection
C. Soluspan
celiac
c. artery
c. axis arteriography
c. disease
c. plexus
c. sprue
cell
A c.
A_1 c.
A_2 c.
acidophilic c.
adenohypophysial corticotroph c.
adrenal cortex c.
adrenocortical c.
adrenomedullary c.
alpha c.
alveolar type II c.
amine precursor uptake and decarboxylation c.
antigen-presenting c. (APC)
antigen-specific suppressor T c.
apical membrane of proximal convoluted tubule c.
APUD c.
argentaffin c.
argyrophil c.
Askanazy c.
c. association
autocrine c.
B c.
c. basement membrane
basophilic c.
beta c.
bone c.
bone-forming c.
bone marrow-derived stromal c.
breast cancer c.
C c.
calcium carbonate oxyphil c.
castration c.
catecholamine-secreting c.
CD4+ T c.
CD8+ T c.
CFU-E c.
chemoreceptive c.
chief c.
Chinese hamster ovary c.
CHO c.
chromaffin c.
chromophilic c.
chromophobic c.
ciliated c.

clear c.
clonal c.
colony-forming unit erythroid c.
compact c.
corticotropic c.
Crooke c.
cuboidal epithelioid c.
c. culture study
cumulus granulosa c.
cycling c.
D c.
delta c.
determined osteoprogenitor c.
ECL c.
electrically excitable c.
endocrine effector c.
endothelial c. (EC)
enterochromaffin c. (EC)
enterochromaffin-like c.
epithelioid giant c.
eukaryotic c.
exocrine c.
F c.
Feryter system endocrine c.
Fischer rat thyroid line-5 c.
foam c.
foamy c.
follicular c.
folliculostellate c.
FRTL-5 c.
G c.
ghost c.
glial c.
goblet c.
gonadectomy c.
gonadotroph c.
granular chromophil c.
granulated c.
granulosa lutein c.
growth hormone c.
growth hormone-expressing c.
growth hormone-prolactin c.
helper T c.
hilar c.
hilus c.
Hofbauer c.
homeobox gene expressed in ES c.'s (HESX1)
hormone-secreting c.
horny c.
host c.
human pluripotent stem c.
Hürthle c.
hybridoma c.
hypochromic microcytic red blood c.
inflammatory c.
insulinoma c.
insulin-producing c.
intercalated c.
islet c.
JG c.
Jurkat c.
juxtaglomerular c.
Kornchenzellen c.
Kulchitsky c.
Kupffer c.
L c.
LAK c.
Langerhans c.
Leydig c.
lipid-laden clear c.
lipoid c.
lutein c.
lymphoid c.
lymphokine-activated killer c.
macula densa c.
mammosomatotroph c.
marrow hematopoietic stem c.
mast c.
medullary c.
melanotropic c.
membrana granulosa c.
mesangial c.
mesenchymal stem c.
mesodermal c.
murine L c.
myelomonocytic c.
myoepithelial c.
myoid c.
natural killer c.
neoplastic adenohypophysial c.
neuroendocrine c.
neuroglia c.
neurohormonal c.
neurosecretory c.
NK c.
noncontractile c.
noncornified c.
nongranular clear chromophobe c.
null c.
osteoblast-like osteosarcoma c.
osteoprogenitor c.
ovarian granulosa c.

C

NOTES

cell *(continued)*
oxyphil c.
pancreatic acinar c.
pancreatic islet beta c.
parabasal c.
paracrine c.
parafollicular calcitonin-producing c.
parathyroid c.
parathyroid hormone-related protein-transfected RIN-141 c.
pathognomonic Askanazy c.
peripheral cytotrophoblast c.
peritubular endothelial c.
pituitary lactotroph c.
pluripotent hematopoietic c.
pluripotential precursor c.
pluripotential stromal c.
pluripotent stem c.
PMN c.
polarized c.
polyclonal B c.
polyclonal T c.
polygonal c.
polyhedral c.
polymorphonuclear c.
polypeptide-producing c.
polyploidic c.
pregnancy c.
primordial germ c. (PGC)
progenitor c.
prokaryotic c.
prolactin hormone-expressing c.
pseudogiant c.
PTHrP-transfected RIN-141 c.
Purkinje c.
red blood c. (RBC)
renal carcinoma c.
resting c.
Schwann c.
secondary interstitial c.
c. senescence
Sertoli c.
Sertoli-Leydig c.
sickle c. (SC)
c. signaling
somatostatin-producing delta c.
somatotroph c.
somatotropic c.
spindle c.
stem c.
stromal c.
suppressor T c.
supraopticohypophysial c.
surrogate beta c.
sympathetic c.
syncytiotrophoblast c.
T c.
tall c.
target c.
Th1 c.
Th2 c.
theca externa c.
theca interna c.
theca interstitial c.
theca lutein c.
T helper c.
T helper 1 c.
T helper 2 c.
thyroidal C c.
thyroid C c.
thyroid deficiency c.
thyroidectomy c.
thyroid epithelial c.
thyroid follicular c.
thyroid parafollicular c.
thyrotroph c.
thyrotropic c.
thyrotropin-stimulating hormone-expressing c.
trophoblast c.
tumor c.
vascular smooth muscle c. (VSMC)
white blood c. (WBC)
zona fasciculata c.
zona glomerulosa c.

cell-bone matrix interaction
cell-cell adhesion molecule (CAM)
CellCept
cell-mediated
c.-m. immunity
c.-m. toxicity

cell-signaling mechanism
cell-specific ablation
cell-surface antigen
cell-to-cell communication
cellular
c. dehydration
c. immunity

cellulitis
necrotizing c.
nonclostridial anaerobic c.
orbital c.
synergistic necrotizing c.

cellulose
c. sodium phosphate
c. sulfate

cellulose-derived matrix
Cel-U-Jec Injection
cement line
cementum
Cenestin
Cenolate
center
aversion c.
central thermoregulatory c.
germinal c.

hypothalamic c.
Joslin Diabetes C.
Memorial Sloan-Kettering Cancer C.
X inactivation c. (Xic)
Center for Human Islet Transplantation
centigray (cGy)
centiMorgan (cM)
central
c. adrenocortical insufficiency
c. diabetes insipidus (CDI)
c. hyperhidrosis
c. hypoadrenalism
c. hypogonadism
c. hypogonadism type IA
c. hypogonadism type IB
c. hypogonadism type IIA
c. hypogonadism type III
c. hypothyroidism
c. necrosis
c. nervous system (CNS)
c. obesity
c. pontine myelinolysis
c. precocious puberty (CPP)
c. scotoma
c. thermoregulatory center
centriole
centripetal obesity
cephalexin
cephalic
c. parenchymography
c. phase
cephalopelvic disproportion
c-erbA
protooncogene c.-e.
c-erbA-beta
c.-e. gene
c.-e. receptor
c.-e. thyroid hormone receptor gene
c-erbA-beta-1 defect
c-erbA-beta-2 defect
cerebellar
c. cortex
c. vermis
cerebelloretinal hemangioblastomatosis
cerebellum
cerebral
c. artery
c. blood flow (CBF)
c. cortex
c. gigantism
c. palsy
c. peduncle
c. salt wasting
c. tetany
c. vein thrombosis
cerebri
acervuli c.
epiphysis c.
pseudomotor c.
pseudotumor c.
cerebrospinal
c. fluid (CSF)
c. fluid ACE level
c. fluid angiotensin-converting enzyme level
c. fluid fistula
c. fluid rhinorrhea
cerebrotendinous xanthomatosis
Ceredase
Cerezyme
cerivastatin
Cerose-DM
Certified Diabetes Educator (CDE)
cerulein
ceruleus
locus c.
ceruloplasmin
cervical
c. factor infertility
c. goiter
c. mucosa
c. mucous plug
c. sensory nerve
cervicodorsal fat pad
cervix uteri
Cesamet
cetylmyristoleate (CMO)
c. II
Cevalin
Cevi-bid
Ce-Vi-Sol
CFA
complete Freund adjuvant
CFC
capillary filtrate collector
CFC BioScanner System
C-fiber pain
c-*fms* oncogene
c-*fos*
c. gene
c. mapping
c. promoter
protooncogene c.

C

NOTES

cFos-cJun heterodimer
CFRD
cystic fibrosis-related diabetes
CFTR
cystic fibrosis transmembrane regulator
CFTR gene
CFU-E
colony-forming unit erythroid
CFU-E cell
CG
chorionic gonadotropin
CGI
glycoprotein crystal growth inhibitor
CGI protein
CGL
chronic granulocytic leukemia
cGMP
cyclic guanosine monophosphate
cyclic 3′,5′-guanosine monophosphate
5′-cyclic guanosine monophosphate
cGMP phosphodiesterase
cGMP-dependent protein kinase
CGMS
continuous glucose monitoring system
CGRH
calcitonin gene-related hormone
CGRP
calcitonin gene-related peptide
cGy
centigray
chain
jugular c.
myosin heavy c. (MHC)
myosin light c. (MLC)
nascent protein c.
oligosaccharide c.
sympathetic c.
challenge
calcium ionophore c.
desferoxamine c.
DFO c.
chamber
hyperbaric c.
change
blood volume c.
Crooke hyaline c.
fluorotic c.
intracytoplasmic oncocytic c.
oxyphilic c.
polyneuropathy, organomegaly, endocrinopathy, monoclonal component, skin c.'s (POEMS)
polyneuropathy, organomegaly, endocrinopathy, M proteins, skin c.'s (POEMS)
rachitic c.
sexual dimorphic physical c.
channel
apical iodide c.
aquaporin-2 water c.
AQ2 water c.
collecting tubule sodium c.
epithelial sodium c. (ENaC)
inward-directed voltage-gated Ca^{2+} c.
inward-rectifying K^+-c. 6.2 ($K_{ir}6.2$)
iodide c.
ion c.
kainate receptor c.
ligand-gated c.
L-type calcium c.
potassium leak c.
T-type calcium c.
voltage-dependent anion c. (VDAC)
voltage-gated Ca^{2+} c.
voltage-gated K^+ c.
voltage-gated Na^+ c.
channel-forming integral protein (CHIP)
CHAOS
coronary artery disease, hypertension, adult-onset diabetes, obesity, and stroke
chaperone
molecular c.
characteristic
chronobiologic c.
charcoal hemoperfusion
Charcot
C. arthropathy
C. joint
Charcot-Marie disease
Charcot-Marie-Tooth
C.-M.-T. disease
C.-M.-T. syndrome
chase incubation
ChAT
choline acetyltransferase
checklist
thyroid symptom c.
Chediak-Higashi syndrome
cheilitis
angular c.
cheiropathy
chelation
chelator
fura-2 fluorescent Ca^{2+} c.
quin-2 fluorescent Ca^{2+} c.
cheloni
Mycobacterium c.
chemical
c. castration
c. gradient
c. messenger
xenobiotic c.

chemiluminescence
c. assay
c. detection
chemiluminescent
c. assay
c. immunoassay (CLIA)
c. reagent
Chemistrip
Micral C.
chemodectoma
chemoembolization
transcatheter arterial c. (TACE)
chemokine
growth factor-inducible c. (FIC)
c. receptor
chemoreceptive cell
chemoreceptor
macula densa c.
chemosis
conjunctival c.
chemosurgery
chemotactic factor
chemotaxis
neutrophil c.
chemotherapy
adjuvant c.
cytotoxic c.
Chemstrip
C. bG
C. MatchMaker blood glucose meter
chest
c. wall lesion
c. wall trauma
Chiari-Frommel syndrome
chiasm
optic c.
chiasmal
c. arachnoiditis
c. compression
c. glioma
c. neuritis
c. syndrome
chiasmapexy
chiasmatic
c. cistern
c. postfixational blindness
c. sulcus
c. syndrome
chiasmatis
cisterna c.
chiasmopathy
chicken ovalbumin upstream promoter-transcription factor (COUP-TF)
chief cell
child
growth hormone-deficient c.
rachitic c.
vitamin D-replete c.
childhood
c. Cushing syndrome
c. Graves disease
c. head and neck irradiation
c. hypothyroidism
Child-Pugh
C.-P. class
C.-P. disease
chimeric
c. protein
c. pseudogene
c. receptor
chimerism
chimerization
Chinese
C. hamster ovary (CHO)
C. hamster ovary cell
CHIP
channel-forming integral protein
Chiron ACS:180 assay
chiropody
Chlamydia trachomatis
chloasma gravidarum
chlorambucil
chloramphenicol acetyl transferase (CAT)
chlorbutanol
chlordiazepoxide
clidinium and c.
chloride
Adrenalin C.
ammonium c.
c. channel gene CLCNKB
methyl c.
thallium c. (TI-201)
^{201}Tl-thallous c.
zinc c.
chloroquine
chlorothiazide
chlorotrianisene
chlorpromazine
chlorpropamide
chlorpyrifos
chlorthalidone

NOTES

CHO
Chinese hamster ovary
CHO cell
Choice
Medi-Jector C.
cholangiography
magnetic resonance c. (MRC)
cholangiopancreatography
endoscopic retrograde c. (ERCP)
magnetic resonance c. (MRCP)
cholecalciferol
cholecystitis
acalculous c.
emphysematous c.
xanthogranulomatous c.
cholecystography
cholecystokinin (CCK)
c. A and cholecystokinin B (CCK-A and CCK-B)
c. A and cholecystokinin B receptor
choledochal cyst
choledochocele
choledochoscopy
percutaneous c.
cholelithiasis
cholera
pancreatic c.
c. toxin
cholerae
Vibrio c.
CholestaGel
cholestane
cholestanol
cholestasis
anicteric c.
intrahepatic c.
cholestatic
c. hepatitis
c. jaundice
c. liver disease
cholesteatoma
cholesterol
c. desmolase
c. desmolase deficiency
c. embolus
c. ester
c. ester hydrolase
c. ester storage disease
c. ester transfer protein
c. ester transfer protein deficiency
lipid c.
c. monohydrate crystal
C. and Recurrent Events (CARE)
C. and Recurrent Events study
c. spike
total c. (TC)
c. transport
cholesteryl
c. ester
c. ester storage disease
c. ester transfer protein
cholestyramine
c. resin
choline
c. acetyltransferase (ChAT)
c. magnesium trisalicylate
c. salicylate
cholinergic
c. effect
c. neuron
c. nicotinic receptor
c. pathway
chondrocalcinosis
chondrocostal junction bulging
chondrocyte
c. proliferation
c. terminal differentiation
chondrocytic
c. growth
c. lineage
chondrodysplasia
Blomstrand lethal c.
Jansen metaphyseal c. (JMC)
c. punctata
Schmid-type metaphyseal c.
chondrodystrophia punctata
chondroitin sulfate
chondroma
pulmonary c.
chondrosarcoma
Chooz
chordoma
sacrococcygeal c.
chorea
Huntington c.
choreiform movement
choreoathetosis
Chorex
choriocarcinoma
primary ovarian c.
testicular c.
chorion
c. frondosum
c. laeve
leafy c.
chorionepithelioma
chorionic
c. gonadotropin (CG)
c. gonadotropin-secreting tumor
c. gonadotropin stimulation test
c. plate
c. sac
c. somatomammotropin (CS)
c. thyrotropin

c. villus
c. villus sampling (CVS)
choristoma
adenohypophysial neuronal c.
intrasellar adenohypophyseal neuronal c.
pituitary adenoma-adenohypophyseal neuronal c. (PANCH)
pituitary adenoma-neuronal c.
choroid
c. artery
c. plexus
choroidal
c. branch
c. fissure
Choron
chromaffin
c. cell
c. granule
c. tissue
c. vesicle
Chromagen OB
chromalum-hematoxylin
Gomori c.-h.
Chroma-Pak
chromatid
sister c.
chromatin
c. derepression
sex c.
supercoiled c.
X c.
Y c.
chromatin-positive seminiferous tubule dysgenesis
chromatofocusing
chromatography
affinity c.
exclusion c.
gas c.
gel filtration c.
high-performance liquid c. (HPLC)
ion exchange c.
chromogen
chromogranin
c. A
c. A, B, C protein
bovine c. A (bCgA)
chromogranin-secretogranin protein
chromophil
chromophilic
c. cell
c. hypophysis
chromophobe
c. adenoma
c. tumor
chromophobic
c. adenoma
c. cell
c. pattern
chromosomal mosaicism
chromosome
c. deletion
c. 7 disorder
c. 12 disorder
c. 20 disorder
c. duplication
heterodisomic c.
isodisomic c.
c. 17p12-13
phosphatase and tensin homologue deleted on c. (PTEN)
phosphate-regulating gene with homologies to endopeptidases found at the HYP locus on the X c. (PEX)
c. 5q31
c. 5q35.3
c. ring
sex-determining region of the Y c. (SRY)
c. translocation
chronic
c. active hepatitis
c. alcoholic pancreatitis (CAP)
c. ambulatory peritoneal dialysis (CAPD)
c. autoimmune thyroiditis
c. calcific pancreatitis of the tropics (CCPT)
c. cystic mastitis
c. dehydration
c. dialysis patient
c. fatigue syndrome
c. fibrous thyroiditis
c. granulocytic leukemia (CGL)
c. granulomatous disease
c. hemodialysis
c. hyperandrogenic anovulation
c. hypercortisolism
c. hypoandrogenic anovulation
c. interstitial nephritis

NOTES

chronic *(continued)*
c. lobular hyperplasia
c. lymphocytic hypophysitis
c. lymphocytic thyroiditis
c. metabolic acidosis
c. myelogenous leukemia (CLL)
c. renal failure (CRF)
c. renal insufficiency (CRI)
c. water intoxication
chronicity
chronobiologic characteristic
chronopharmacologic
chronopharmacology
chronopharmacotherapy
chronotherapy
chronotropic
CHUK
conserved helix-loop-helix ubiquitous kinase
chupatti flour
Chvostek
C. sign
C. test
chylomicron
c. retention disease
chylomicronemia syndrome
chylomicrons
chymotrypsin
ciamexone
Cibacalcin
ciglitazone
ciliary neurotrophic factor (CNTF)
ciliated cell
cimetidine
cinereum
hamartoma of tuber c.
tuber c.
cingulate
c. cortex
c. gyrus
cingulum
ciprofloxacin
circadian
c. clock
c. gating
c. hormonal rhythm
c. locomotor output cycles kaput (CLOCK)
c. oscillator
c. pattern
c. rhythm of hormone secretion
c. variation
circadian/diurnal hormonal rhythm
circannual
c. rhythm
c. rhythmicity of steroid
circle of Willis
circulating
c. blood
c. calcium
c. estrogen level
c. lipolytic enzyme
circulation
enterohepatic c.
fetomaternal c.
hypophysial-portal c.
hypophysial stalk c.
portal c.
circulatory shock
circumferential lamella
circumoral numbness
circumscripta
calcinosis c.
osteoporosis c.
circumventricular organ (CVO)
CIRP
cold-inducible ribonucleic acid-binding protein
cold-inducible RNA-binding protein
cirrhosis
primary biliary c.
cis
c. element
c. Golgi network
c. mechanism
cis-acting
c.-a. DNA element
c.-a. factor
cisapride
***cis*-clomiphene citrate**
cisplatin
cistern
basilar c.
chiasmatic c.
interpeduncular chiasmatic c.
suprasellar c.
cisterna, pl. **cisternae**
c. chiasmatis
endoplasmic reticulum cisternae
cisternography
contrast c.
Citracal
citrate
buffered c.
calcium c.
cis-clomiphene c.
clomiphene c.
fentanyl c.
gallium c. (Ga-67)
c. ion
potassium c.
ranitidine bismuth c.
sildenafil c.
c. synthase

trans clomiphene c.
Zuclomiphene c.
citrated blood
citric
c. acid
c. acid cycle
Citrobacter diversus
citrullinemia
citrus fruit
CJD
Creutzfeldt-Jakob disease
cJun
c. gene
c. molecule
c-*jun* promoter
CK
creatine kinase
clamp
Babcock c.
Crile c.
endoscope holding c.
euglycemic insulin c.
hyperglycemic glucose c.
Kelly c.
Ochsner c.
clarithromycin
Clark oxygen electrode
class
c. I major histocompatibility complex molecule
c. I MHC molecule
c. II major histocompatibility complex molecule
c. II MHC molecule
c. III major histocompatibility complex molecule
c. III MHC molecule
c. 1B cardiac antiarrhythmic agent
Child-Pugh c.
c. II HLA locus
c. II human leukocyte antigen locus
classical
c. hydroxylase deficiency
c. XO karyotype
classic homocystinuria
classification
diabetes mellitus c.
TNM c.
tumor/node/metastases c.
White c.
clathrin
clathrin-coated
c.-c. pit
c.-c. vesicle
clavicular fat pad
claw-toe deformity
CLCNKB
chloride channel gene C.
clear
c. cell
c. cell metaplasia
c. cytoplasm
c. zone
clearance
cortisol c.
creatinine c.
free water c.
insulin c.
iron c.
osmolar c.
cleavage
collagenase c.
ether-link c.
c. product
proteolytic c.
P450 side chain c. (P450SCC)
side chain c. (SCC)
cleft
hypophysial c.
c. of the Rathke pouch
synaptic c.
cleidocranial dysplasia
Cleocin
C. HCl Oral
C. Pediatric Oral
C. Phosphate Injection
C. Vaginal
CLI
corpus luteum insufficiency
CLIA
chemiluminescent immunoassay
clidinium and chlordiazepoxide
climacteric
male c.
Climara
C. transdermal
climax
female c.
clindamycin
Clindex
clinical
c. hypothyroidism

C

NOTES

clinical *(continued)*
c. insulin sensitivity
c. obesity
clinically
c. euthyroid
c. hyperthyroid
c. nonfunctioning pituitary adenoma (CNFA)
c. silent tumor
clinodactyly
clinoid process
Clinoril
CLIP
corticotropin-like intermediate lobe peptide
clitoridis
frenulum c.
glans c.
clitoris
clitoromegaly
clitoroplasty
clival
c. indentation
c. portion
clivus
upper c.
CLL
chronic myelogenous leukemia
CLOCK
circadian locomotor output cycles kaput
Clock gene
CLOCK protein
clock
circadian c.
clodronate
clofibrate
Clomid
clomiphene
c. citrate
c. citrate challenge test (CCCT)
clonal
c. anergy
c. cell
c. deletion
c. expansion
c. neoplasm
c. rejection
clonality
cloned steroid acute respiratory protein
clonidine
c. gel
c. hydrochloride
c. suppression test
Clonorchis sinensis
Clopra
clorgyline
closed-loop insulin delivery system
clostridia
Clostridium septicum
closure
epiphyseal c.
clotting
c. factor II
c. factor V
c. factor VII
c. factor X
clouded sensorium
clozapine
cluster
consanguineous c.
Clyde mood scale
cM
centiMorgan
CMO
cetylmyristoleate
corticosterone methyl oxidase
CMO I deficiency
CMO II deficiency
CMO deficiency
CMO I
CMO II
c-*mpl*
c. ligand
CMV
cytomegalovirus
c-myc
c.-m. oncogene
c.-m. protein
c.-m. protooncogene
CNFA
clinically nonfunctioning pituitary adenoma
CNP
C-type natriuretic peptide
CNS
central nervous system
CNTF
ciliary neurotrophic factor
CO
cardiac output
CO_3^{2-}
carbonate
CoA
coenzyme A
coactivator
AIB1 c.
amplified in breast-1 c.
glucocorticoid receptor-interacting protein 1 c.
GRIP 1 c.
NCoA-1 c.
NCoA-2 c.
p/CIP c.
c. protein
receptor-associated c. 3 (RAC3)
SRC-1 c.

TIF2 c.
TRAM-1 c.
coactivators
p160 family of c.
coagulability
red cell c.
coagulation
disseminated intravascular c. (DIC)
red cell c.
coagulator
#8 suction monopolar c.
coalesce
tubuli recti c.
coarsened facial feature
coast
c. of California smooth margin
c. of Maine irregular margin
coated pit
cobalamin metabolism
cobalt-knife radiosurgery
Cobex
COC
combined oral contraceptive
cocaine
c. and amphetamine regulated transcript (CART)
c. and amphetamine-responsive transcript
Coccidioides
C. immitis
C. immitis thyroiditis
coccidioidomycosis
coccidioidomycosis-induced thyroiditis
Cockayne syndrome
Codamine
codeine
acetaminophen and c.
aspirin and c.
bromodiphenhydramine and c.
brompheniramine, phenylpropanolamine, and c.
butalbital compound and c.
Capital and c.
Empirin with c.
Fiorinal With C.
Phenergan VC with c.
Phenergan With c.
terpin hydrate and c.
Tylenol With C.
codfish vertebra
codon
c. 12
c. 13
c. 61
AUG c.
glutamic acid c. (GAA)
premature top c. (TAA)
Codoxy
coelomic epithelium
coenzyme A (CoA)
cofactor
mahogany c.
plasma ristocetin c.
Coffin-Lowry syndrome
Co-Gesic
cognate antigen
coherence therapy
coil spring
colchicine
cold
c. mass
c. naïve
c. nodule
cold-inducible
c.-i. ribonucleic acid-binding protein (CIRP)
c.-i. RNA-binding protein (CIRP)
cold-shock protein
colestipol
colestyramine
coli
Escherichia c.
colic
biliary c.
renal c.
collagen
carboxyterminal cross-linked telopeptide of type I c. (ICTP)
c. cross-link
C-telopeptide of c.
C-terminal telopeptide of type I c.
c. fiber
c. fibril
c. gene
c. molecule
c. monomer
N-telopeptide c.
N-terminal telopeptide of type I c.
c. synthesis
type I c.
c. type I
type II c.
type IX c.
type X c.

NOTES

collagenase
c. cleavage
collagenoma
collagenosis
Collagraft
collecting
c. tubule
c. tubule sodium channel
collection
24-hour urine c.
urine c.
collector
capillary filtrate c. (CFC)
colli
pterygium c.
colliculus
c. seminalis
superior c.
Collier sign
collimation
converging hole c.
parallel hole c.
pinhole c.
collimator
flat-field c.
pinhole c.
colloid
c. adenoma
c. droplet
eosinophilic c.
c. goiter
c. osmotic pressure
c. stage
thyroid c.
viscous c.
colloidal
c. gold-198
c. yttrium-91
coloboma, pl. **colobomata**
c. dysplasia
retinal c.
uveal c.
colobomatous dysplasia
colocalize
colon carcinoma
colony-forming
c.-f. unit erythroid (CFU-E)
c.-f. unit erythroid cell
colony morphology
colony-stimulating
c.-s. factor
c.-s. factor-1
color
c. Doppler scan
c. Doppler ultrasonography (CDU)
c. duplex ultrasonography
c. vision
colorimetric
c. assay
c. method
colostrum
column
intermediolateral cell c.
intermediolateral gray c.
trophoblastic cell c.
coma
acidotic c.
diabetic ketoacidosis-related c.
hyperglycemic c.
hyperosmolar nonketotic c.
hypoglycemic c.
myxedema c.
nonketotic hyperosmolar c.
Combantrin
Combid
combination assay
combined
c. hyperlipidemia
c. immunodeficiency
c. oral contraceptive (COC)
c. pituitary hormone deficiency (CPHD)
c. therapy
CombiPatch
Combivent
comedone
commissure
anterior c.
habenular c.
common bile duct (CBD)
communicating artery
communication
cell-to-cell c.
comorbid
compact
c. bone
c. cell
Companion 2 self blood glucose monitoring device
comparator element
compartment
abluminal c.
basal c.
early endosomal c.
extramitochondrial c.
hematopoietic c.
interstitial fluid c.
intramitochondrial c.
intravascular c.
luminal c.
transcellular fluid c.
compartmentalization
Compazine

compensated
c. euthyroidism
c. iodine deficiency
compensation
respiratory c.
compensatory
c. feedback
c. hyperparathyroidism
c. hypertrophy
c. ligand-induced upregulation of tissue receptor
competitive
c. insulin autoantibody
c. zona binding assay
complement
c. defect
c. level
complementary
c. deoxyribonucleic acid (cDNA)
c. DNA (cDNA)
complement-fixing thyroid antibody
complete
c. androgen sensitivity
c. autoinfarction
c. blood count (CBC)
c. Freund adjuvant (CFA)
c. hydatidiform mole
c. hypopituitarism
c. precocious puberty
c. testicular feminization
complex
acquired immunodeficiency syndrome-related c.
actin-myosin c.
AIDS-related c. (ARC)
aminoacyl-tRNA c.
aromatase enzyme c.
axonemal c.
beta-gamma c.
calcium c.
c. carbohydrate
Carney c.
C-cell c.
corepressor c.
glycine cleavage c.
Golgi c.
G-protein trimeric c.
GTP-dependent regulatory protein c.
guanosine triphosphate-dependent regulatory protein c.
hormone receptor-ligand c.
c. hyperthyroxinemia
hypothalamohypophyseal c.
immune c.
iron dextran c.
150-kDa ternary c.
ligand-receptor c.
major histocompatability c. (MHC)
NeoVadrin B C.
nuclear pore c.
polysaccharide-iron c.
receptor-ligand c.
19S cap c.
ternary c.
thyroperoxidase-iodide c.
transthyretin-ligand c.
transthyretin thyroid hormone analogue c.
TTR-ligand c.
TTR-thyroid hormone analogue c.
tubular bulbo c.
vitamin B c.
complexed calcium
compliance
vascular c.
complication
Epidemiology of Diabetes Interventions and C.'s (EDIC)
sinonasal c.
component
group-specific c. (Gc)
intrathoracic goitrous c.
RI regulatory c.
RII regulatory c.
Composite Cultured Skin
composition
body c.
side-chain c.
water c.
compound
c. B
calcimimetic c.
calcium phosphate c.
catechol c.
dihydrocodeine c.
gadolinium-chelated c.
glutahione c.
c. heterozygosity
iodolipid c.
lanthanum-containing c.
pentazocine c.
c. S
SH c.
sulfhydryl c.

NOTES

compound *(continued)*
thiourea c.
thyromimetic c.
zirconium-containing c.
compression
chiasmal c.
c. neuropathy
spinal cord c.
compressive
c. mononeuropathy
c. neuropathy
computed
c. tomography (CT)
c. tomography under endoscopic retrograde pancreatography (ERP-CT)
computer
c. tomographic methods of axial skeleton (axial QCT)
c. tomographic methods of peripheral skeleton (pQCT)
computer-aided sperm analysis (CASA)
computer-assisted semen analysis (CASA)
COMT
catechol-*O*-methyltransferase
concanavalin-A
concentration
apo A-I c.
blood glucose c.
calcium ion c.
dialysate calcium c.
glucose c.
inactive renin c.
insulin c.
intrathyroid iodide c.
ionized calcium c.
leptin c.
midnight plasma cortisol c.
minimal detectable c. (MDC)
plasma aldosterone c. (PAC)
plasma glucose c.
platelet lipid peroxide c.
postprandial glucose c.
postprandial insulin c.
salivary cortisol c.
serum albumin c.
serum cholesterol c.
serum 18-hydroxycorticosterone c.
serum IGF-1 c.
serum IGFBP-3 c.
serum insulinlike growth factor-1 c.
serum insulinlike growth factor binding protein-3 c.
serum ionized calcium c.
serum leptin c.
tissue c.
total serum calcium c.
urine c.
conchal type sphenoid sinus
concretion
prostatic c.
condition
anestrous c.
autosomal dominant c.
diabetes associated with certain c.'s
pathophysiological c.
conductivity
total body electrical c. (TOBEC)
conduit
aortic allograft c.
confabulation
confinement
estimated date of c. (EDC)
confluence
superior mesenteric-portal vein c. (SP-PVC)
conformational dependent epitope
congenita
adrenal hypoplasia c. (AHC)
arthrogryposis multiplex c.
congenital
c. abnormality
c. adrenal dysplasia
c. adrenal hyperplasia (CAH)
c. androgen insensitivity
c. anorchia
c. aplasia of the parathyroid
c. bilateral absence of the vas deferens (CBAVD)
c. bilateral aplasia
c. bone defect
c. bone disorder
c. cretinism
c. cytomegalovirus infection
c. erythropoietic porphyria
c. facial diplegia
c. forebrain anomaly
c. GH resistance syndrome
c. growth hormone resistance syndrome
c. hereditary lymphedema
c. hyperinsulinism
c. hyperthyroidism
c. hypoaldosteronism
c. hypophosphatemia
c. hypothyroidism
c. ichthyosis
c. intrathyroidal cyst
c. lipoatrophic diabetes
c. lipoid adrenal hyperplasia
c. lipoid adrenal hypoplasia
c. rubella syndrome (CRS)
c. thymic aplasia
c. virilizing adrenal hyperplasia

Congest
Congo red stain
Congressional Diabetes Caucus
conical lobe
conjugate
  glucuronide c.
  sulfate c.
conjugated
  c. bilirubin
  c. equine estrogen (CEE)
  c. equine estrogen plus norgestrel (CEEP)
conjunctival
  c. chemosis
  c. edema
conjunctivitis
connecting peptide
connection
  corticohypothalamic c.
  intracavernous venous c.
connective
  c. tissue
  c. tissue disease
connexin-37 (Cx37)
connexin-43 (Cx43)
connexin protein
Conn syndrome
conotruncal anomaly
consanguineous
  c. cluster
  c. parents
consanguinity
consensus
  c. sequence
  c. TATA box
consensus-response element
conserved helix-loop-helix ubiquitous kinase (CHUK)
consolidation
  bone c.
constant
  equilibrium association c. (K_a)
  equilibrium dissociation c. (K_d)
  Faraday c.
  universal gas c.
constitutional
  c. delay
  c. delay in growth and adolescence (CDGA)
  c. precocious puberty
constitutive
  c. heterochromatin
  c. secretion
constriction
  hourglass c.
consumption
  platelet c.
contact
  desmose-like c.
content
  forearm and lumbar spine bone mineral c.
  keratin c.
  phosphorus c.
  sialic acid c.
contiguous gene syndrome
continuous
  c. ambulatory peritoneal dialysis (CAPD)
  c. ambulatory radiolucent cyst
  c. capillary endothelium
  c. glucose monitoring system (CGMS)
  c. hormone replacement therapy
  c. positive airway pressure (CPAP)
  c. regional arterial infusion (CRAI)
  c. subcutaneous insulin infusion (CSII)
continuous-combined hormone replacement therapy (ccHRT)
contraception
  postcoital c.
contraceptive
  combined oral c. (COC)
  postcoital c.
contractile protein
contraction
  Braxton-Hicks c.
  ipsilateral c.
  premature ventricular c.
  tonic muscle c.
contraction-associated protein (CAP)
contracture
  Dupuytren c.
contrainsulin hormone
contralateral lobe
contrasexual
  c. precocity
  c. pubertal development
contrast
  c. cisternography

NOTES

contrast *(continued)*
c. dynamic study
nonionic iodinated c.
control
anticipatory c.
feedback c.
glycemic c.
hypothalamic-pituitary c.
metabolic c.
neuroendocrine c.
conventional radiotherapy
converging hole collimation
convertase
prohormone c.
prohormone c. 1 (PC1)
prohormone c. 2 (PC2)
prohormone c. 3 (PC3)
proprotein c. (PC)
Cooley anemia
cool nodule
Cooper
suspensory ligaments of C.
copeptin
Cope syndrome
Cophene XP
copolymer
ethylene-vinyl acetate c.
copper deposition
Co-Pyronil 2 Pulvules
CoR
corepressor
cord
tethered c.
cordocentesis
coregulator
c. molecule
corepressor (CoR, CoRs)
c. complex
nuclear receptor c.
core promoter
Cor Flow
coronary blood flow
Corgonject
Cori
C. cycle
C. disease
corneal
c. arcus
c. leukoma
c. ulceration
Cornelia de Lange syndrome
coronal
c. plane
c. postgadolinium study
c. slice
corona radiata
coronary
c. artery
c. artery disease, hypertension, adult-onset diabetes, obesity, and stroke (CHAOS)
c. blood flow (Cor Flow, Cor Flow)
corpus, pl. **corpora**
c. albicans
corpora amylacea
corpora arenacea
c. callosum
c. cavernosum
c. hemorrhagicum
c. luteum
c. luteum insufficiency (CLI)
c. spongiosum
c. uteri
corpuscle
Hassall c.
corrodens
Eikenella c.
CoRs
corepressor
Cortef Oral
cortex, pl. **cortices**
adrenal c.
adult adrenal c.
cerebellar c.
cerebral c.
cingulate c.
ovarian c.
c. pancreas
piriform c.
thickening of c.
cortical
c. amygdaloid nucleus
c. androgen-stimulating hormone (CASH)
c. atrophy
c. bone
c. collecting duct (CCD)
c. nephron
corticalis
hyperostosis c.
cortices (*pl. of* cortex)
corticohypothalamic connection
corticoid-induced osteopenia
corticomedullary osmotic gradient
corticopupillary osmolality gradient
corticorelin ovine triflutate
corticospinal tract dysfunction
corticostatin
corticosteroid
high-dose c.
c. receptor
c. therapy
corticosteroid-binding globulin (CBG)
corticosterone
c. methyl oxidase (CMO)

c. methyl oxidase deficiency
c. methyl oxidase II
c. methyl oxidase II deficiency
serum c.
corticotrope
pituitary c.
corticotroph
c. adenoma
c. cell hyperplasia
c. hyperplasia
c. stimulation test
c. tumor
corticotropic cell
corticotropin
corticotropin-dependent Cushing syndrome
corticotropin-like intermediate lobe peptide (CLIP)
corticotropinoma
pituitary c.
corticotropin-releasing
c.-r. factor (CRF)
c.-r. hormone (CRH)
c.-r. hormone-binding protein (CRH-BP)
c.-r. hormone-R1 (CRH-R1)
c.-r. hormone 1R (CRH1R)
c.-r. hormone 2R (CRH2R)
c.-r. hormone test
corticotropin-secreting adenoma
cortisol (F)
adrenal c.
c. assay
basal plasma c.
c. biosynthesis
c. clearance
fetal adrenal c.
fetal plasma c.
free c.
24-hour urine free c.
morning c.
c. nadir
plasma c.
postcosyntropin plasma c.
random c.
c. resistance syndrome
salivary c.
c. secreting lesion
c. secretion
urinary free c.
urine free c. (UFC)
cortisol-binding globulin (CBG)
cortisol-producing cortical adenoma
cortisol-secreting adenoma
cortisone
c. acetate
Cortone Acetate
Cortrosyn
C. stimulation test
C. stimulation testing
Corynebacterium
cosecrete
cosmesis
cosmid
cosyntropin
c. stimulation test
Cotazym
Cotazym-S
cotransporter
bumetanide-sensitive sodium-postassium-2 chloride c.
Na^+-phosphate c.
sodium glucose c. (SGLT)
sodium-potassium-2 chloride c. (NKCC2)
Cottle elevator
cotton pledget packing
cotton-wool appearance
cotyledon
coumestan
coumestrol
counseling
genetic c.
preconception c.
count
complete blood c. (CBC)
counter
Geiger c.
whole body c.
counterion
counterregulation
impaired glucose c.
c. mechanism
counterregulatory hormone
countertransport system
counting
^{40}K c.
coupled amplification and sequencing technique
coupling
c. domain
c. factor
iodothyronine c.
iodotyrosine c.

NOTES

coupling *(continued)*
c. phase
receptor-effector c.
stimulus-secretion c.
synthesis-secretion c.
COUP-TF
chicken ovalbumin upstream promoter-transcription factor
COUP-TF thyroid hormone receptor auxillary protein
Cowden
C. disease
C. syndrome
Cowper
bulbourethral gland of C.
C. gland
COX
cyclooxygenase
COX-1
cyclooxygenase-1
COX-2
cyclooxygenase-2
coxsackievirus
c. A9
c. B
group B c.
cox vara
COZ
cranioorbitozygomatic osteotomy
CPAP
continuous positive airway pressure
C-peptide
C.-p. level
C.-p. suppression test
CPHD
combined pituitary hormone deficiency
CPP
central precocious puberty
CPTI
carnitine palmitoyltransferase I
CPTI deficiency
CPTII
carnitine palmitoyltransferase II
CPTII deficiency
CRAI
continuous regional arterial infusion
cranial
c. irradiation
c. nerve palsy
c. neuropathy
c. sclerosis
craniodiaphysial dysplasia
craniofacial abnormality
craniomegaly
craniometaphyseal dysplasia
cranioorbitozygomatic osteotomy (COZ)
craniopharyngeal
c. canal
c. duct
craniopharyngioma
adamantinomatous c.
cystic c.
papillary c.
pituitary c.
craniostenosis
craniosynostosis
nonsyndromic coronal c.
primary c.
craniotabes
craniotomy
bifrontal c.
frontal c.
temporal c.
craving
salt c.
CRE
cAMP-response element
C-reactive protein (CRP)
cream
Amino-Cerv Vaginal C.
dehydroepiandrosterone c.
DHEA c.
0.2% fluocinolone acetonide c.
Locilex pexiganan acetate c. 1%
Locilex topical c.
Medrol Veriderm C.
VANIQA c.
creatine kinase (CK)
creatinine
c. clearance
urinary c.
creatinuria
CREB
cAMP response element-binding
cyclic adenosine 3′,5′-monophosphate response element-binding
CREB-binding protein (CBP)
CREM
cAMP-response element modulator
cremasteric fascia
cremaster muscle
Creme
Gormel C.
Creon
C. 10
C. 20
Creo-Terpin
crest
mammary c.
neural c.
vagal neural c.
cretin
athyreotic c.

cretinism
congenital c.
endemic c.
goitrous c.
myxedematous c.
myxedematous endemic c.
neurologic endemic c.
Creutzfeldt-Jakob disease (CJD)
CRF
chronic renal failure
corticotropin-releasing factor
CRH
corticotropin-releasing hormone
placental CRH
CRH stimulation test
CRH-binding protein (CRH-BP)
CRH-BP
corticotropin-releasing hormone-binding protein
CRH-binding protein
CRH-mRNA transcript
CRH1R
corticotropin-releasing hormone 1R
CRH-R1
corticotropin-releasing hormone-R1
CRH-R1 receptor
CRH2R
corticotropin-releasing hormone 2R
CRI
chronic renal insufficiency
cribriform plate
cricoarytenoid
lateral c.
posterior c.
cricoid cartilage
cricothyroid
c. joint
c. membrane
c. muscle
cri du chat syndrome
Crile clamp
Crinone bioadhesive progesterone gel
crinophagy
crisis
acute addisonian c.
addisonian c.
adrenal c.
bone c.
carcinoid c.
fetal/neonatal adrenal c.
hypoglycemia c.
parathyroid c.
salt-losing c.
salt-wasting c.
thyroid c.
thyrotoxic c.
cristae
tubular c.
criteria
Age, Metastases, Extent and Size risk c.
AMES risk c.
National Cholesterol Education Program c.
NCEP c.
Crk
cytokinin-regulated kinase
Crk protein
CrkI
cytokinin-regulated kinase I
CrkI protein
CrkII
cytokinin-regulated kinase II
CrkII protein
CrkL
cytokinin-regulated kinase L
CrkL protein
Crohn disease
Crolom
cromolyn sodium
Crooke
C. cell
C. hyaline change
C. hyalinization
crossed test
crossing nasal retinal fiber
Crosslaps immunoassay
cross-link
collagen c.-l.
pyridinium c.-l.
pyridinoline c.-l.
total deoxypyridinoline c.-l.
trifunctional pyridinium c.-l.
urinary N-telopeptide collagen c.-l.
cross-reactive
trophoblast-lymphocyte c.-r. (TLX)
cross-talk
transcriptional c.-t.
Crouzon
C. disease
C. syndrome
CRP
C-reactive protein

NOTES

CRS
congenital rubella syndrome
crus, gen. **cruris**
diaphragmatic c.
c. penis
ulcus cruris
cryoglobulin
c. level
cryptic
c. hydroxylase deficiency
c. hyperandrogenemia
cryptococcal
c. antigen
c. infection
cryptococcosis
Cryptococcus
C. neoformans
cryptomenorrhea
cryptorchidism
cryptorchism
crystal
apatite c.
calcium oxalate dihydrate c.
calcium oxalate monohydrate c.
calcium phosphate c.
cholesterol monohydrate c.
cystine c.
hydroxyapatite c.
Reinke c.
struvite c.
uric acid c.
crystallographic
c. stone analysis
crystallography
x-ray c.
crystalloid
Reinke c.
crystalluria
Crystamine
CS
chorionic somatomammotropin
CSF
cerebrospinal fluid
CSF rhinorrhea
CSII
continuous subcutaneous insulin infusion
c-*src*
protooncogene c.
CSS
cavernous sinus sampling
CT
calcitonin
computed tomography
dynamic CT
dynamic spiral CT
helical CT
spiral CT
CT-1
cardiotropin-1
C-telopeptide of collagen
C-terminal
C.-t. assay for parathyroid hormone
C.-t. assay for PTH
C.-t. propeptide
C.-t. telopeptide of type I collagen
C.-t. type I collagen telopeptide
C-termini
CT-guided fine-needle aspiration
CTL
cytotoxic T lymphocyte
CTLA-4
cytotoxic lymphocyte antigen-4
C-type natriuretic peptide (CNP)
cube
porous calcium phosphate c.
cubitus valgus
cuboidal epithelioid cell
cue
nonphotic c.
Cullen sign
culture
monolayer c.
semen c.
cumulus
c. adherens
c. granulosa cell
c. oophorus
Cunninghamella
Cupid bow
cuprophane dialysis membrane
curette, curet
Hardy ring c.
straight bone c.
Curretab Oral
curve
growth c.
growth hormone dose-response c.
Cushing
C. disease
C. disease of the omentum
C. forceps
C. procedure
C. syndrome
Cushing-Landolt speculum
custom-healing orthotic
cutaneous
c. adnexa
c. flushing
c. hamartoma
c. hyperpigmentation
c. lupus
c. myxoma
c. photoaging
c. pigmentation
c. vasodilation

cutis
aplasia c.
c. verticis
c. verticis gyrata
cuvette
CV 205-502
CVO
circumventricular organ
CVS
chorionic villus sampling
Cx37
connexin-37
Cx43
connexin-43
cyanide-nitroprusside
cyanocobalamin
cyanogen bromide
cyanogenic glucoside
cyanoglucoside
5-cyano group
Cyanoject
cyclase
adenyl c.
adenylate c.
adenylyl c.
guanylate c.
guanylyl c.
thyroid adenylate c.
cycle
alanine c.
c. amplitude
annual c.
anovulatory c.
Basic Rest-Activity C. (BRAC)
citric acid c.
Cori c.
dark-light c.
endometrial c.
estrous c.
free-running melatonin c.
futile c.
glucose-fatty acid c.
menstrual c.
ornithine c.
ovarian c.
ovulatory c.
prolactin secretion during menstrual c.
Randle c.
remodeling c.
sleep-wake c.
substrate c.
urea c.
Vollman c.
cycler
thermal c.
cyclic
c. adenosine monophosphate (cAMP)
c. 3′,5′-adenosine monophosphate (cAMP)
c. adenosine 3′,5′-monophosphate-response element
c. adenosine 3′,5′-monophosphate response element-binding (CREB)
c. AMP (cAMP)
c. AMP response-element binding protein
c. arginine monophosphate (cAMP)
c. arginine monophosphate response element-binding
c. conjugated estrogen
c. endoperoxide prostaglandin G_2
c. GMP
c. guanosine monophosphate (cGMP)
c. 3′,5′-guanosine monophosphate (cGMP)
5′-c. guanosine monophosphate (cGMP)
c. guanosine 3′,5′-monophosphate-dependent protein kinase
c. guanosine monophosphate-phosphodiesterase
c. hyperthermia
c. hypothermia
c. nucleotide phosphodiesterase
c. porphyria
cyclical
c. Cushing disease
c. ethinyl estradiol
c. hormone replacement therapy
c. supplementation
cyclicity
endogenous c.
cyclin
c. D gene
c. D1 protein
cyclin-dependent kinase (CDK, Cdk)
cycling cell
cyclocephaly
cyclodextrin
testosterone c.
cycloheximide

NOTES

Cyclo(His-Pro)
Cyclomen
cyclooxygenase (COX)
c. pathway
cyclooxygenase-1 (COX-1)
cyclooxygenase-2 (COX-2)
cyclophosphamide
cycloplegic refraction
cyclosporin A
cyclosporine
c. A-induced osteopenia
c. A-induced resorption
cyclotron
Cycrin Oral
cylooxygenase
Cyomin
CYP
cytochrome P450 enzyme
cytochrome pigment
cytochrome protein
CYP19
cytochrome P450 enzyme 19
CYP19 gene
CYP27
cytochrome P450 enzyme 27
CYP1A1
cytochrome P450 enzyme 1A1
CYP1A1 gene
CYP11A
cytochrome P450 enzyme 11A
CYP11A gene
CYP11B1
11-beta-hydroxylase
CYP21B
cytochrome P450 enzyme 21B
CYP21B deficiency
CYP21B1
21-beta-hydroxylase
cypionate
testosterone c.
cyproheptadine
c. hydrochloride
cyproterone
c. acetate
cyst
arachnoid c.
arrested follicular c.
c. aspiration
atretic follicular c.
benign pituitary c.
choledochal c.
congenital intrathyroidal c.
continuous ambulatory radiolucent c.
dermoid c.
endolymphatic c.
epidermal c.
epidermoid c.
follicular c.
intrasellar hydatid c.
luteal c.
microphthalmic c.
multiple luteinized theca c.
nabothian c.
ovarian endometriosis c.
parathyroid c.
pars intermedia c.
pituitary c.
pleuropericardial c.
Rathke cleft c.
Rathke pouch c.
sellar c.
subchondral c.
suprasellar epidermoid c.
thin-walled simple c.
thyroglossal duct c.
cystadenocarcinoma
ductectatic-type mucinous c.
mucinous c.
cystadenoma
epididymal c.
mucinous c.
cystathionase
cystathionine
c. synthase
c. synthase deficiency
cystathioninuria
cysteine
c. aminopeptidase
c. endopeptidase
cysteine-penicillamine
cystic
c. acne
c. bone lesion
c. craniopharyngioma
c. fibrosis
c. fibrosis-related diabetes (CFRD)
c. fibrosis transmembrane regulator (CFTR)
c. fibrosis transmembrane regulator gene
c. hygroma
c. hyperplasia
c. mastitis
c. neurilemoma
c. nodule
c. ovary
cystica
osteitis fibrosa c.
cysticercosis
Cysticercus
cystine
c. crystal
c. knot
c. renal stone

cystinosis
adult c.
benign c.
infantile c.
juvenile c.
nephropathic c.
cystinuria
cystinuric
homozygous c.
cystitis
cystogastrostomy
cystometrogram
cystosarcoma phylloides
cystoscopy
Cystospaz
Cystospaz-M
cytoarchitectonically
cytochemical bioassay (CBA)
cytochrome
c. C oxidase deficiency
c. oxidase
c. P450
c. P450 aromatase
c. P450 enzyme (CYP)
c. P450 enzyme 19 (CYP19)
c. P450 enzyme 27 (CYP27)
c. P450 enzyme 1A1 (CYP1A1)
c. P450 enzyme 11A (CYP11A)
c. P450 enzyme 21B (CYP21B)
c. P450 family of enzymes
c. P450 hemoprotein
c. pigment (CYP)
c. protein (CYP)
cytodiagnosis
cytodifferentiation
cytokeratin
cytokine
activating c.
bone-resorbing c.
c. gene
inflammatory c.
osteoporotic c.
c. production
proinflammatory c.
tumor necrosis factor-related activation-induced c. (TRANCE)
cytokine-induced thyroiditis
cytokinin-regulated
c.-r. kinase (Crk)
c.-r. kinase I (CrkI)
c.-r. kinase I protein
c.-r. kinase II (CrkII)
c.-r. kinase II protein
c.-r. kinase L (CrkL)
c.-r. kinase L protein
c.-r. kinase protein
Cytolex
cytologic atypia
cytology
brush c.
cytomegalic-type congenital adrenal hypoplasia
cytomegalovirus (CMV)
Cytomel
C. Oral
C. suppression test
Cytopathology
Papanicolaou Society of C.
cytoplasm
clear c.
dark c.
perikaryal c.
cytoplasmic
c. bridge
c. Ca^{2+}
c. calcium
c. estrogen
c. islet-cell antibody
c. pseudopod
c. receptor
cytoreductive surgery
cytosine arabinoside
cytosine-guanine dinucleotide
cytoskeleton
cytosol
neuronal c.
cytosolic
c. enzyme
c. free calcium
c. osmolality
Cytotec
cytotoxic
c. chemotherapy
c. lymphocyte antigen-4 (CTLA-4)
c. T lymphocyte (CTL)

NOTES

cytotoxicity
antibody-dependent cell c. (ADCC)
antibody-dependent cell-mediated c.
antibody-dependent cellular c. (ADCC)
immune cell-mediated c.

cytotrophoblast
Langhans c.
villous c.

Cytoxan

cytsol

D
D apolipoprotein
aspartic endopeptidase cathepsin D
cathepsin D
D cell
hypervitaminosis D
immunoglobulin D (IgD)
phospholipase D (PLD)
D1
type 1 deiodinase
D2
$T_4$5′-deiodinase type 2
type 2 deiodinase
D3
type 3 deiodinase
D_1
vitamin D_1
D_{28K}
calbindin D_{28K}
D_2
D_2 agonist
prostaglandin D_2 (PGD_2)
vitamin D_2
D_{9K}
calbindin D_{9K}
D_3
active vitamin D_3
1-alpha-hydroxyvitamin D_3
1,25-dihydroxyvitamin D_3
labile previtamin D_3
previtamin D_3
vitamin D_3
D_4
leukotriene D_4 (LTD_4)
D_β
total body bone mineral density
d_{FF}
density of the fat mass
d_{FFM}
density of the fat-free mass
DA
dopamine
D4-A
androstenedione
dacarbazine (DTIC)
d'accoucheur
main d.
daclizumab
dactinomycin
DAG
diacylglycerol
daidzein
Dalgan
Dalrymple sign
dalton
damage
oxidative d.
Damason-P
Dana Diabecare insulin pump
danazol
Dandy-Walker syndrome
Danocrine
dantrolene
DAO
diamine oxidase
Dapa
Dapacin
Darbid
Darier sign
dark cytoplasm
dark-light cycle
Darvocet-N
Darvocet-N 100
Darvon
D. Compound-65 Pulvules
Darvon-N
daunomycin
daunorubicin
dawn phenomenon
DAX-1 gene
Day
Acutrim Late D.
Daypro
daytime somnolence
Dayto Himbin
DAZ
deleted in azoospermia
DAZH
DAZ-homologue
deleted in azoospermia-homologue
DAZ-homologue (DAZH)
DAZLA
DAZ-like autosomal
deleted in azoospermia-like autosomal
DAZ-like autosomal (DAZLA)
DBD
DNA-binding domain
db gene
DBH
dopamine beta-hydroxylase
DBP
vitamin D-binding protein
DC
Bromanate DC
DCCT
Diabetes Control and Complications Trial
D-chiro-inositol
DCT
distal convoluted tubule

D

DDAVP
desamino D-arginine vasopressin
DDD
dichlorodiphenyldichloroethane
DDT
dichlorodiphenyltrichloroethane
de
d. Lange syndrome
d. Morsier syndrome
d. novo synthesis
d. Quervain nonsuppurative thyroiditis
deacetylation
histone d.
deaf mutism
deafness
diabetes insipidus, diabetes mellitus, optic atrophy, and d. (DIMOAD)
diabetes insipidus, diabetes mellitus, progressive bilateral optic atrophy, and sensorineural d. (DIDMOAD)
maternally inherited diabetes and d. (MIDD)
sensorineural d.
deaminase
adenosine d. (ADA)
adenosine monophosphate d. 1 (AMPD1)
polyethylene glycol-adenosine d. (PEG-ADA)
deaminate
adenosine deaminase d.
death
granulosa cell d.
debridement
minor mechanical d.
debris
calcified desquamated d.
Debrisan
debulked
debulking
transsphenoidal d.
d. of tumor
Decadron
D. Injection
D. Oral
Decadron-LA
Deca-Durabolin
Decaject
Decaject-LA
decanoate
Hybolin D.
nandrolone d.
decapacitation factor
decapeptide
antigonadotropic d. (AGD)
decarboxylase
antiglutamic acid d. (anti-GAD)
aromatic L-amino acid d.
branch chain 2-ketoacid d.
dihydroxyphenylalanine d.
DOPA d.
glutamic acid d. (GAD)
ornithine d. (ODC)
decarboxylation
amine precursor uptake and d. (APUD)
decidua
d. basalis
d. capsularis
d. parietalis
decidualization
decline
response curve d.
Declomycin
decompression
gastric d.
deconvolution
decorin
decorticate
d. rigidity
decreased
d. flare reaction
d. lean mass
d. libido
d. mineral apposition rate
d. oxygen tension
d. thyroid reserve
dedifferentiation
deepening of voice
deep tendon reflex
defect
acquired organification d.
alcohol-induced birth d.
bitemporal d.
cecocentral d.
c-erbA-beta-1 d.
c-erbA-beta-2 d.
complement d.
congenital bone d.
enzyme d.
granulosa cell d.
hemianopic d.
thyroid hormonogenesis d. II b
insulin secretory d.
iodide transport d.
iodine organification d.
iodine-trapping d.
iodotyrosine coupling d.
iodotyrosine dehalogenase d.
luteal phase d.
mineralization d.
mitochondrial d.
monocular temporal arcuate d.
organification d.
osmoregulatory d.
pupillary d.

rachitic-like skeletal d.
rake d.
regulatory gene d.
structural gene d.
superotemporal hemianoptic d.
thyroglobin synthesis d.
thyroid hormone receptor d.
ventricular septal d. (VSD)
visual field d.

defensin

deferens, pl. **deferentia**
ampulla of the vas d.
congenital bilateral absence of the vas d. (CBAVD)
ductus d.
vas d.

deferoxamine (DFO)
d. test
d. therapy

deficiency
absolute leptin d.
acetyl-CoA d.
acid cholesteryl ester hydrolase d.
acid phosphatase d.
acquired immune d.
adenine phosphoribosyltransferase d.
adenosine monophosphate deaminase d.
adenylosuccinate lyase d.
adrenal androgen d.
aldosterone synthase d.
alpha-antitrypsin d.
alpha-1 antitrypsin d.
17-alpha-hydroxylase d.
17-alpha-hydroxylase/17,20-lyase d.
17-alpha-hydroxylase/17,20-lyase (p450c17) d.
ankyrin d.
anti-müllerian hormone d.
apolipoprotein d. A-I
apolipoprotein d. B
apolipoprotein d. E
aromatase d.
11-beta-hydroxylase d.
3-beta-hydroxysteroid dehydrogenase d.
beta-ol-dehydrogenase d.
biotin cofactor d.
bone d.
CA II d.
calcitriol d.
calcium d.
carbamoyl phosphate synthetase I d.
carbonic anhydrase II d.
carnitine acylcarnitine translocase d.
carnitine palmitoyltransferase d.
carnitine palmitoyltransferase I d.
carnitine palmitoyltransferase II d.
cholesterol desmolase d.
cholesterol ester transfer protein d.
classical hydroxylase d.
CMO d.
CMO I d.
CMO II d.
combined pituitary hormone d. (CPHD)
compensated iodine d.
corticosterone methyl oxidase d.
corticosterone methyl oxidase II d.
CPTI d.
CPTII d.
cryptic hydroxylase d.
CYP21B d.
cystathionine synthase d.
cytochrome C oxidase d.
20,22-desmolase (P450scc) d.
dihydrobiopterin synthase d.
dihydropteridine reductase d.
enzyme d.
estrogen d.
factor IX d.
factor VIII d.
familial glucocorticoid d. (FGD)
follicle-stimulating hormone d.
FSH d.
galactose-l-phosphate uridyltransferase d.
α-galactosidase d.
glucocerebrosidase d.
glucocorticoid receptor d.
glucose-6-phosphatase d.
glycerol kinase d.
glycoprotein neuraminidase d.
glycosylasparaginase d.
gonadotropin d.
gonadotropin-releasing hormone d.
growth hormone d.
hepatic lipase d.
heterozygous cystathione beta synthase d.
HPRT d.
hydroxylase d.
11-hydroxylase d.

NOTES

deficiency *(continued)*
17-hydroxylase d.
21-hydroxylase d.
3-hydroxy-3-methylglutaryl-CoA carboxylase d.
hypothalamic gonadotropin-releasing hormone d.
hypoxanthine-guanine phosphoribosyltransferase d.
insulin d.
iodide d.
iodine d.
isolated gonadotropin d.
isolated growth hormone d. (IGHD)
isolated growth hormone d., type II (IGHD-II)
isolated growth hormone d., type III (IGHD-III)
isomerase dehydrogenase d.
17-ketosteroid reductase d.
3-ketothiolase d.
late onset hydroxylase d.
LCAD d.
LCAT d.
LCHAD d.
LDL d.
leptin d.
LHRH d.
lipoprotein lipase d.
long chain acyl-CoA dehydrogenase d.
long chain 3-hydroxyacyl-CoA dehydrogenase d.
low-density lipoprotein d.
luteal phase d.
luteinizing hormone-releasing hormone d.
magnesium d.
MCAD d.
medium chain acyl-CoA dehydrogenase d.
3-methylcrotonyl-CoA carboxylase d.
mineral d.
multiple anterior pituitary hormone d.
multiple pituitary hormone d.
multiple sulfatase d.
nonclassical hydroxylase d.
nonclassical 21-hydroxylase d.
nonclassic 21-hydroxylase d.
ornithine transcarbamylase d.
OTC d.
P450 aromatase (placental) d.
partial 21-hydroxylase d.
P450c17 d.
P450c21 d.
peripheral glucocorticoid d.
PGK d.
phosphate d.
phosphoglycerate kinase d.
phosphoglycerate mutase d.
pituitary d.
placental aromatase d.
placental hormone d.
placental sulfatase d.
pluriglandular endocrine d.
plurihormonal d.
PNP d.
polyglandular endocrine d.
primary immune d. (PID)
prolactin d.
pseudocholinesterase d.
purine nucleoside phosphorylase d.
red-green d.
reductase d.
5-reductase d.
relative leptin d.
salt-losing d.
short chain acyl-CoA dehydrogenase d. (SCAD)
side chain cleavage d.
single hormone d.
somatotropin d.
StAR d.
steroid acute regulatory protein d.
steroid acute respiratory protein d.
steroid 5-alpha-reductase d.
steroidogenic acute regulatory protein d.
steroid sulfatase d.
TBG d.
TH beta-receptor d.
thyroid-stimulating hormone d.
thyroxine-binding globulin d.
TSH d.
very long chain acyl-CoA dehydrogenase d.
vitamin D receptor d.
xanthine oxidase d.

deficiency/resistance
leptin d.

deficit
free water d.
pancreatic exocrine d.
pituitary hormone d.

definitive placenta

deformans
osteitis d.

deformity
barrel d.
bilateral pes cavus d.
claw-toe d.
Erlenmeyer flask d.
Madelung d.
rachitic d.
skeletal d.

Degas

degeneration
macular d.
sarcomatous d.
wallerian d.
degenerative enthesopathy
deglutition
deglycosylated
deglycosylation
degradation
calcium d.
hormone d.
receptor d.
T-lymphocyte insulin binding and d.
45-degree angled Jannetta microdissector
dehalogenase
iodotyrosine d.
dehiscence
wound d.
dehydration
cellular d.
chronic d.
extracellular fluid d.
dehydroalanine (DHA)
dehydroandrosterone sulfate rhythm
7-dehydrocholesterol
11-dehydrocorticosterone (DHC)
dehydroepiandrosterone (DHEA)
d. cream
d. sulfate (DHEAS, DHEA-S)
d. supplement
dehydroestrone
dehydrogenase
alcohol d.
aldehyde d.
alpha-glycerophosphate d.
3-alpha-hydroxysteroid d. (3-alpha-HSD)
3-beta-hydroxysteroid d. (3-beta-HSD)
11-beta-hydroxysteroid d. (11-beta-HSD)
17-beta-hydroxysteroid d. (17-beta-HSD)
17-beta-hydroxysteroid d. type 1 (17-beta-HSD1)
17-beta-hydroxysteroid d. type 2 (17-beta-HSD2)
17-beta-hydroxysteroid d. type 3 (17-beta-HSD3)
17-beta-hydroxysteroid d. type 4 (17-beta-HSD4)
17-beta-hydroxysteroid d. type 5 (17-beta-HSD5)
glucose-6-phosphate d. (G6PD, G6PDH)
glyceraldehyde-3-phosphate d.
glycerol-3-phosphate d.
hydroxysteroid d. (HSD)
11-hydroxysteroid d.
isovaleryl-CoA d.
lactate d. (LDH)
lactic d.
long chain acyl-CoA d. (LCAD)
long chain 3-hydroxyacyl-CoA d. (LCHAD)
lysine d.
medium chain acyl-CoA d. (MCAD)
pyrroline-5-carboxylate d.
pyruvate d. (PDH)
sarcosine d.
very long chain acyl-CoA d. (VLCAD)
deiodinase
d. enzyme
iodothyronine d.
iodotyrosine-specific d.
type 1 d. (D1)
type 2 d. (D2)
type 3 d. (D3)
deiodinate
deiodination
sequential d.
Deknatel tape
Deladumone
Delalutin
Delatestryl
D. Injection
delay
constitutional d.
neurodevelopmental d.
delayed
d. bone age
d. brain radionecrosis
d. epiphyseal fusion
d. gastric emptying (DGE)
d. puberty
deleted
d. in azoospermia (DAZ)
d. in azoospermia-homologue (DAZH)

NOTES

deleted *(continued)*
d. in azoospermia-like autosomal (DAZLA)
deletion
chromosome d.
clonal d.
gene d.
germline d.
somatic d.
delipidation
delirium
toxic d.
delivery
amino acid d.
portal insulin d.
salt d.
Delphian lymph node
Delsym
delta-5-desaturase enzyme
delta-6-desaturase enzyme
delta cell
Delta-Cortef Oral
Delta-D
deltanoid
Deltasone
Del-Vi-A
Demadex
demeclocycline
dementia
dialysis d.
Demerol
demineralization
Demulen
demyelinating disorder
demyelination
d. injury
osmotic d.
demyelinative neuropathy
denaturation
denaturing gradient gel electrophoresis (DGGE)
dendrite
Purkinje cell d.
denervation
pancreatic d.
portohepatic d.
dengue fever
DENIS
Deutsch Nicotinamide Diabetes Intervention Study
densa
macula d.
dense
d. LDL
d. staining of adenoma
densitometer
Hologic QDR 4500 DXA bone d.
densitometry
body d.
bone d.
density
bone mass d.
bone mineral d. (BMD)
endothelin receptor d.
d. of the fat-free mass (d_{FFM})
d. of the fat mass (d_{FF})
femoral neck bone d.
low bone d.
lumbar spine bone d.
total body bone mineral d. (D_β, TBBMD)
dental
d. lamina
d. papilla
dentatorubral-pallidoluysian atrophy (DRPLA)
Dent disease
dentin
radicular d.
dentinal tubule
dentine
dentinogenesis imperfecta
Denver shunt
Denys-Drash syndrome
21-deoxidation
21-deoxyaldosterone
deoxycorticosterone (DOC)
11-deoxycorticosterone (DOC)
deoxycorticosterone-producing tumor
deoxycortisol
11-deoxycortisol
21-deoxycortisol
2-deoxyglucose
deoxyinosine triphosphate (dITP)
deoxynucleotide triphosphate (dNTP)
17-deoxy pathway
deoxypyridinoline (DPD)
deoxyribonucleic
d. acid (DNA)
d. acid-binding domain
17-deoxysteroid
depAndrogyn
depAndro Injection
dependency
type 1 autosomal recessive vitamin D d. (ARVDD-1)
depGynogen Injection
dephosphorylate
depigmentation
progressive d.
depletion
hypertonic volume d.
magnesium d.
phosphate d.

potassium d.
volume d.
depMedalone Injection
Depo-Estradiol Injection
Depogen Injection
Depoject Injection
depolarization
Depo-Medrol Injection
Depopred Injection
Depo-Provera
D.-P. Injection
deposit
aluminum d.
amyloid d.
metastatic d.
deposition
β_2-microglobulin amyloid d.
calcium d.
copper d.
glycosaminoglycan d.
iron d.
retroorbital fat d.
deposteroid
depot
Androcur D.
Lupron D.
d. medroxyprogesterone
d. medroxyprogesterone acetate (DMPA)
Nutropin D.
Sandostatin LAR D.
Testoviron D. 50
Testoviron D. 100
Depo-Testadiol
Depotest Injection
Depotestogen
Depo-Testosterone
D.-T. Injection
Depot-Ped
Lupron D.-P.
deprenyl
depression
major d.
postpartum d.
depressive disorder
deprivation
estrogen d.
water d.
depth
erosion d. (EDe)
d. perception
derangement
derepression
chromatin d.
derivative
androstane d.
ergoline d.
Ergot Alkaloid and D.
estrane d.
fibric acid d.
imidazole d.
müllerian d.
pregnane d.
proopiomelanocortin d.
dermal papilla
dermatan sulfate
dermatitidis
Bacteroides d.
Blastomyces d.
dermatitis
eczematoid d.
d. herpetiformis
lichenified d.
perioral d.
dermatofibrosis lenticularis disseminata
dermatomyositis
dermatosis
acquired perforating d. (APD)
dermoid cyst
dermopathy
d. of Graves disease
infiltrative d.
pretibial d.
thyroid d.
DES
diethylstilbestrol
1-desamino-8-d arginine vasopressin
desamino-cys-D-arg-vasopressin
desamino D-arginine vasopressin (DDAVP)
desArg
d. bradykinin
d. kallidin
desAsp-heptapeptide
desaturase
stearoyl acyl-CoA d.
desensitization
adenylate cyclase d.
postreceptor d.
receptor d.
desethylamiodarone
desferoxamine challenge
desferrioxamine therapy
desialylation

NOTES

desiccated thyroid
designer estrogen
desipramine hydrochloride
desmolase
cholesterol d.
20,22-desmolase
20,22-d. (P450scc) deficiency
desmoplastic stroma
desmopressin
d. acetate
intranasal d.
desmose-like contact
desmosome
desmosterol
Desogen
desogestrel
ethinyl estradiol and d.
desoxycorticosterone
Desoxyn
destruction
beta cell d.
osteoarticular d.
destruction-induced thyrotoxicosis
destructive
d. arthropathy
d. thyrotoxicosis
desynchronization
desynchrony
detachment
retinal d.
detection
bioluminescence d.
carrier d.
chemiluminescence d.
liquid chromatography with electrochemical d. (LCED)
sex-determining region Y gene d.
SRY d.
Y chromosome d.
Detection of Ischemia in Asymptomatic Diabetics (DIAD)
detector
cadmium telluride d.
Detensol
determinant
immunodominant serologic d.
ligand binding d.
determined osteoprogenitor cell
Deutsch Nicotinamide Diabetes Intervention Study (DENIS)
devascularization
development
ambisexual d.
brain d.
breast d.
contrasexual pubertal d.
isosexual pubertal d.
pubertal d.
device
Accu-Chek SoftClix lancet d.
accuDEXA bone mineral assessment d.
Autoclix fingerstick d.
Autolet fingerstick d.
Companion 2 self blood glucose monitoring d.
endoscope cleaning d.
Genotropin Pen 5 growth hormone delivery d.
GlucoWatch glucose monitoring d.
intrauterine d. (IUD)
Lasette laser lancing d.
levonorgesterol-releasing intrauterine d.
levonorgestrel-releasing intrauterine d.
Monojector fingerstick d.
O_2 disposable boot d.
oxygen disposable boot d.
Progestasert intrauterine d.
Select-Lite lancing d.
steroid-releasing intrauterine d.
vacuum tumescence d.
DEXA
dual-energy x-ray absorptiometry
DEXA scan
Dex-A-Diet
Maximum Strength D.-A.-D.
dexamethasone
d. suppression test
d. suppression therapy
dexamethasone-suppressed
d.-s. corticotropin-releasing hormone stimulation
d.-s. CRH stimulation
d.-s. ovine corticotropin-releasing hormone
dexamethasone-suppressible hyperaldosteronism
Dexasone
D. L.A.
Dexatrim
Maximum Strength D.
D. Pre-Meal
Dexedrine
dexfenfluramine
DexFerrum
Dexone
D. LA
dextran
parenteral iron d.
dextranomer
dextroamphetamine
d. and amphetamine
dextrose
dialysate d.

Dextrostix
Dey-Dose
D.-D. isoproterenol
D.-D. metaproterenol
Dey-Lute isoetharine
dezocine
DFEN
D-fenfluramine
D-fenfluramine (DFEN)
DFO
deferoxamine
DFO challenge
DFO test
DGAT
diacylglyceroacyl transferase
DGE
delayed gastric emptying
DGGE
denaturing gradient gel electrophoresis
DHA
dehydroalanine
docosahexaenoic acid
DHC
11-dehydrocorticosterone
Duradyne DHC
DHC Plus
DHEA
dehydroepiandrosterone
DHEA cream
DHEA sulfate
DHEAS, DHEA-S
dehydroepiandrosterone sulfate
DHPG
dihydroxyphenylglycol
DHT
dihydrotestosterone
DHT gel
Diabenal
diabesity
Diab II
DiaBeta
diabetes
adrenal d.
adult-onset d.
d. associated with certain conditions
d. associated with certain syndrome
atypical d.
autoimmune d.
brittle d.
bronze d.
congenital lipoatrophic d.
D. Control and Complications Trial (DCCT)
cystic fibrosis-related d. (CFRD)
Diabetes Prevention Trial of Type 1 D. (DPT-1)
drug-induced d.
D. in Early Pregnancy Study
European Association for the Study of D.
familial autoimmunity in d. (FAD)
fibrocalculous pancreatic d. (FCPD)
gestational d.
D. Hypoglucose capsule
idiopathic d.
immune-mediated d. (IMD)
d. insipidus
d. insipidus, diabetes mellitus, optic atrophy, and deafness (DIMOAD)
d. insipidus, diabetes mellitus, progressive bilateral optic atrophy, and sensorineural deafness (DIDMOAD)
insulin-dependent d. (IDD)
J-type d.
juvenile-onset d. (JOD)
lipoatrophic d.
lipotrophic d.
maturity-onset d. (MOD)
d. mellitus
d. mellitus classification
D. Mellitus Insulin-Glucose Infusion in Acute Myocardial Infection (DIGAMI)
D. Mellitus Insulin-Glucose Infusion in Acute Myocardial Infection study
d. mellitus, pregnancy classification, class A, B, C, D, E, F
nephrogenic d.
occult d.
ocular complications of d.
pancreatic d.
pituitary d.
pregestational d.
D. Prevention Program (DPP)
D. Prevention Trial (DPT-1)
D. Prevention Trial research study
protein-deficient pancreatic d.
renal d.
D. Retinopathy Study (DRS)
d. self-management
small bowel d.

NOTES

diabetes *(continued)*
steroid-induced d.
type 1 d.
type 2 d.
virus-induced d.
diabetes-deafness syndrome
diabetic
d. amyotrophy
d. autonomic neuropathy
d. cardiomyopathy
Detection of Ischemia in Asymptomatic D.'s (DIAD)
d. diarrhea
d. dyslipidemia
d. enteropathy
d. foot syndrome
d. gastroparesis
d. ketoacidosis (DKA)
d. ketoacidosis-related coma
d. lipoatrophy
d. lipohypertrophy
d. microangiopathy
d. mononeuropathy
d. myocardial infarction
d. nephropathy
d. neuropathic arthropathy
nonobese d.
d. retinopathy
D. Tussin
D. Tussin Allergy Relief
D. Tussin Children's Formula
D. Tussin DM Maximum Strength Cough Suppressant/Expectorant
D. Tussin EX
d. vasculopathy
diabeticorum
bullosis d.
bullous d.
necrobiosis lipoidica d. (NLD)
scleredema d.
diabetic vasculopathy
DiabetiDerm
DiabetiSweet
D. sugar substitute
diabetogenecity
diabetogenesis
diabetogenic
d. effect
d. haplotype
d. hormone
d. locus
d. stimulus
diabetologist
Diab II
Diabinese
diacetate
ethinyl estradiol and ethynodiol d.
ethynodiol d.
progestin ethynodiol d.
diacylglyceroacyl transferase (DGAT)
diacylglycerol (DAG)
DIAD
Detection of Ischemia in Asymptomatic Diabetics
DIAD study
diagnosis
prenatal d.
presymptomatic d.
diagnostant
pancreatic functioning d. (PFD)
diagnostic imaging
Dialume
dialysate
aluminum-contaminated d.
d. calcium concentration
d. dextrose
high-calcium d.
low-calcium d.
dialysis
chronic ambulatory peritoneal d. (CAPD)
continuous ambulatory peritoneal d. (CAPD)
d. dementia
equilibrium tracer d.
d. membrane
d. modality
peritoneal d. (PD)
dialysis-associated amyloidosis
dialysis-related amyloidosis (DRA)
dialytic therapy
dialyzable factor
diameter
myofiber d.
Diamicron
diamine oxidase (DAO)
Diamyd
Dianabol
Diane-35
Dianette
diapedesis
diaphoresis
diaphragm
urogenital d.
diaphragma
d. sella
diaphragmal opening
diaphragmatic crus
diaphyseal, diaphysial
d. cortical hyperostosis
d. dysplasia
d. sclerosis
diaphysis
diarrhea
diabetic d.

osmotic d.
toxin-induced d.
Diasensor
D. 2000 glucose monitor
D. 1000 sensor
diastase
diastrophic
d. dystrophia (DTD)
d. dystrophia gene
diathesis
hemorrhagic d.
diazoxide
dibasic
d. aminoaciduria
d. calcium phosphate
dibenzodiazepine
tricyclic d.
Dibenzyline
dibromochloropropane
dibutyryl
d. cAMP
d. cyclic arginine monophosphate
DIC
disseminated intravascular coagulation
Dicarbosil
dicarboxylic acid
dichlorodiphenyldichloroethane (DDD)
dichlorodiphenyltrichloroethane (DDT)
diclofenac
DIDMOAD
diabetes insipidus, diabetes mellitus, progressive bilateral optic atrophy, and sensorineural deafness
Didrex
Didronel
DIDS
4,4′-di-isothiocyanatostilbene-2,2′-disulfonic acid
diencephalic
d. cachexia
d. epilepsy
d. syndrome
d. syndrome of infancy
diencephalon
dienogest
progestin d.
diet
acid ash d.
animal protein d.
cafeteria d.
HCF d.
high-carbohydrate high-fiber d.
high glycemic index d.
high-phosphorus d.
high-salt d.
hypocaloric d.
isocalorically substituted d.
low glycemic index d.
low-phosphorus d.
phenylalanine-restricted d.
step 2 d.
very low calorie d.
dietary
d. calcium intake
d. phosphorus
d. protein
diethylpropion
diethylstilbestrol (DES)
diet-induced obesity
dieting
inappropriate d.
difference
arteriovenous d.
differentiated
d. thyroid carcinoma
d. thyroid carcinoma, intermediate type
differentiation
carcinoma with thymus-like d. (CASTLE)
chondrocyte terminal d.
morphologic d.
prechondrocyte d.
sexual d.
spindled and epithelial tumor with thymus-like d. (SETTLE)
differentiation-inhibiting activity
diffuse
d. endocrine system
d. idiopathic skeletal hyperostosis (DISH)
d. neuroendocrine system (DNES)
d. renal ischemia
d. toxic goiter
diffuse papillomatosis
diffusion
proton d.
diflunisal
DIGAMI
Diabetes Mellitus Insulin-Glucose Infusion in Acute Myocardial Infection
DIGAMI study
Di-Gel
DiGeorge syndrome

NOTES

D

Digepepsin
Digess 8000
DigiScope
digital
d. subtraction angiography (DSA)
d. vasospasm
digitalis
digitonin
digoxin
dihomo-gamma-linoleic acid
dihydrobiopterin
d. synthase deficiency
d. synthetase
dihydrocodeine compound
dihydroequilenin
dihydrogen phosphate
dihydropteridine
d. reductase
d. reductase deficiency
dihydropyridine
d. antagonist
dihydrotachysterol
dihydrotestosterone (DHT)
d. gel
dihydroxyacetone
dihydroxyaluminum sodium carbonate
2′4-dihydroxybenzoic acid
1,25-dihydroxycholecalciferol
5,6-dihydroxyindole
dihydroxymandelic acid (DOMA)
dihydroxyphenylacetic acid (DOPAC)
dihydroxyphenylalanine (DOPA)
d. decarboxylase
dihydroxyphenylglycol (DHPG)
dihydroxyvitamin
d. D
1,25-d. D (1,25$(OH)_2$-VitD)
1,25-d. D_3
Dihyrex Injection
diiodinated tyrosine (DIT)
diiodotyrosine (DIT)
3,5-d. (DIT)
diketopiperazine
Dilantin
dilatation
aortic root d.
d. of aortic root
fusiform d.
dilated fundus examination
dilation
triventricular d.
Dilaudid
D. Injection
D. Oral
D. suppository
Dilaudid-HP Injection
Dilor
diltiazem
diluent
dilution
isotope d.
dimenhydrinate
dimer
glucocorticoid receptor d.
type II regulatory d. (RII)
type I regulatory d. (RI)
dimercaptosuccinate
pentavalent d. (DMSA)
^{99m}Tc-pentavalent d.
dimercaptosuccinic acid (DMSA, DMSA-V-Tc99-m)
dimeric form
dimerization
estrogen receptor d.
Dimetabs Oral
3,5-dimethyl-3′-isopropyl-L-thyronine (DIMIT)
dimethyl triazeno imidazole carboxamide-Dome (DTIC-Dome)
diminished ovarian reserve
DIMIT
3,5-dimethyl-3′-isopropyl-L-thyronine
DIMOAD
diabetes insipidus, diabetes mellitus, optic atrophy, and deafness
DIMOAD syndrome
dimorphic
sexually d.
dimorphism
sexual d.
dimorphous
Dinate Injection
2,4-dinitrophenylhydrazine test
dinucleotide
cytosine-guanine d.
nicotinamide-adenine d. (NAD)
Dioval Injection
dioxin
d. receptor
dioxolone
imidazole d.
dioxygenase
4-hydroxyphenylpyruvate d.
2,3-dioxygenase
indoleamine 2,3-d. (IDO)
dipalmitoylphosphatidylcholine (DPPC)
dipeptidyl
d. carboxypeptidase
d. peptidase
Diphenhist
diphenoxylate
diphenyl
d. ether linkage
d. ether moiety
diphenylhydantoin

diphosphate
adenosine 5′ d. (ADP)
guanosine 5′ d. (GDP)
inositol d.
uridine 5′-d.
diphosphate-binding
guanosine d.-b.
1,3-diphosphoglycerate
diphosphonate
diphtheroid
diplegia
congenital facial d.
Diplococcus pneumoniae
diplopia
diplosome
diplotene
dipsogenic
d. diabetes insipidus
d. stimulus
dipyridamole
Disalcid
disc
morning glory d.
neovascularization of d. (NVD)
discharge
discontinuous capillary endothelium
disease
acquired von Willebrand d. (AvWD)
Addison d.
adrenal medullary d.
adult polycystic kidney d.
adynamic bone d.
Albers-Schönberg d.
aluminum bone d.
aluminum-related bone d.
Alzheimer d.
anemia of end-stage renal d.
aplastic bone d.
autoimmune endocrine d.
autoimmune thyroid d. (AITD)
autosomal recessive d.
Ayala d.
Basedow d.
B-cell autoimmune thyroid d.
benign nodular d.
bilateral adrenal d.
bovine viral diarrhea mucosal d. (BVD-MD)
brittle-bone d.
broad beta d.
bronze d.
Brown-Schilder d.
Bruton d.
bubble boy d.
Camurati-Engelmann d.
Canavan d.
Castleman d.
celiac d.
Charcot-Marie d.
Charcot-Marie-Tooth d.
childhood Graves d.
Child-Pugh d.
cholestatic liver d.
cholesterol ester storage d.
cholesteryl ester storage d.
chronic granulomatous d.
chylomicron retention d.
connective tissue d.
Cori d.
Cowden d.
Creutzfeldt-Jakob d. (CJD)
Crohn d.
Crouzon d.
Cushing d.
cyclical Cushing d.
Dent d.
dermopathy of Graves d.
ductus-dependent congenital heart d.
Dupuytren d.
endocrine d.
end-stage renal d. (ESRD)
Engelmann d.
Erdheim-Chester d.
euthyroid Graves d.
extrathyroidal manifestation of Graves d.
Fabry d.
Farber d.
fibrocystic breast d.
fulminant Letterer-Siwe d.
Gagel d.
Gaucher d.
gestational trophoblastic d.
Gierke d.
Glanzmann d.
glomerular d.
glucagon storage d.
glycogen storage d. types I/1a, II, III, IV, V, VI, VII, VIII
granulomatous d.
Graves d.
Gull d.
GVH d.
Hand-Schüller-Christian d.
Hansen d.

NOTES

disease *(continued)*
Hashimoto d.
hepatic d.
Hirschsprung d.
Hodgkin d.
Huntington d.
hyaline membrane d.
hyperabsorptive hypercalciuric stone d.
hyperparathyroid bone d.
hypophosphatemic bone d.
hypothalamic-pituitary d.
I-cell d.
idiopathic Addison d.
inclusion cell d.
iron storage d.
Jod-Basedow d.
Kearns-Sayre d.
Kennedy d.
Krabbe d.
kwashiorkor d.
Kyrle d.
Laron d.
Leigh d.
Lesch-Nyhan d.
Letterer-Siwe d.
Lhermitte-Duclos d.
liver d.
Lowe d.
low-turnover d.
Lyme d.
macrovascular d.
mad cow d.
maple syrup urine d.
marble bone d.
Meige d.
Menkes d.
metabolic bone d.
micronodular adrenal d.
microvascular d.
Milroy d.
Modification of Diet in Renal D. (MDRD)
monostotic d.
neurodegenerative d.
Newcastle bone d.
Niemann-Pick d.
node-based malignant lymphoproliferative d.
nonendocrine d.
nonthyroid d.
Norrie d.
obstructive intestinal d.
ophthalmic Graves d.
Osler-Rendu-Weber d.
Paget d.
Parkinson d.
Parry d.
pathologic parathyroid d.
Pelizaeus-Merzbacher d.
pelvic inflammatory d.
peptic ulcer d.
peripheral arterial d. (PAD)
Peyronie d.
pigmented nodular adrenocortical d. (PPNAD)
pituitary Cushing d.
pituitary-dependent Cushing d.
Plummer d.
plurihormonal Cushing d.
polycystic kidney d.
polycystic ovarian d.
polycystic ovary d. (PCOD)
polyostotic Paget d.
Pompe d.
Pompe glycogen storage d. type II
postpartum thyroid d. (PPTD)
predominant hyperparathyroid bone d.
Pyle d.
rachitic d.
Recklinghausen d.
renovascular d.
Ribbing d.
Riedel d.
runt d.
Salla d.
Sandhoff d.
SC d.
Schindler d.
sellar d.
severe combined immunodeficiency d. (SCID)
sialic acid storage d.
sickle cell d.
Simmonds d.
stigmata of Cushing d.
suprasellar d.
Swiss cheese d.
Tangier d.
Tay-Sachs d.
thyrocardiac d.
thyroid eye d.
thyroid inflammatory d.
thyrotoxic Graves d.
trophoblastic d.
tubulointerstitial renal d.
type I von Willebrand d.
unilateral adrenal d.
unstable Cushing d.
van Buchem d.
venous thromboembolic d.
VHL d.
von Basedow d.
von Gierke d.
von Hippel-Lindau d.
von Recklinghausen d.

von Willebrand d.
wasting d.
Whipple d.
Wilson d.
Wolman d.
X-linked lymphoproliferative d.

Disetronic
D. Diaport pump
D. Dihedi 25 insulin pump
D. D-Tron insulin pump
D. H-Tron pump
D. Pen

DISH
diffuse idiopathic skeletal hyperostosis

disk pallor

Diskus
Serevent D.

dismutase
superoxide d.

disodium
edetate d.
etidronate d.
d. etidronate
tiludronate d.

disomy
uniparental d.

disorder
adipsic d.
adynamic bone d.
aplastic bone d.
attention-deficit hyperactivity d.
autoimmune neuromuscular junction d.
autoimmune thyroid d. (AITD)
autosomal dominant d.
autosomal karyotypic d.
autosomal recessive d.
cardiovascular d.
chromosome 7 d.
chromosome 12 d.
chromosome 20 d.
congenital bone d.
demyelinating d.
depressive d.
dysbaric d.
eating d.
endocrine d.
familial lipid d.
glucocorticoid-resistant depressive d.
growth d.
heredofamilial d.
hyperprolactinemic d.
hypodipsic d.
hypothalamic-pituitary d.
infiltrative d.
International Council for Control of Iodine Deficiency D. (ICCIDD)
iodine-deficiency d. (IDD)
ketoacid d.
late luteal phase d.
lymphoproliferative d.
major depressive d. (MDD)
monogenic d.
multihormonal system d.
neuromuscular junction d.
neuropsychiatric d.
nonsyndromic autosomal recessive d.
pancreatic d.
paroxysmal pain d.
peroxisomal d.
pituitary d.
posttransplantation lymphoproliferative d. (PTLD)
posttraumatic stress d.
premenstrual dysphoric d. (PMDD)
Riedel d.
seasonal affective d. (SAD)
sperm transport d.
vocal cord d.

disordered water metabolism

disproportion
cephalopelvic d.

dissection
en bloc d.

dissector
Hardy spoon d.
McCabe nerve d.

disseminata
dermatofibrosis lenticularis d.

disseminated
d. fat necrosis
d. histiocytosis X
d. intravascular coagulation (DIC)
d. mucormycosis
d. strongyloidosis

disseminatum
xanthoma d.

distal
d. anhidrosis
d. convoluted tubule (DCT)
d. Golgi apparatus
d. motor axonal loss
d. renal tubular acidosis type 4

NOTES

distal *(continued)*
d. sensory polyneuropathy
d. subtotal pancreatectomy
d. symmetric diabetic neuropathy
d. symmetric sensorimotor polyneuropathy
distalis
pars d.
distant metastasis
distemper
canine d.
distention
adrenal capsular d.
distichiasis
distinct nodule
distress
epidermic d.
distribution
android fat d.
glove-and-stocking d.
gynoid fat d.
phosphorus d.
disturbance
visual field d.
disulfide
d. bridge
carbon d.
d. isomerase
d. loop
disuse atrophy
DIT
diiodinated tyrosine
diiodotyrosine
3,5-diiodotyrosine
Dital
dITP
deoxyinosine triphosphate
Diucardin
diuresis
osmotic d.
pressure d.
solute d.
spontaneous d.
water d.
diuretic
loop d.
osmotic d.
potassium-sparing d.
d. therapy
thiazide d.
Diurigen
Diuril
diurnal rhythm
divalent
d. ion
diversus
Citrobacter d.
diverticulitis
diverticulum, pl. **diverticula**
epiphrenic d.
posterior gastric d.
thyroid d.
division
meiotic d.
parvocellular d.
divisum
pancreas d.
dizygotic twins
DKA
diabetic ketoacidosis
DLP
dyslipoproteinemia
D-Med Injection
D-methylmalonyl-CoA
DMN
dorsomedial nucleus
D-Modem and insulin pump therapy
DMPA
depot medroxyprogesterone acetate
DMSA
dimercaptosuccinic acid
pentavalent dimercaptosuccinate
rhenium-188 DMSA
DMSA-V-Tc99-m
dimercaptosuccinic acid
DNA
deoxyribonucleic acid
antidouble-stranded DNA
complementary DNA (cDNA)
mitochondrial DNA
putative regulatory sequence DNA
DNA-binding domain (DBD)
DNES
diffuse neuroendocrine system
dNTP
deoxynucleotide triphosphate
DOC
deoxycorticosterone
11-deoxycorticosterone
docking protein
docosahexaenoic acid (DHA)
Döderlein bacillus
Doehle body
Dolacet
Dolene
dolichol
d. phosphate carrier
dolichostenomelia
dolichyl phosphate
Dolobid
Dolophine
Dolorac
DOMA
dihydroxymandelic acid

domain
amino terminal d.
coupling d.
deoxyribonucleic acid-binding d.
DNA-binding d. (DBD)
extracellular d.
hexameric d.
hormone-binding d. (HBD)
kringle d.
leucine-zipper d.
ligand-binding d. (LDB)
phosphotyrosine-binding d. (PTB)
pleckstrin homology d.
pleiotropic d.
recognition d.
Src homology 2 d.
trans-activation d. (TAD)
transmembrane d.
dominant
d. follicle
d. thyroid nodule
domperidone
Donnamar
Donnan effect
Donnatal
Donnazyme
DOPA
dihydroxyphenylalanine
DOPA decarboxylase
L-dopa
DOPAC
dihydroxyphenylacetic acid
dopamine (DA)
d. agent
d. agonist therapy
d. beta-hydroxylase (DBH)
d. enzyme
d. receptor
d. receptor agonist
dopaminergic
d. agonist
d. blocker
d. drug
d. neuron
d. receptor
d. system
d. tone
Dopar
Dopram
d'orange
Dorcol
Dorello canal
Dormarex 2 Oral
Dormin Oral
dornase alfa
dorsal
d. motor nucleus
d. pancreatic artery
dorsalis
tabes d.
dorsocervical fat pad
dorsomedial
d. nucleus (DMN)
d. nucleus of the hypothalamus
dorsum
d. sella
dosage-sensitive
d.-s. sex (DSS)
d.-s. sex reversal
d.-s. sex reversal gene
dose
growth hormone d.
intravaginal d.
steroid d.
supraphysiologic d.
dosimetric scheme
dosimetry
dosing
pulse d.
Dospan
Tenuate D.
Dostinex
D. tablet
double-duct sign
double-labeling technique
double strength (DS)
Douglas
rectouterine recess of D.
dowager hump
down
milk let d.
downgaze
impaired d.
downregulate
downregulation
insulin-induced receptor d.
Down syndrome
doxapram
doxazosin
doxercalciferol
doxorubicin
doxycycline
DPC4 gene

NOTES

DPD
deoxypyridinoline
D-penicillamine
DPP
Diabetes Prevention Program
DPPC
dipalmitoylphosphatidylcholine
DPRHP
duodenum-preserving pancreatic head resection
DPT-1
Diabetes Prevention Trial
Diabetes Prevention Trial of Type 1 Diabetes
DPT-1 research study
DQ
D. allele
D. alpha sequence
DR4 allele
DRA
dialysis-related amyloidosis
drag
solvent d.
DR allele
Dramamine Oral
Dramilin Injection
drill
high-speed microsurgical d.
Midas Rex d.
dripping-candle-wax appearance
Drisdol
droepiandrosterone
droloxifene
dronabinol
droperidol
d. and fentanyl
droplet
colloid d.
drops
ADEKs pediatric d.
Fer-In-Sol d.
Multi Vit D.
rose bengal d.
vitamin C d.
DRPLA
dentatorubral-pallidoluysian atrophy
DRS
Diabetes Retinopathy Study
drug
antiestrogen d.
antithyroid d. (ATD)
aphrodisiac d.
Ca^{2+} ionophore d.
calcimimetic d.
carbamide d.
dopaminergic d.
lipophilic d.
methylxanthine d.
nitrous oxide-donor d.
NO-donor d.
nonsteroidal antiinflammatory d. (NSAID)
sulfonylurea hypoglycemic d.
sympatholytic d.
sympathomimetic d.
thionamide antithyroid d.
thiourea d.
drug-induced
d.-i. diabetes
d.-i. lupus
DS
double strength
Gas-Ban DS
Tolectin DS
DSA
digital subtraction angiography
DSS
dosage-sensitive sex
DSS gene
DSS reversal
D-stix
DTD
diastrophic dystrophia
DTD gene
D-thyroxine
DTIC
dacarbazine
DTIC-Dome
dimethyl triazeno imidazole carboxamide-Dome
dual-energy x-ray absorptiometry (DEXA, DXA)
dual-phase spiral computed tomography
dual-photon absorptiometry
dual-x-ray absorptiometry
Dubovitz syndrome
Duchenne-Becker muscular dystrophy
Duchenne muscular dystrophy
duct
bile d. (BD)
common bile d. (CBD)
cortical collecting d. (CCD)
craniopharyngeal d.
d. ectasia
ejaculatory d.
excretory d.
extrahepatic bile d.
intrahepatic bile d.
intralobular d.
ipsilateral paramesonephric d.
lactiferous d.
main pancreatic d. (MPD)
medullary collecting d. (MCD)
müllerian d.
parafollicular d.
paramesonephric d.

prostatic d.
thyroglossal d.
wolffian d.
ductectatic-type mucinous cystadenocarcinoma
ductule
efferent d.
ductuli efferentes
ductus
d. deferens
d. epididymis
ductus-dependent congenital heart disease
Duet glucose control monitor
dulcitol
Dull-C
dumbbell-shaped tumor
dumping syndrome
DuoCet
Duo-CVP
Duo-Cyp
duodenal intubation test
duodenography
hypotonic d.
duodenum-preserving pancreatic head resection (DPRHP)
DuPan-2 antibody
duplication
chromosome d.
Dupuytren
D. contracture
D. disease
dura
lamina d.
Duradyne DHC
Duragesic transdermal
dural microclip
Duralone Injection
Duramorph Injection
Duratest Injection
Duratestrin
Durathate Injection
Duratuss-G
Duricef
Durrax Oral
Duvoid
dwarf
Levi-Lorain d.
dwarfism
camptomelic d.
emotional deprivation d.
Laron d.
Laron-type d. (LTD)
osteodysplastic primordial d.
pituitary d.
psychosocial d.
Seckel bird-headed d.
short-limbed d.
d. of Sindh
DX
Naldecon Senior DX
DXA
dual-energy x-ray absorptiometry
dydrogesterone
dye
iodinated contrast d.
oral cholecystographic d.
radiopaque d.
dye-diluting technique
Dymelor
Dymenate Injection
DynA
dynorphin A
dynamic
d. computed tomography
d. CT
d. equilibrium
d. histomorphometry
d. spiral CT
dynamometer
isokinetic d.
dynein
dynorphin
d. A (DynA)
d. system
dyphylline
Dyrexan-OD
dysalbuminemia
familial d.
dysalbuminemic hyperthyroxinemia
dysarthria
dysautonomia
familial d.
dysbaric disorder
dysbetalipoproteinemia
familial d.
gas d.
dysembryogenesis
branchial pouch d.
dysesthesia
dysfunction
adrenal d.
autonomic d.
corticospinal tract d.

NOTES

dysfunction *(continued)*
endothelial cell d.
erectile d. (ED)
exocrine pancreatic d.
extraocular muscle d.
gonadal d.
G protein d.
luteal d.
maternal postpartum thyroid d.
neonatal thyroid d.
ovarian steroidogenic d.
parathyroid gland d.
pilosebaceous d.
pituitary d.
postpartum thyroid d.
sphincter of Oddi d.
transient neonatal thyroid d.
dysgammaglobulinemia
dysgenesis
chromatin-positive seminiferous tubule d.
d. of corpus callosum
epiphyseal d.
gonadal d.
incomplete XY gonadal d.
mixed gonadal d.
ovarian d.
seminiferous tubule d.
thyroid d. (TD)
45,X gonadal d.
46,XX gonadal d.
46,XY gonadal d.
dysgenetic gonad
dysgerminoma
pineal d.
primary suprasellar d.
dysgeusia
dysglycemic macroangiopathy
dyshomogenesis
dyshormonogenesis
thyroid d.
dyshormonogenetic goiter
dysinsulinism
dyskinesia
dyslipidemia
diabetic d.
dyslipidosis
dyslipoproteinemia (DLP)
dysmenorrhea
dysmorphic facies
dysmotility
ocular d.
dysosteosclerosis
dysostosis multiplex
dyspareunia
dysphagia
dysphonia
spasmodic d.
dysplasia
camptomelic d.
cleidocranial d.
coloboma d.
colobomatous d.
congenital adrenal d.
craniodiaphysial d.
craniometaphyseal d.
diaphyseal d.
fibrous d.
Kniest d.
Kniest-Stickle d.
mammary d.
mesometric d.
metaphyseal d.
Mondini d.
oculodentoosseous d.
polyostotic fibrous d. (PFD)
primary pigmental nodular adrenal d.
primary pigmented nodular adrenal d.
progressive diaphyseal d.
Schmid-type metaphyseal d.
septooptic d.
spondyloepiphyseal d. (SED)
spondylometaphyseal d.
Strudwick-type spondyloepimetaphyseal d.
thanatophoric d. I, II
X-linked hypohidrotic ectodermal d.
dyspnea
recumbent d.
dyspraxia
speech d.
dysproteinemia
angioimmunoblastic lymphadenopathy with d. (AILD)
dysregulation
blood pressure d.
hypothalamic d.
theca interstitial cell d.
thecal d.
dysthyroid orbitopathy
dystocia
dystonia type 1
dystonic reaction
dystopia
pituitary d.
dystrophia
diastrophic d. (DTD)
dystrophica
myotonia d.
dystrophic calcification
dystrophy
adiposogenital d.
autoimmune polyendocrinopathy-candidiasis-ectodermal d. (APECED)

Duchenne-Becker muscular d.
Duchenne muscular d.
fascioscapulohumeral muscular d.
mixed sclerosing bone d.
muscular d.
myotonic d.
oculopharyngeal muscular d.
reflex sympathetic d.

NOTES

E
apolipoprotein E
E apolipoprotein
Aquasol E
carboxypeptidase E
hemoglobin E
hepatitis E
immunoglobulin E (IgE)
E1
1/35E
Norethin 1/35E
E2
E_1
estrone
prostaglandin E_1 (PGE_1)
E_3
estriol
prostaglandin E_3
E_2
estradiol
E_2 agonist
prostaglandin E_2 (PGE_2)
E_2 receptor
E_4
leukotriene E_4 (LTE_4)
EAAT2 protein
EAE
experimental allergic autoimmune encephalitis
early
e. collecting tubule
e. endosomal compartment
e. hypocalcemia
e. pregnancy factor (EPF)
e. pubertal hyperandrogenism
e. satiety
early-onset
e.-o. idiopathic chronic pancreatitis
e.-o. uterine leiomyoma
Early Treatment Diabetic Retinopathy Study (ETDRS)
Easprin
easy satiety
EAT
experimental autoimmune thyroiditis
eating disorder
EBV
Epstein-Barr virus
EC
endothelial cell
enterochromaffin cell
E-cadherin
E.-c. protein
ecchymosis
eccrine sweat gland
ecdysone receptor
ECF
extracellular fluid
ECG
electrocardiogram
Echinococcus
E. granulosus
echo
fast asymmetric spin e. (FASE)
echogenic
e. ovarian stroma
echogenicity
echotexture
echovirus
e. 6
ECL
enterochromaffin-like
ECL cell
ECL cell hyperplasia
eclosion hormone
E-Complex-600
***Eco*RI**
Ecotrin
ectasia
duct e.
ecthyma gangrenosis
ectoderm
stomodeal e.
ectodermal anomaly
ectoenzyme
thyroid-releasing hormone-degrading e.
TRH-degrading e. (TRH-DE)
ectohormone
ectopia lentis
ectopic
e. acromegaly
e. ACTH-secreting tumor
e. ACTH secretion
e. ACTH syndrome
e. adrenal adenoma
e. adrenocorticotropic hormone secretion
e. adrenocorticotropic hormone syndrome
e. calcification
e. corticotropin-releasing hormone syndrome
e. CRH syndrome
e. Cushing syndrome
e. endometrium
e. expression
e. growth hormone-releasing hormone secretion
e. hormone production

E

ectopic *(continued)*
e. hormone receptor
e. hormone syndrome
e. intrapancreatic protease activation
e. neuroendocrine tumor
e. paraneoplastic ACTH production
e. pinealoma
e. pituitary adenoma
e. pregnancy
e. thyroid
e. thyroid tissue
ectoplasmic specialization
eczematoid dermatitis
ED
erectile dysfunction
EDAX
energy-dispersive x-ray analysis
EDC
estimated date of confinement
EDe
erosion depth
Edecrin
edema
brawny e.
conjunctival e.
hereditary angioneurotic e.
interstitial e.
macular e.
neurogenic pulmonary e.
periorbital e.
Reinke e.
type 1 angioneurotic e.
type 2 angioneurotic e.
edetate disodium
edetic acid
EDF
erythroid differentiation factor
EDIC
Epidemiology of Diabetes Interventions and Complications
Edinger-Westphal nucleus
Edmonton Protocol
EDRF
endothelium-derived relaxing factor
ED-SPAZ
EDTA
ethylenediaminetetraacetic acid
Educator
Certified Diabetes E. (CDE)
EFA
essential fatty acid
effect
acute Wolff-Chaikoff e.
allosteric e.
alpha-adrenergic e.
aluminum e.
anticholinergic side e.
antilipolytic e.
antimitotic e.
antirachitic e.
antirachitogenic e.
antiserotoninergic e.
antistress e.
base-substitution e.
beta-adrenergic e.
bone e.
calcemic e.
cardiovascular e.
cholinergic e.
diabetogenic e.
Donnan e.
endocrine e.
estrogenic e.
extrahepatic e.
gastrointestinal e.
growth hormone protein-sparing e.
hair e.
hepatic e.
hormone-dependency e.
hydrogen-bonding e.
ileal-brake e.
immunoregulatory e.
incretin e.
insulinomimetic e.
Jod-Basedow e.
K_m e.
maternotoxic e.
metabolic e.
multiplier e.
muscle e.
neuropsychiatric e.
nongenomic e.
paracrine e.
physiologic e.
piezoelectric e.
ring-substitution e.
Somogyi e.
stalk section e.
Staub-Traugott e.
vitamin D e.
Wolff-Chaikoff e.
effective
e. circulating volume
e. half-life
e. osmolality
effector
allosteric e.
bihormonal e.
e. organ
efferent
e. arteriole
e. ductule
e. system
efferentes
ductuli e.

effluent
thyroid venous e.
efflux
calcium e.
hepatic glucose e.
iodide e.
net e.
parathyroid hormone-mediated calcium e.
PTH-mediated calcium e.
eflornithine hydrochloride
Efudex
EFV
extracellular fluid volume
EGF
epidermal growth factor
heparin-binding EGF
EGF receptor
EGF-like growth factor
EGP
endogenous glucose production
Ehlers-Danlos syndrome types I, II, III, IV, VII
EIA
enteroinsular axis
enzyme immunoassay
eicosanoid
e. synthesis
eicosapentaenoic acid (EPA)
Eikenella corrodens
ejaculation
retrograde e.
ejaculatory duct
ejection
milk e.
EKG
electrocardiogram
elastase
plasma polymorphonuclear e. (PMN-3)
elastase-1 level
elastin
elastography
magnetic resonance e. (MRE)
Eldercaps
electrical gradient
electrically excitable cell
electrocardiogram (ECG, EKG)
electrochemical
e. glucose sensor
e. gradient
electroconvulsive therapy
electrode
amperometric glucose oxidase e.
Clark oxygen e.
H_2O_2 amperometric e.
ion-selective e.
platinum e.
electrogenic
electroimmunoassay
electrolyte
e. flux
electromyography (EMG)
electronic barostat
electron transport flavoprotein (ETF)
electroosmotic sampling procedure
electrophoresis
denaturing gradient gel e. (DGGE)
gel e.
hydrolink gel e.
polyacrylamide gel e.
electrovaporization of the prostate
eledoisin
element
activator protein-1 e.
anamnestic e.
AP-1 e.
basal promoter e. (BPE)
bone marrow e.
cAMP-response e. (CRE)
cis e.
cis-acting DNA e.
comparator e.
consensus-response e.
cyclic adenosine 3′,5′-monophosphate-response e.
estrogen-receptor e. (ERE)
estrogen-response e. (ERE)
glucocorticoid response e. (GRE)
glucocorticoid-responsive e. (GRE)
hormone response e. (HRE)
inhibitory response e. (IRE)
laminin B1 e.
lysozyme F_2 e.
negative T_3 response e. (TRE)
negative triiodothyronine response e.
NF-kappa-B e.
nuclear factor-kappa B e.
response e.
steroid hormone-receptor hormone-response e.
steroid hormone-response e.
thyroid hormone-response e. (TRE)

NOTES

E

element *(continued)*
T_3 responsive e. (T_3RE)
vitamin D-regulatory e.
vitamin D-response e. (VDRE)
xenobiotic-response e. (XRE)
Z e.
element-binding
cAMP response e.-b. (CREB)
cyclic adenosine 3′,5′ monophosphate response e.-b.
cyclic arginine monophosphate response e.-b.
elephantiasic
elephantiasis
elevated
e. intracranial pressure
e. radioactive iodine uptake
e. RAIU
e. waist-to-hip ratio
elevation
spurious e.
elevator
Cottle e.
Freer e.
elfin
e. facies
e. facies syndrome
ELISA
enzyme-linked immunosorbent assay
Elixir
Lycolan E.
Elixomin
Elixophyllin
elliptocytosis
Ellis-van Creveld syndrome
Eltroxin
EM-652
emaciation
embedding
bone e.
embolization
fat e.
hepatic artery e.
superselective microcoil e.
transcatheter celiac artery e.
embolus
cholesterol e.
embryogenesis
embryologic development end-organ ovarian failure
embryonal
e. adenoma
e. carcinoma
e. path
embryonic testicular regression syndrome
embryotoxic
embryotoxicity
embryo transfer (ET)
emergency
hypocalcemic e.
EMG
electromyography
EMH
extramedullary hematopoiesis
eminence
infundibular e.
infundibulum e.
median e.
emissary vein
emission
nocturnal e.
emollient
Ponaris nasal e.
emotional deprivation dwarfism
emphysematous
e. cholecystitis
e. pyelonephritis
Empirin
E. with codeine
empty
e. sella
e. sella syndrome
emptying
delayed gastric e. (DGE)
gastric e.
en
e. bloc dissection
e. face
ENaC
epithelial sodium channel
enalapril
enanthate
testosterone e.
encapsulated
e. angioinvasive carcinoma
e. islet transplant
encephalitis
experimental allergic autoimmune e. (EAE)
e. pandemic
St. Louis e.
encephalocele
basal e.
forebrain basal e.
frontoethmoidal e.
sphenoethmoidal e.
sphenoorbital e.
transethmoidal basal e.
transsphenoidal e.
encephalopathy
Hashimoto e.
hypertonic e.
hyponatremic e.
hypoxic e.

spongiform e.
Wernicke e.
endemia
goiter e.
endemic
e. colloid goiter
e. cretinism
e. fluorosis
e. iodine-deficiency goiter
ending
terminal nerve e.
ENDIT
European Nicotinamide Diabetes Intervention Trial
endobone
endochondral
e. bone formation
e. bone maturation
e. ossification
endocrine
e. abnormality
e. anomaly
e. axis
e. disease
e. disorder
e. effect
e. effector cell
e. gene
e. gland
e. hyperfunction
e. hypertension
e. ophthalmopathy
e. pancreas
pulmonary neuroepithelial e. (PNEE)
e. remission
e. rhythm
e. therapy
e. tumor
e. tumor syndrome
endocrine-inactive pituitary adenoma
endocrinologic
endocrinologist
American Association of Clinical E.'s
endocrinoma
endocrinopathy
autoimmune polyglandular e.
hyperprolactinemic e.
secondary e.
endocytose
endocytosis
absorptive e.
receptor-mediated e.
endoderm
endodermal sinus tumor
endo-exocrine tumor
endogenous
e. circadian pacemaker
e. cyclicity
e. estrogen bioassay
e. fecal calcium
e. glucose production (EGP)
e. gonadal hormone
e. growth hormone
e. hypercortisolism
e. insulin
e. morphine
e. opioid
e. opioid peptide (EOP)
e. rhythm
e. testosterone
endoglycosidase H
endolymph
endolymphatic cyst
endometrial
e. cancer
e. cavity
e. cycle
e. gland
e. stroma
e. thickness
endometrioid tumor
endometrioma
leaking e.
endometriosis
endometriotic implant
endometritis
tuberculous e.
endometrium
ectopic e.
eutopic e.
uterine e.
endomysial connective tissue
endonasal
e. endoscopic pituitary surgery
e. endoscopic technique
endoneurial blood vessel
endopeptidase
cysteine e.
neutral e.
endoplasmic
e. reticulum (ER)

NOTES

endoplasmic *(continued)*
e. reticulum cisternae
e. reticulum-Golgi network
endoprotease
aspartyl e.
serum e.
subtilisin-related e.
endorectal
e. magnetic resonance imaging
e. MRI
end-organ
e.-o. resistance
e.-o. response
endorphin
endoscope
e. cleaning device
e. holding clamp
rigid sinonasal e.
e. shaft
endoscopic
e. pituitary surgery technique
e. retrograde cholangiopancreatography (ERCP)
e. sphincterotomy (ES)
e. transsphenoidal hypophysectomy
e. ultrasound (EUS)
Endoscrub
endosome
endosonography
endostatin
endosteal
e. envelope
e. fibrosis
e. hyperostosis
e. membrane
endosteum
endothelial
e. cell (EC)
e. cell dysfunction
e. cell-stimulating angiogenesis factor (ESAF)
e. layer
e. PAS-domain protein-1 (EPAS1)
endothelin (ET)
e. immunostaining
e. isopeptide
e. level
e. receptor
e. receptor density
e. receptor expression
e. release
endothelin-1 (ET-1)
endothelin-induced protein synthesis
endothelium
capillary e.
continuous capillary e.
discontinuous capillary e.
fenestrated capillary e.
luminal e.
endothelium-derived relaxing factor (EDRF)
endotoxemia
endotoxin
endotracheal tube
endozepine
end-stage renal disease (ESRD)
end-systolic
e.-s. stress
e.-s. volume
Enduron
Enemol
Ener-B
energy
activation e.
e. pathway
energy-dispersive x-ray analysis (EDAX)
Engelmann disease
englitazone
engraftment
enhanced proximal tubular salt absorption
enhancer
pleiotrophin/midkine growth e. (PTN/MK)
Enisyl
enkephalin
leucine e. (LE)
methionine e. (ME)
Met and Leu e.
e. system
enlargement
acral e.
facial feature e.
hand e.
pituitary e.
stromal e.
enolase
e. enzyme
neuron-specific e.
enophthalmos
Enovid
enoxaparin
ENS
enteric nervous system
Ensure Glucerna OS
enteral aluminum absorption
enteric
e. fever
e. hyperoxaluria
e. nervous system (ENS)
enteric-coated sodium fluoride
enteritidis
Salmonella e.

Enterobacter
enterochromaffin cell (EC)
enterochromaffin-like (ECL)
e.-l. cell
e.-l. cell hyperplasia
enterocolitica
Yersinia e.
enteroglucagon
enterohepatic
e. circulation
e. tumor
enteroinsular axis (EIA)
enterokinase
enteropathy
diabetic e.
Entero-Vioform
enterovirus
Enterra therapy
enthesopathy
degenerative e.
entrainment
nonphotic e.
photic e.
entropy
approximate e. (ApEn)
enucleation
enuresis
envelope
endosteal e.
glial e.
periosteal e.
Schwann e.
environment
photoperiodic e.
enzootic goiter
enzyme
acrosomal e.
amidating e.
angiotensin-converting e. (ACE)
brush-border alpha-glucosidase e.
carbonic anhydrase e.
cathepsin B e.
circulating lipolytic e.
cytochrome P450 e. (CYP)
cytochrome P450 e. 19 (CYP19)
cytochrome P450 e. 27 (CYP27)
cytochrome P450 e. 1A1 (CYP1A1)
cytochrome P450 e. 11A (CYP11A)
cytochrome P450 e. 21B (CYP21B)
cytochrome P450 family of e.'s
cytosolic e.
e. defect
e. deficiency
deiodinase e.
delta-5-desaturase e.
delta-6-desaturase e.
e. DNase I
dopamine e.
enolase e.
e. expression
extrapancreatic digestive e.
furin e.
galactosyltransferase e.
e. glucokinase
glycolytic e.
guanylate cyclase e.
hepatocellular e.
hexokinase e.
11-hydroxylase e.
e. immunoassay (EIA)
insulin-degrading e. (IDE)
insulin-sensitive e.
intracellular effector e.
iodinase e.
laminin e.
lipogenic e.
liver e.
e. lysyl oxidase
malic e.
mitochondrial e.
muscle e.
oligosaccharide transferase e.
pancreatic e.
phosphatase e.
phospholipase C e.
phosphorylase e.
prolyl hydroxylase e.
proteolytic e.
P450SCC e.
P450 side chain cleavage e.
*Pst*I restriction e.
pulmonary angiotensin I converting e. (PACE)
restriction e.
SCC e.
side chain cleavage e.
steroidogenic e.
sulfotransferase e.
*Taq*I restriction e.
telomerase e.

NOTES

E

enzyme *(continued)*
tyrosine aminotransferase e.
e. urease
enzyme-linked
e.-l. immunoassay
e.-l. immunosorbent assay (ELISA)
EOP
endogenous opioid peptide
EORTC
European Organization for Research and Treatment of Cancer
eosin
e. stain
eosinopenia
eosinophil
eosinophilia
e. myalgia syndrome
eosinophilic
e. colloid
e. pancreatitis
EPA
eicosapentaenoic acid
EPAS1
endothelial PAS-domain protein-1
ependymoma
EPF
early pregnancy factor
ephedra
ephedrine
EPI
epinephrine
exocrine pancreatic insufficiency
epiandrosterone
epiblast
epicanthus
epidemic hemorrhagic fever
Epidemiology of Diabetes Interventions and Complications (EDIC)
epidermal
e. cyst
e. growth factor (EGF)
e. growth factor receptor
e. hyperplasia
e. necrolysis
epidermic distress
epidermidis
Staphylococcus e.
epidermoid cyst
epidermolysis bullosa
epididymal cystadenoma
epididymis, pl. **epididymides**
caput e.
ductus e.
epididymitis
epididymoorchitis
epilepsy
catamenial e.
diencephalic e.
epilepticus
status e.
epileptiform activity
EPILOG
Evaluation of PTCA to Improve Long-Term Outcome by C7E3 GpIIb/IIIa Receptor Blockade
EPILOG trial
epinephrine (EPI)
e. provocation test
epinephrine-to-norepinephrine ratio
epinephros
epineurial blood vessel
epiphenomenon
epiphrenic diverticulum
epiphyseal
e. closure
e. dysgenesis
e. fusion
e. growth plate
e. maturation
epiphysis, pl. **epiphyses**
e. cerebri
fused e.
stippled e.
episode
metabolic stress e.
myopathy, encephalopathy, lactic acidosis, stroke-like e.'s (MELAS)
EPISTENT
Evaluation of Platelet IIb-IIIa Inhibitors for Stenting
EPISTENT trial
epitaxial
e. crystal proliferation
e. growth
epithalamic region
epithelial
e. sodium channel (ENaC)
e. thyroid carcinoma
epithelioid giant cell
epithelium
coelomic e.
germinal e.
hormone-responsive e.
maceration of e.
pseudostratified stereociliated columnar e.
seminiferous e.
squamous follicular e.
epitode
epitope
antibody e.
conformational dependent e.
T-cell e.
Eplerenone
EPO
erythropoietin

epoetin alfa
Epogen
epostane
epoxymextrenone
Epstein-Barr
E.-B. transformed lymphocyte
E.-B. virus (EBV)
equation
Goldman-Hodgkin-Katz e.
Harris-Benedict e.
Henderson-Hasselbalch e.
Nernst e.
equilenin
Equilet
equilibrium
e. association constant (K_a)
e. dissociation constant (K_d)
dynamic e.
osmotic e.
e. tracer dialysis
equilin
equine
e. conjugated estrogen
equol
ER
endoplasmic reticulum
estrogen receptor
ER alpha
ER beta
erb
e. B2/HER2 ligand
***erb* oncogene**
ERCP
endoscopic retrograde cholangiopancreatography
Erdheim-Chester disease
ERE
estrogen-receptor element
estrogen-response element
erectile
e. dysfunction (ED)
e. impairment
e. impotence
e. tissue
erect penile length
ergocalciferol
ergogenic acid
ergoline
e. derivative
ergonovine
Ergoset
E. tablet
ergosterol
ergot
e. alkaloid
E. Alkaloid and Derivative
ergotamine
erigentes
parasympathetic nervi e.
ERK
extracellularly regulated kinase
extracellular signal-regulated kinase
Erlenmeyer flask deformity
erosio interdigitalis blastomycetica
erosion
e. depth (EDe)
e. surface per bone surface (ES/BS)
ERP-CT
computed tomography under endoscopic retrograde pancreatography
error
ERT
estrogen replacement therapy
eruption
acneiform e.
erythema
e. multiforme
necrolytic migratory e. (NME)
e. nodosum
erythematosus
lupus e.
systemic lupus e. (SLE)
erythrasma
erythroblastosis fetalis
erythrocyte sedimentation rate (ESR)
erythrocytosis
erythrogenin
erythroid
colony-forming unit e. (CFU-E)
e. differentiation factor (EDF)
e. hyperplasia
e. precursor
e. series
erythroleukemia
erythromelalgia
erythromycin
erythropoiesis
erythropoietin (EPO)
recombinant e.
serum e.
erythrosin
ES
endoscopic sphincterotomy

NOTES

ES *(continued)*
extra strength
Pertussin ES
Vicodin ES
ESAF
endothelial cell-stimulating angiogenesis factor
ES/BS
erosion surface per bone surface
escalator
mucous e.
escape
aldosterone e.
e. phenomenon
eschar
pathognomonic black e.
Escherichia coli
Esclim transdermal
escutcheon
E-selectin ligand
Esidrix
esmolol
esodeviation
esophageal stethoscope
esophagography
barium contrast e.
esotropia
ESR
erythrocyte sedimentation rate
ESRD
end-stage renal disease
essential
e. fatty acid (EFA)
e. hypernatremia
e. hypertension
EST
expressed sequence tag
ester
cholesterol e.
cholesteryl e.
L-nitro-L-arginine methyl e.
plant stanol e.
retinyl fatty acid e.
testosterone e.
esterification
esterified
e. estrogen
e. estrogen-methyltestosterone
estimated date of confinement (EDC)
Estinyl
Estrace
E. Oral
Estracomb TTS
Estraderm
E. transdermal
Estraderm-TTS
estradiol (E_2)
17B e.
cyclical ethinyl e.
ethinyl e.
e. matrix
micronized e.
nonestrogenic stereoisomer 17-alpha e.
e. and norethindrone
e. peak
serum e.
e. and testosterone
transdermal e.
estradiol/norethindrone acetate
estradiol-norethisterone phase
estradiol/norgestimate
estradiol/testosterone ratio
Estra-L Injection
estrane derivative
Estratab
Estratest H.S.
Estring
E. vaginal insert
estriol (E_3)
Estro-Cyp Injection
estrogen
conjugated equine e. (CEE)
e. C_{19} steroid
cyclic conjugated e.
cytoplasmic e.
e. deficiency
e. deprivation
designer e.
equine conjugated e.
esterified e.
intravaginal e.
low-dose vaginal e.
e. and medroxyprogesterone
menopausal e.
e. metabolism
e. monotherapy
noncontraceptive e.
nonsteroidal e.
e. receptor (ER)
e. receptor alpha
e. receptor antihormone
e. receptor beta
e. receptor B-variant
e. receptor dimerization
e. receptor phosphorylation
e. receptor-positive breast cancer
e. replacement therapy (ERT)
e. synthase
e. synthesis
synthetic conjugated e.
systemic e.
e. therapy
transdermal e.
unopposed e. (UNE)
estrogen/androgen therapy

estrogenic effect
estrogenization
estrogen-methyltestosterone
esterified e.-m.
estrogen-producing tumor
estrogen-receptor
e.-r. element (ERE)
e.-r. modulator
estrogen-response element (ERE)
estrone (E_1)
e. hypothesis
serum e.
e. sulfate
estropipate
estroprogestin
Estrostep 21
Estrostep Fe
estrous cycle
ET
embryo transfer
endothelin
ET-1
endothelin-1
ETDRS
Early Treatment Diabetic Retinopathy Study
ETF
electron transport flavoprotein
ethacrynic acid
ethanol
e. hypoglycemia
ethaverine
ether
e. bridge substitution
ethinyl estradiol-3-methyl e.
ether-link cleavage
ether-stimulation test
ethinyl, ethynyl
e. estradiol
e. estradiol and desogestrel
e. estradiol and ethynodiol diacetate
e. estradiol and levonorgestrel
e. estradiol-3-methyl ether
e. estradiol and norethindrone
e. estradiol and norgestimate
e. estradiol and norgestrel
e. testosterone
ethinylestradiol
Ethiofos
ethionamide
ethmoidal
e. rongeur
e. scissors
ethylene
e. glycol
e. thiourea
ethylenediaminetetraacetic acid (EDTA)
ethylene thiourea
ethylene-vinyl acetate copolymer
ethynodiol
e. diacetate
ethynyl (*var. of* ethinyl)
etidronate
disodium e.
e. disodium
etiocholanedoine
etiocholanolone
etodolac
etomidate
etoposide
etrogenic
eucalcemic
euchromatin
eucortisolemic
eucortisolism
Euflex
Euglucon
euglycemia
euglycemic
e. glucose clamp technique
e. insulin clamp
eugonadal
e. infertility
eugonadism
eugonadotrophic anovulation
eukaryote
eukaryotic cell
Eulexin
eumelanin
eumenorrheic
e. hirsute woman
eumetabolic
e. state
eunuchism
female e.
hypothalamic e.
eunuchoidal body proportion
eunuchoid body habitus
eunuchoidism
euphoria
Euro-Ficoll solution

NOTES

European
E. Association for the Study of Diabetes
E. Nicotinamide Diabetes Intervention Trial (ENDIT)
E. Organization for Research and Treatment of Cancer (EORTC)
EUS
endoscopic ultrasound
euthyroid
biochemically e.
e. brain glucose transporter
clinically e.
e. diffuse goiter
e. Graves disease
e. hyperthyroxinemia
e. nodular goiter
e. ophthalmopathy
e. sick
e. sick syndrome
e. state
euthyroidism
compensated e.
Euthyrox
eutopic
e. endometrium
euvolemic
e. patient
Evaluation
Acute Physiology and Chronic Health E. (APACHE, APACHE II)
Heart Outcome Prevention E. (HOPE)
E. of Platelet IIb-IIIa Inhibitors for Stenting (EPISTENT)
E. of Platelet IIb-IIIa Inhibitors for Stenting trial
E. of PTCA to Improve Long-Term Outcome by C7E3 GpIIb/IIIa Receptor Blockade (EPILOG)
E. of PTCA to Improve Long-Term Outcome by C7E3 GpIIb/IIIa Receptor Blockade Trial
evening primrose oil
Events
Cholesterol and Recurrent E. (CARE)
Everone Injection
Evista
E-Vitamin
EX
Diabetic Tussin EX
Naldecon Senior EX
Ex
Touro Ex
ExacTech blood glucose meter
examination
dilated fundus e.
funduscopic e.
histomorphometric e.
PPJ cytologic e.
pure pancreatic juice cytologic e.
visual e.
excavatum
Excedrin
E., Extra Strength
E. IB
E. P.M.
Excel
E. GE
E. GE electrochemical glucose monitoring test strip
excess
e. acral growth
adrenal androgen e.
androgen e.
apparent mineralocorticoid e. (AME)
glucocorticoid e.
glucocorticoid-suppressible mineralocorticoid e.
LH-dependent androgen e.
luteinizing hormone-dependent androgen e.
mineralocorticoid e.
parathyroid hormone e.
prolactin e.
sodium e.
syndrome of apparent mineralocorticoid e.
TBG e.
thyroxine-binding globulin e.
unilateral aldosterone e.
vasopressin e.
excessive
e. body odor
e. seborrhea
e. stature
e. sweating
exchange
plasma e.
exchanger
urate-hydroxyl e.
urate-lactate e.
excitability
membrane e.
excitable tissue
excitatory
e. amino acid
e. input
e. transmitter
exclusion chromatography

excretion
aldosterone e.
basal 24-hour UFC e.
basal 24-hour urine free cortisol e.
24-hour urinary aldosterone e.
increased aldosterone e.
renal e.
urinary genistein e.
urinary hydroxyproline e.
urinary pyridinoline cross-link e.
urine phosphorus e.
excretory duct
excurrent duct system
excursion
postprandial glucose e.
exemption
humanitarian device e. (HDE)
exercise-related amenorrhea
exhaustion atrophy
exocrine
e. cell
e. gland
e. pancreas
e. pancreatic dysfunction
e. pancreatic insufficiency (EPI)
e. response
exocytosis
misplaced e.
exodeviation
exogenous
e. glucocorticoid
e. glucocorticoid therapy
e. gonadotropin
e. hypercortisolism
e. hyperinsulinemia
e. thyroid hormone
e. thyrotoxicosis
exon
XL-alpha-s e.
exopeptidase
e. dipeptidyl peptidase I
e. dipeptidyl peptidase II
exophthalmic
e. cachexia
e. goiter
exophthalmometer
Hertel e.
Luedde e.
exophthalmos
idiopathic e.
exostosis, pl. **exostoses**
bony e.
metaphyseal e.
exotropia
expansion
clonal e.
retrobulbar tissue e.
expenditure
resting energy e. (REE)
experimental
e. allergic autoimmune encephalitis (EAE)
e. autoimmune thyroiditis (EAT)
exposure keratitis
expressed sequence tag (EST)
expression
aberrant e.
biallelic e.
calcitonin gene e.
cardiac gene e.
ectopic e.
endothelin receptor e.
enzyme e.
growth factor e.
monoallelic e.
protooncogene e.
ras gene protooncogene e.
receptor e.
surfactant protein gene e.
thyroglobulin e.
thyroid-stimulating hormone receptor e.
TSH receptor e.
extension
alar-like e.
extrathyroidal e.
MacFee e.
suprasellar e.
externa
membrana limitans e.
theca e.
external
e. beam radiation
e. ophthalmoplegia
e. subcutaneous insulin infusion pump
extirpate
extirpation
surgical e.
extorsion
extraadrenal
e. paraganglioma
e. pheochromocytoma

NOTES

extracellular
e. calcification
e. cathepsin action
e. domain
e. fluid (ECF)
e. fluid dehydration
e. fluid osmolarity
e. fluid volume (EFV)
e. iodide pool
e. matrix
e. pH
e. receptor
e. signal-regulated kinase (ERK)
e. signal related kinase
extracellularly regulated kinase (ERK)
extracellular-regulated kinase
extracorporeal
e. ultrafiltration
extract
soy phytoestrogen e. (SPE)
thyroid e.
extraction
testicular sperm e. (TESE)
extradural space
extraembryonic somatic mesoderm
extraglandular lesion
extraglomerular mesangium
extragonadal
e. site
extrahepatic
e. bile duct
e. effect
extrahypophyseal portal vessel
extrahypothalamic
e. nervous system
e. site
extramedullary hematopoiesis (EMH)
extramitochondrial compartment
extraneuronal amine transport system
extraocular muscle dysfunction
extrapancreatic digestive enzyme
extrapituitary
e. prolactin
extrasellar
extraskeletal calcification
extrasplanchnic area
extra strength (ES)
extrathyroidal
e. extension
e. immunological process
e. manifestation of Graves disease
e. primary
extrathyroid autoantigen
extravascular
extravillus
extreme insulin resistance
extrusion
granule e.
supradiaphragmatic e.
exuberant
e. neutrophilic infiltrate
e. thrombosis
eye
Orphan Annie e.
Ezide

F
cortisol
F body
F cell
hepatitis F
$F_{2\alpha}$
prostaglandin $F_{2\alpha}$ ($PGF_{2\alpha}$)
$F_{1\alpha}$
prostaglandin $F_{1\alpha}$
FA
Natabec FA
Pramet FA
Pramilet FA
FA-1
fertilization antigen-1
Fab
fragment antigen binding
FABP
fatty acid-binding protein
FABP2
fatty acid-binding protein 2
$FABP_{pm}$
plasma membrane fatty acid binding protein
Fabry disease
face
en f.
moon f.
myxedematous f.
facial
f. feature enlargement
f. hirsutism
f. plethora
facies
adenoid f.
bird-like f.
dysmorphic f.
elfin f.
moon f.
plethoric f.
triangular f.
facilitative glucose transporter
factitia
thyrotoxicosis f.
factitial hypoglycemia
factitious
f. hyperthyroidism
f. hypoglycemia
factor
abiotic environmental f.
acidic fibroblast growth f. (aFGF)
activated Hageman f.
activating f.
amplification f.
androgen-induced growth f. (AIGF)
atrial natriuretic f. (ANF)
autocrine motility f. (AMF)
azoospermia f. (AZF)
basic fibroblast growth f. (bFGF)
basic helix-loop-helix transcription f.
B-cell growth f. (BCGF)
beta-nerve growth f.
bHLH transcription f.
bone-derived growth f. (BDGF)
brain-derived neurotropic f. (BDNF)
calcium homeostatic f.
C/EBP transcription f.
chemotactic f.
chicken ovalbumin upstream promoter-transcription factor (COUP-TF)
ciliary neurotrophic f. (CNTF)
cis-acting f.
clotting f. V
colony-stimulating f.
corticotropin-releasing f. (CRF)
coupling f.
decapacitation f.
dialyzable f.
early pregnancy f. (EPF)
EGF-like growth f.
endothelial cell-stimulating angiogenesis f. (ESAF)
endothelium-derived relaxing f. (EDRF)
epidermal growth f. (EGF)
erythroid differentiation f. (EDF)
fibroblast growth f. (FGF)
fibroblastic growth f. (FGF)
genetically predisposing f.
GH-releasing f. (GRF)
glia-activating f. (GAF)
glial cell line-derived neurotrophic f. (GDNF)
glia maturation f. (GMF)
glycosylation-inhibiting f. (GIF)
G&M colony-stimulating f. (GM-CSF)
granulocyte colony-stimulating f. (G-CSF)
granulocyte-macrophage colony-stimulating f. (GM-CSF)
growth differentiation f. (GDF)
growth hormone-releasing f. (GRF)
Hageman f.
hematopoietic cell growth f.
heparin-binding epidermal growth f.
heparin-bound growth f.
hepatocyte growth f. (HGF)
hepatocyte nuclear f. (HNF)
hepatocyte nuclear f.-3 (HNF3)

F

factor *(continued)*
hepatocyte nuclear f.-4 (HNF4)
f. Hesx1
HNF3 transcription f.
HNF4 transcription f.
homeodomain f.
humoral f.
hypophysiotropic f.
hypothalamic-releasing f.
f. II mutation
inhibitory f.
insulin gene transcription f.
insulin growth f.
insulinlike growth f. (IGF)
interleukin growth f. I (IGF-I)
invasion suppressive f.
f. IX
f. IX deficiency
juxtacrine f.
Kaposi sarcoma human growth f. (hFGF)
keratinocyte growth f. (KGF)
leukemia-inhibiting f. (LIF)
leukemia inhibitory f. (LIF)
luteinization-inhibiting f.
macrophage-activating f.
macrophage colony-stimulating f. (M-CSF)
macrophage migration-inhibiting f.
macrophage migration inhibitory f.
melanocyte-stimulating f. (MRF)
migration inhibitory f. (MIF)
myeloid leukemia inhibitory f.
nerve growth f. (NGF)
neurotrophic f.
NF-1 transcription f.
nongenomic f.
nonsuppressible insulinlike activity f.
nuclear transcription f.
octamer-binding transcription f.
Oct-1 transcription f.
oocyte maturation-inhibiting f.
opioid growth f. (OGF)
osteoclast differentiation f. (ODF)
osteoclastogenesis inhibitory f. (OCIF)
osteoprotegerin f. (OPGF)
ovarian growth f. (OGF)
paracrine f.
PAX8 f.
pelvic infertility f.
peptide growth f.
permissive f.
platelet-activating f. (PAF)
platelet-derived growth f. (PDGF)
POU-homeodomain transcription f.
predisposing f.
prolactin-inhibiting f. (PIF)
prolactin inhibitory f.
prolactin-releasing f. (PRF)
prophet of Pit-1 transcription f.
PROP-1 transcription f.
Rathke pouch homeobox transcription f. (Rpx)
recombinant human insulinlike growth f. (rhIGF)
recombinant insulinlike growth f. I
renal erythropoietic f.
rheumatoid f.
satiety f.
schwannoma-derived growth f.
serum thymic f.
signal transducer and activator of transcription-4 transcription f.
signal transducer and activator of transcription-5 transcription f.
somatotropin release f. (SRF)
somatotropin release-inhibiting f. (SRIF)
SP-1 transcription f.
SRY transcription f.
Stat4 transcription f.
Stat5 transcription f.
stem cell f. (SCF)
sulfation f.
T-cell growth f. (TCGF)
testis-determining f. (TDF)
thyroid transcription f. (TTF)
thyroid transcription f. 1 (TTF-1)
thyroid transcription f. 2 (TTF-2)
thyrotroph embryonic f. (TEF)
thyrotropin release f. (TRF)
tissue necrosis f. (TNF)
trans-acting f.
transactivation f. (TAF)
transcriptional intermediary f. 2 (TIF2)
transforming growth f. (TGF)
trophic f.
T-suppressor f. (TsF)
tumor necrosis f. (TNF)
tumor necrosis factor receptor-associated f. (TRAF)
vaccinia virus growth f.
vascular endothelial growth f. (VEGF)
vascular permeability f. (VPF)
f. V deficiency Leiden mutation
f. VIII
f. VIII deficiency
f. VIII-related antigen
f. VIII ristocetin cofactor antigen
vitamin D-binding protein macrophage-activating f.
f. V Leiden gene
von Willebrand f. (vWF)

Wilms tumor 1 transcription f.
WTI transcription f.
f. XI
f. XIIa

factor-1
adipocyte determination and differentiation f. (ADD1)
antifertility f. (AF-1)
colony-stimulating f.
hepatocyte transcription f.
human stomach cancer-transforming f. (hst-1)
insulinlike growth f. (IGF1)
insulin promoter f. (IPF-1)
pituitary-specific transcription f. (Pit-1)
preadipocyte f. (Pref-1)
serum insulinlike growth f.
steroidogenic f. (SF-1)

factor-2
heparin-binding growth f. (HBGF-2)
human stomach cancer-transforming f. (hst-2)
insulinlike growth f. (IGF2)

factor-9
growth differentiation f. (GDF-9)

factor-4a
hepatocyte nuclear f. (HNF-4a)

factor-alpha
tumor necrosis f. (TNF-alpha)

factor-1-alpha
hypoxia-inducible f. (HIF-1alpha)

factor-κB
nuclear f. (NF-kappa-B)

factor-beta
tumor necrosis f.-b. (TNF-beta)

factor-I
insulinlike growth f.-I (IGF-I)

factor-II
insulinlike growth f.-II

factor-kB
nuclear f.-k.

factor XI

Factrel

facultative
f. heterochromatin
f. thermogenesis

FAD
familial autoimmunity in diabetes

fadrozole

***fa* gene**

failure
adult Leydig cell f.
autoimmune polyglandular f.
cartilage calcification f.
chronic renal f. (CRF)
embryologic development end-organ ovarian f.
glucocorticoid-induced growth f.
gonadal f.
hepatic f.
hypoglycemia-associated autonomic f.
liver f.
mild thyroid f.
ovarian f.
polyglandular endocrine f.
premature gonadal f.
premature ovarian f.
primary adrenal f.
primary gonadal f.
regulatory f.
renal f.
secondary gonadal f.
f. to thrive (FTT)
type II multiple endocrine glandular f.

falciform
f. fold
f. ligament

Falck-Hillarp histofluorescence method

falling height velocity

fallopian tube

Fallot
tetralogy of F.

familial
f. adenomatous polyposis
f. adrenoleukodystrophy
f. amyloidotic polyneuropathy
f. amyloid polyneuropathy (FAP)
f. atypical multiple mole-melanoma (FAMMM)
f. atypical multiple mole-melanoma syndrome
f. autoimmunity in diabetes (FAD)
f. C-cell hyperplasia
f. central diabetes insipidus
f. cerebral ataxia
f. colorectal cancer
f. combined hyperlipidemia (FCH)
f. defective apolipoprotein B100
f. Down syndrome
f. dysalbuminemia

NOTES

familial *(continued)*
f. dysalbuminemic hyperthyroxinemia (FDH)
f. dysalbuminemic hypertriiodothyroninemia
f. dysautonomia
f. dysbetalipoproteinemia
f. expansile osteolysis (FEO)
f. gastric cancer
f. glucocorticoid deficiency (FGD)
f. glucocorticoid resistance
f. hyperaldosteronism
f. hypercholesterolemia (FH)
f. hyperinsulinism
f. hyperkalemia
f. hyperphosphatasemia
f. hypertriglyceridemia
f. hypoalphalipoproteinemia
f. hypocalciuric hypercalcemia (FHH)
f. hypoparathyroidism
f. hypophosphatemic rickets
f. hypospadias
f. isolated primary hyperparathyroidism (FIHP, FIPH)
f. lipid disorder
f. male-limited gonadotrophin-independent sexual precocity
f. male precocious puberty
f. Mediterranean fever
f. medullary thyroid cancer (FMTC)
f. medullary thyroid carcinoma (FMTC)
f. multiple endocrine neoplasia
f. multiple endocrine neoplasia type 1
f. nephrogenic diabetes insipidus
f. nonautoimmune hyperthyroidism
f. oculoleptomeningea amyloidosis
f. ovarian cancer
f. periodic paralysis
f. pheochromocytoma
f. testitoxicosis
f. X-linked hypophosphatemic rickets

family
G_q f.
helix-loop-helix f.
leucine zipper gene f.
T-box gene f.

FAMMM
familial atypical multiple mole-melanoma
FAMMM syndrome

famotidine

Fanconi
F. anemia
F. syndrome

Fanconi-type idiopathic hypercalcemia

FAP
familial amyloid polyneuropathy

Faraday constant

Farber disease

Farré
line of F.

FAS
fatty acid synthetase
fetal alcohol syndrome

Fas
F. ligand (Fas-L)
F. receptor

fascia
cremasteric f.
pectoralis f.
prethyroidal f.
superficial f.

fasciculata
adrenal zona f.
f. reticularis
zona f.

fasciculation

fasciculus
mammillary f.
mammillotegmental f.
medial longitudinal f.

fasciitis
necrotizing f.
nodular f.

fascioscapulohumeral muscular dystrophy

FASE
fast asymmetric spin echo
FASE sequence

Fas-L
Fas ligand

fast
f. asymmetric spin echo (FASE)
f. asymmetric spin echo sequence
protein-sparing modified f.
f. spin-echo technique
f.-twitch muscle fiber

fast-acting insulin

Fastin

fasting
f. blood glucose (FBG)
f. growth hormone
f. hyperglycemia
f. hypoglycemia
f. hypophosphatemia
f. plasma glucose (FPG)

FastTake blood glucose monitoring system

FAT
fatty acid translocase

fat
brown f.
f. catabolism

f. embolization
f. maldigestion/malabsorption
f. mass (FM)
f. necrosis
orbital f.
perinephric f.
perithymic f.
sparse body f.
fat-free mass (FFM)
fatigue
quadriceps f.
FATP
fatty acid transport protein
fatty
f. acid
f. acid-binding protein (FABP)
f. acid-binding protein 2 (FABP2)
f. acid oxidation
f. acid synthase
f. acid synthetase (FAS)
f. acid translocase (FAT)
f. acid transport protein (FATP)
f. acylcarnitine
f. liver
FBG
fasting blood glucose
FBP
fructose-bisphosphatase
FCH
familial combined hyperlipidemia
FCPD
fibrocalculous pancreatic diabetes
FDG
fluorodeoxyglucose
FDG-F-18
^{18}F-labeled fluorodeoxyglucose
FDG-PET
^{18}F-fluorodeoxyglucose positron emission tomography
FDG-PET study
FDH
familial dysalbuminemic hyperthyroxinemia
FE
Fe
iron
Estrostep Fe
Slow Fe
feature
acromegalic f.
coarsened facial f.
histomorphic f.
tinctorial f.
ultrastructural f.
fecal chymotrypsin test
fecundability
fecundity
Federation
International Diabetes F.
feedback
compensatory f.
f. control
f. inhibition
long-loop f.
f. loop
monofollicular f.
monoovarial f.
negative f.
positive f.
short-loop f.
tubuloglomerular f. (TGF)
ultrashort-loop f.
feeding artery
feet
insensate f.
Feldene
Felig insulin pump
female
f. climax
f. eunuchism
f. infertility
f. orgasm
f. phenotype
f. pseudohermaphrodite
f. pseudohermaphroditism
f. sperm
Femara
FemHRT
feminization
complete testicular f.
incomplete testicular f.
testicular f.
feminizing
f. adrenal syndrome
f. testis
Femiron
Femogen
femora
femoral neck bone density
FemPatch
FemSeven
FemSoy
Fenesin
fenestra

NOTES

fenestrated
f. capillary endothelium
fenestration
fenofibrate
fenoprofen
fentanyl
f. citrate
droperidol and f.
Fentanyl Oralet
fenugreek
FEO
familial expansile osteolysis
Feosol
Feostat
Ferancee
Feratab
Fergon
Ferguson reflex
Fer-In-Sol drops
Fer-Iron
Fero-Grad 500
Fero-Gradumet
Ferospace
Ferralet
Ferralyn Lanacaps
Ferra-TD
ferredoxin
renal f.
ferric chloride test
Ferriman-Gallwey score
Ferriman scale of hirsutism
ferritin
ferromagnetic
Ferro-Sequels
ferrous
f. fumarate
f. gluconate
f. salt and ascorbic acid
f. sulfate
f. sulfate, ascorbic acid, and vitamin B-complex
f. sulfate, ascorbic acid, vitamin B complex, and folic acid
fertile
f. eunuch syndrome
f. eunuch variant
fertilization
f. antigen-1 (FA-1)
in vitro f. (IVF)
Fertinex
Feryter system endocrine cell
fetal
f. adenoma
f. adrenal cortisol
f. alcohol syndrome (FAS)
f. allograft
f. catecholamine
f. endocrine rhythm
f. hormone rhythm
f. hyperthyroidism
f. hypothyroidism
f. hypothyroxinemia
f. hypoxemia
f. macrosomia
f. mineral homeostasis
f. pancreas transplant
f. plasma cortisol
f. steroid rhythm
f. T_4
f. zone
fetal-hypothalamic-pituitary-adrenal axis
fetalis
erythroblastosis f.
fetal/neonatal
f. adrenal crisis
f. rhythm
fetectomy
fetomaternal circulation
fetoplacental
f. blood flow
f. unit
fever
dengue f.
enteric f.
epidemic hemorrhagic f.
familial Mediterranean f.
rheumatic f.
Feverall
FFA
free fatty acid
^{18}F-fluorodeoxyglucose
^{18}F-f. positron emission tomography (FDG-PET)
^{18}F-f. positron emission tomography study
FFM
fat-free mass
FGD
familial glucocorticoid deficiency
FGF
fibroblast growth factor
fibroblastic growth factor
FGFR
fibroblast growth factor receptor
FH
familial hypercholesterolemia
FHA
functional hypothalamic amenorrhea
FHH
familial hypocalciuric hypercalcemia
FHIT
fragile histidine triad
FHIT gene
fiber
angiotensinergic f.
atriopeptidergic f.

f. atrophy
collagen f.
crossing nasal retinal f.
fast-twitch muscle f.
GABAergic f.
gamma-aminobutyric acidergic f.
glutamatergic f.
f. hypertrophy
f. pebble
postganglionic sympathetic f.
preganglionic sympathetic nerve f.
reciprocal peptidergic f.
secretomotor f.
slow-twitch oxidative f.
soluble f.
temporal f.
terminal nerve f.
type 1 f.
type 2 f.
type II muscle f.
unmyelinated nerve f.
urocortin f.
vasopressinergic f.
viscous dietary f.

fiberoptic headlight

fibric
f. acid
f. acid derivative

fibril
actin f.
amyloid f.
birefringent collagen f.
collagen f.
hydrolyzed lithostathine f.

fibrillar collagen strip

fibrillary gliosis

fibrillation
ventricular f.

fibrin glue

fibrinogen

fibrinolysin

fibrinolysis
increased f.

fibrinolytic activity

fibroadenoma
benign prostatic f.
mammary f.

fibroadenomatous hyperplasia of breast

fibroblast
f. growth factor (FGF)
f. growth factor receptor (FGFR)
orbital f.
perimysial f.
SV40-transformed human f.

fibroblastic
f. growth factor (FGF)
f. phenotype

fibrocalculous
f. pancreatic diabetes (FCPD)
f. pancreatopathy

fibrocystic breast disease

fibrodysplasia ossificans progressiva (FOP)

fibrogenesis
f. imperfecta
f. imperfecta ossium

fibroglandular tissue

fibrolipoma

fibromatosis

fibromyalgia
F. Impact Questionnaire (FIQ)

fibromyositis

fibronectin
f. gene
f. peptide isoform
serum f.

fibroneuroma

fibroplasia

fibrosa
osteitis f.

fibrosarcoma

fibrosclerosis

fibrosis
cardiac f.
cystic f.
endosteal f.
hypocellular marrow without f.
interlobular f.
intralobular f.

fibrous
f. atrophy
f. dysplasia
f. dysplasia of bone

FIC
growth factor-inducible chemokine

field
Goldmann visual f.
Humphrey visual f.

FIHP
familial isolated primary hyperparathyroidism

filament
actin f.

filarial infection

F

NOTES

Filmtabs
Cefol F.
Surbex-T F.
Surbex With C F.
fimbria
ovarian f.
finasteride
fine-needle
f.-n. aspiration (FNA)
f.-n. aspiration biopsy (FNAB)
fine needle
finger
steroid hormone receptor zinc f.
zinc f.
finger-stick blood sugar
Finochietto retractor
Fiorinal With Codeine
FIPH
familial isolated primary hyperparathyroidism
FIQ
Fibromyalgia Impact Questionnaire
fire
St. Anthony f.
firefly luciferase
firm goiter
first-generation agent
first messenger
first-passage phenomenon
first-phase
f.-p. insulin release
f.-p. insulin response (FPIR)
first-year growth velocity response
Fischer
F. rat thyroid line-5 (FRTL-5)
F. rat thyroid line-5 cell
FISH
fluorescence in situ hybridization
FISH method
fissure
choroidal f.
lid f.
f. of Santorini
widened palpebral f.
fistula
biliary f.
cerebrospinal fluid f.
intestinal f.
Fitzgerald trait
FK506
FK-binding
F.-b. protein (FKBP)
F.-b. protein 12 (FKBP12)
FKBP
FK-binding protein
FKBP-rapamycin-associated protein (FRAP)
FKBP12
FK-binding protein 12
^{18}F-labeled fluorodeoxyglucose (FDG-F-18)
flaccid penile length
flagellar movement
flagellum
Flagyl Oral
flame
osteolytic f.
f. photometry
FLAP
5-lipoxygenase activating protein
flap
Karydakis f.
right frontal osteoplastic f.
flare
tumor f.
flashes
hot f.
flat-field collimator
flat spring
flattened lumbar spine
flattening
posterior skull f.
Flatulex
Flaujeac trait
flavone
flavonoid
flavoprotein
electron transport f. (ETF)
f. NADPH-cytochrome P450 reductase
f. nicotinamide adenine dinucleotide phosphate-cytochrome P450 reductase
Flavorcee
flavum
ligamentum f.
flavus
Aspergillus f.
Fleet Phospho-Soda
FlexiGard
floating beta band
Florical
Florida Sexual Questionnaire
Florinef
F. Acetate
flour
chupatti f.
flow
anterograde f.
cerebral blood f. (CBF)
Cor F.
coronary blood flow
coronary blood f. (Cor Flow, Cor Flow)
f. cytometric analysis

fetoplacental blood f.
hepatofugal f.
hepatopetal f.
placental blood f.
renal plasma f. (RPF)
uteroplacental blood f.

flowmetry
laser Doppler f.

flow-volume loop spirometry
floxuridine
fluasterone
fluconazole
flucytosine
fludarabine
fludrocortisone
f. replacement therapy

flufenemic acid
fluid
amniotic f.
bloody f.
bone f.
cerebrospinal f. (CSF)
extracellular f. (ECF)
follicular f.
f. intake
interstitial f. (ISF)
intracellular f. (ICF)
nonpurulent f.
pancreatitis-associated ascites f. (PAAF)
perilymph f.
peritoneal f. (PF)
preseminal f.
f. shear stress
subarachnoid f.
testicular f.
tubule f.
turbid f.
xanthochromic f.

flunisolide
flunitrazepam
fluochrome
fluocinolone
0.2% f. acetonide cream

fluorescein
fluorescein-labeled
f.-l. pea agglutinin
f.-l. peanut agglutinin

fluorescence
f. imaging
f. microlymphography
f. polarization
f. quencing spectroscopy
f. in situ hybridization (FISH)

fluorescent
f. iodide
f. in situ hybridization method

fluoride
bioavailable f.
enteric-coated sodium f.
serum f.
skeletal f.
sodium f.
sustained-release sodium f. (SR-NaF)

fluorine
fluorochrome
fluorodeoxyglucose (FDG)
^{18}F-labeled f. (FDG-F-18)
f. uptake

fluoroscopic C-arm
fluorosis
endemic f.

fluorotic change
fluorouracil
5-fluorouracil (5-FU)
fluoxetine
f. hydrochloride

fluoxymesterone
fluphenazine
flurbiprofen
flush
vasomotor f.

flushing
cutaneous f.

flutamide
fluvastatin
fluvoxamine
flux
calcium f.
electrolyte f.
mineral f.
transmucosal calcium f.

fly
tsetse f.

FM
fat mass

FMTC
familial medullary thyroid cancer
familial medullary thyroid carcinoma

FNA
fine-needle aspiration
FNA biopsy

NOTES

F

FNAB
fine-needle aspiration biopsy
foam
f. cell
f. cell formation
foamy cell
focal
f. dermal hypoplasia
f. epithelial hyperplasia
f. glomerulitis
f. segmental glomerulosclerosis (FSGS)
f. tumor necrosis
foci
anechoic f.
focusing
isoelectric f.
fodrin
foenum-graecum
Trigonella f.-g.
fold
falciform f.
urogenital f.
foliaceus
toxic pemphigus f.
folic acid
follicle
androgenic f.
antral f.
dominant f.
graafian f.
hair f.
lymphoid f.
mature f.
ovarian f.
ovulatory f.
preantral f.
preovulatory f.
primary f.
primordial f.
secondary f.
tertiary f.
thyroid f.
vesicular f.
follicle-stimulating
f.-s. hormone (FSH)
f.-s. hormone-beta gene
f.-s. hormone deficiency
f.-s. hormone receptor
f.-s. hormone-releasing hormone (FSH-RH)
follicular
f. adenoma
f. arrest
f. atresia
f. cell
f. cyst
f. fluid
f. hyperthecosis
f. lumen
f. mucinosis
f. neoplasm
f. phase
f. stage
f. stimulating hormone (FSH)
f. thyroid cancer
f. thyroid carcinoma
folliculi
liquor f.
theca f.
folliculogenesis
folliculostatin
folliculostellate cell
follistatin
Follistim
follitropin (FSH)
f. alpha
f. beta
Follutein
Folvite
Fontana-Masson procedure
fontanelle
open posterior f.
food
thermic effect of f.
food-dependent Cushing syndrome
food-related hypercortisolism
FOP
fibrodysplasia ossificans progressiva
foramen, pl. **foramina**
f. caecum linguae
f. cecum
foramina of Magendie and Luschka
f. of Monro
f. ovale
f. rotundum
f. spinosum
force
Starling f.
forceps
Cushing f.
transsphenoidal bipolar f.
forearm and lumbar spine bone mineral content
forebrain
f. basal encephalocele
foregut
form
alimentary f.
dimeric f.
gadolinium in chelated f. (Gd-EDTA)
monostotic f.
non-histocompatibility locus antigen-associated f.
non-HLA-associated f.

nonhuman leukocyte antigen associated f.
polyostotic f.
formation
brainstem reticular f.
endochondral bone f.
foam cell f.
hippocampal f.
marrow cavity f.
osteoblast-mediated bone f.
pseudopapillary f.
thrombus f.
formation-stimulating agent
formation-stimulation agent
formed visual hallucination
formes fruste
formestane
formication
forming-unit
formononetin
formula
Diabetic Tussin Children's F.
isoosmolar semielemental f.
fornix, pl. **fornices**
vaginal f.
forskolin
adenylyl cyclase agonist f.
Forte
Norgesic F.
Rexigen F.
Robinul F.
Vicon F.
fortuitum
Mycobacterium f.
Fosamax
foscarnet
f. therapy
***FOS* gene**
fossa
interpeduncular f.
pituitary f.
superior orbital f.
Foundation
Insulin-Free World F.
Juvenile Diabetes F. (JDF)
National Osteoporosis F. (NOF)
Osteogenesis Imperfecta F.
four-compartment model
Fournier gangrene
FPG
fasting plasma glucose
FPIR
first-phase insulin response
FQ
nociceptin/orphanin FQ (N/OFQ)
fraction
oxytocic f.
S-phase f.
very low density lipoprotein f.
VLDL f.
fractional shortening
fractionated
f. linear accelerator-based irradiation
f. radiation therapy
f. urinary catecholamine
fracture
stress f.
fragile
f. histidine triad (FHIT)
f. X-E (FRAXE)
f. X-E syndrome
f. X syndrome
fragilis
Bacteroides f.
fragment
f. antigen binding (Fab)
Klenow f.
luteinizing hormone beta core f.
major proglucagon f. (MPF)
fragmentation
osseous f.
frame
Leksell model G stereotactic f.
open reading f. (ORF)
relocatable stereotactic f.
frank
f. basilar impression
f. necrosis
FRAP
FKBP-rapamycin-associated protein
Frasier syndrome
Frataxin gene
FRAXE
fragile X-E
FRAXE syndrome
free
f. Ca^{2+}
f. cortisol
f. hormone
f. levothyroxine
f. Mg^{2+}
f. radical
f. T_3

NOTES

F

free *(continued)*
f. T_4
f. testosterone
f. testosterone level
f. thyroxine (FT_4)
f. thyroxine index (FTI, FT4I, FT_4I, FT4i)
f. T_4 index (FT_4I)
f. triiodothyronine (FT_3)
f. water clearance
f. water deficit
Freedom
Accu-Chek II F.
free fatty acid (FFA)
Freeman-Sheldon syndrome
free-radical
f.-r. scavenger
Freer elevator
free-running melatonin cycle
freeze-dried allograft
#7 French suction cannula
frenulum
f. clitoridis
frequency
gonadotropin-releasing hormone pulse f.
pulse f.
frequent blood sampling
Frey operation
friable
Friedewald calculation
Friedreich ataxia
frog skin sauvagine
Fröhlich syndrome
frondosum
chorion f.
front
mineralization f.
frontal
f. bossing
f. craniotomy
f. neocortex
frontoethmoidal encephalocele
frontooccipital prominence
frontotemporal
f. balding
f. headache
FRTL-5
Fischer rat thyroid line-5
FRTL-5 cell
fructosamine
f. test
fructose
f. intolerance
fructose-bisphosphatase (FBP)
fructose-2,6-bisphosphate
fructose-6-phosphate
fruit
Caribbean f.
citrus f.
fruste
formes f.
F-scan
FSGS
focal segmental glomerulosclerosis
FSH
follicle-stimulating hormone
follicular stimulating hormone
follitropin
FSH-beta gene
FSH deficiency
FSH receptor
urinary FSH (uFSH)
FSH-RH
follicle-stimulating hormone-releasing hormone
FT_3
free triiodothyronine
FT_4
free thyroxine
FTI
free thyroxine index
FT4I
free thyroxine index
FT_4I
free thyroxine index
free T_4 index
FT4i
free thyroxine index
FTT
failure to thrive
5-FU
5-fluorouracil
fuchsin
aldehyde f.
fucose
fucosidosis
fucosylation
fuel
f. homeostasis
f. metabolism
f. reservoir
Fujiwara trait
fullness
supraclavicular f.
full pulse
fulminant
f. hyperthermia
f. Letterer-Siwe disease
fumarate
ferrous f.
fumarylacetoacetate
f. hydrolase type Ia
Fumasorb
Fumerin

fumigatus
Aspergillus f.
function
anterior pituitary f.
B-cell f.
bone marrow f.
gastric reservoir f.
HPA f.
hypophysiotropic hormonal f.
hypothalamic-pituitary-adrenal f.
intracellular f.
iodide trapping f.
juxtaglomerular f.
osteoclastic f.
phosphorylated rhodopsin f.
pituitary f.
pituitary-adrenal f.
pituitary-gonadal f.
pituitary hormone f.
pituitary-thyroid f.
pleiotropic f.
renal f.
steroidogenic enzyme f.
target gland f.
thyroid f.
transactivation f. 1
transactivation f. 2
functional
f. hypoglycemia
f. hypothalamic amenorrhea (FHA)
f. hypothalamic hypogonadism
f. impotence
f. ovarian hyperandrogenism
f. sensitivity
functionale
stratum f.
functioning nodule
funduscopic examination
fungal septicemia
fungiform papilla
fungus, pl. **fungi**
fura-2 fluorescent Ca^{2+} **chelator**
furin
f. enzyme
furosemide
furunculosis
fused epiphysis
fusiform dilatation
fusion
delayed epiphyseal f.
epiphyseal f.
f. gene
futile cycle
fuzzy logic model
Fyn protein

NOTES

F

γ (*var. of* gamma)
G
G band
G cell
immunoglobulin G (IgG)
G inhibiting protein (G_i)
G&M colony-stimulating factor (GM-CSF)
G protein
G protein activation
G protein-coupled receptor (GPCR)
G protein dysfunction
protein kinase G (PKG)
G protein-linked receptor
G spot
G_2
cyclic endoperoxide prostaglandin G_2
prostaglandin G_2 (PGG_2)
G_i
G inhibiting protein
G_s
G-stimulating protein
Ga-67
gallium citrate
GAA
glutamic acid codon
GABA
gamma-aminobutyric acid
GABA/BZD
gamma-aminobutyric acid/benzodiazepine
GABA/BZD system
GABAergic
G. fiber
G. projection
gabapentin
gabexate
^{67}Ga-citrate
GAD
glutamic acid decarboxylase
gadolinium
g. in chelated form (Gd-EDTA)
gadolinium-chelated compound
gadolinium-diethylenetriaminepentaacetic acid contrast medium
gadolinium-enhanced MRI
GAF
glia-activating factor
GAG
glycosaminoglycan
Gagel disease
gain
weight g.
gain-of-function
g.-o.-f. alteration
g.-o.-f. mutation
gait
g. ataxia
waddling g.
galactitol
galactocele
galactopoiesis
galactorrhea
idiopathic g.
galactorrhea-amenorrhea
g.-a. syndrome
galactosamine
galactose
g. intolerance
galactose-l-phosphate uridyltransferase deficiency
galactosemia
galactosialidosis
α-galactosidase deficiency
galactosyltransferase
4-g. (GalTase)
g. enzyme
4-g. isoenzyme II
galanin
Galen loop
gallium
g. citrate (Ga-67)
g. nitrate
G_s-alpha-coupled receptor
GALT
gut-associated lymphoid tissue
GalTase
4-galactosyltransferase
GalTase isoenzyme II
gamete
g. intrafallopian transfer (GIFT)
gametogenesis
Gamma
G. Knife
G. Knife beam radiotherapy
gamma, γ
g. camera
g. glutaryl transferase
neuropeptide g.
g. unit
gamma-aminobutyric
g.-a. acid (GABA)
g.-a. acid/benzodiazepine (GABA/BZD)
g.-a. acid/benzodiazepine system
g.-a. acidergic fiber
g.-a. acidergic projection
g.-a. acid transaminase inhibitor

gamma-carboxyglutamic
g.-c. acid (GLA, Gla)
g.-c. acid protein
gamma-carboxylated glutamic acid
gamma-carboxylation
gamma-emitter
gamma-glutamylcysteine
gamma-glutamyltranspeptidase
gamma-hydroxybutyrate (GHB)
gamma-linolenic acid (GLA)
gamma-melanocyte-stimulating hormone (gamma-MSH)
gamma-MSH
gamma-melanocyte-stimulating hormone
Gammaplan software
gamma-preprotachykinin A
ganciclovir
ganglia
basal g.
sympathetic g.
gangliocytoma
adenohypophysial g.
intrasellar g.
gangliocytoma-pituitary adenoma
ganglioglioma
ganglioneuroblastoma
ganglioneuroma
ganglionic synapse
ganglioside
gangliosidosis
GM1 g.
gangrene
acute streptococcal g.
Fournier g.
hospital g.
major g.
gangrenosis
ecthyma g.
gantry tilt
GAP
GnRH-associated peptide
GTPase-activating protein
guanosine triphosphate-activating protein
gap
anion g.
g. junction
osmolar g.
Gardnerella vaginalis
Gardner syndrome
gargoylism
garment
gradient pressure g.
GAS
gene-activating sequence
gas
g. chromatography
g. chromatography of plasma
g. dysbetalipoproteinemia
Gas-Ban DS
gas-containing abscess
gastric
g. achlorhydria
g. acid secretion
g. atony
g. banding
g. bypass
g. carcinoid variant syndrome
g. decompression
g. emptying
g. epithelioid leiomyosarcoma
g. impedance measurement
g. inhibitory peptide (GIP)
g. inhibitory polypeptide (GIP)
g. myoelectric abnormality
g. prokinetic agent
g. resection
g. reservoir function
gastrin
g. analog
g. receptor
gastrinoma
g. triangle
gastrin-releasing peptide (GRP)
gastritis
atrophic g.
Gastrocrom
gastroduodenal artery
gastrohepatic ligament
gastrointestinal (GI)
g. autonomic neuropathy
g. calcium absorption
g. effect
g. hamartoma
g. hormone
g. mucormycosis
g. polyposis
g. signal
gastroparesis
diabetic g.
gastroplasty
vertical banded g.
vertical ring g.
gastroprokinetic
Gastrosed
gate
biochemical g.
gating
circadian g.
Gaucher disease
Gaur method
Gaviscon-2 Tablet
Gaviscon Tablet
gaze
impaired medial g.
GC300
GluControl G.

Gc
  group-specific component
GCRH
  glucose counterregulatory hormone
G-CSF
  granulocyte colony-stimulating factor
Gd-EDTA
  gadolinium in chelated form
GDF
  growth differentiation factor
GDF-9
  growth differentiation factor-9
GDM
  gestational diabetes mellitus
GDNF
  glial cell line-derived neurotrophic factor
GDP
  guanosine 5′ diphosphate
GE
  Excel GE
ge
  Novolin g.
Gee
  Gee G.
Geiger counter
gel
  aluminum g.
  clonidine g.
  Crinone bioadhesive progesterone g.
  DHT g.
  dihydrotestosterone g.
  g. electrophoresis
  g. filtration chromatography
  H.P. Acthar G.
  Regranex g.
  transdermal 1% hydroalcoholic g.
gelastic seizure
Gelfilm
Gelfoam
  G. sponge
Gelpirin
gelsolin
gemcitabine
gemfibrozil
Genahist Oral
Genapap
Genatuss
Gencalc 600
gender assignment
gender identity
gene
  AIRE g.
  AKR g.
  aldo-keto reductase g.
  androgen receptor g.
  antibiotic resistance g.
  apolipoprotein B g.
  aromatase g.
  ataxia telangiectasia mutated g.
  ATM g.
  autoimmune regulator g.
  beta-thyroid-stimulating hormone g.
  beta-TSH g.
  BRCA g.
  BRCA1 g.
  BRCA2 g.
  breast cancer g.
  Bruton tyrosine kinase g.
  BTK g.
  CA II g.
  calcitonin g.
  carbonic anhydrase II g.
  catecholamine receptor g.
  cathepsin K g.
  cationic trypsinogen g.
  c-erbA-beta g.
  c-erbA-beta thyroid hormone receptor g.
  c-*fos* g.
  CFTR g.
  cJun g.
  Clock g.
  collagen g.
  cyclin D g.
  CYP19 g.
  CYP1A1 g.
  CYP11A g.
  cystic fibrosis transmembrane regulator g.
  cytokine g.
  DAX-1 g.
  db g.
  g. deletion
  diastrophic dystrophia g.
  dosage-sensitive sex reversal g.
  DPC4 g.
  DSS g.
  DTD g.
  endocrine g.
  fa g.
  factor V Leiden g.
  FHIT g.
  fibronectin g.
  follicle-stimulating hormone-beta g.

NOTES

gene *(continued)*
FOS g.
Frataxin g.
FSH-beta g.
fusion g.
GH-1 g.
GH-2 g.
GH-releasing hormone receptor g.
GHRH-R g.
glucokinase g.
GNAS g.
GNAS1 g.
gonadotropin g.
growth hormone-1 g.
growth hormone-2 g.
H19 g.
hemochromatosis g.
hexokinase B g.
hexokinase II g.
histocompatibility complex g.
hKGK1 g.
housekeeping g.
Hoxa3 homeobox g.
human growth hormone g.
human kidney glandular kallikrein-1 g. (hKGK1)
human proCHR g.
human prokaryotic chromosome g.
human X chromosome, g. 1
21-hydroxylase g.
Ig g.
IGF2 g.
IGF-II g.
IGF-IIR g.
immunoglobulin G g.
immunoglobulin V g.
insulin g.
insulinlike growth factor-II g.
insulinlike growth factor-II receptor g.
insulin receptor g.
integration g. 2 (int2)
KAL g.
Kallmann syndrome interval g. 1 (KALIG-1)
KCNJ1 g.
Knudson model of tumor suppression g.
Krev-1 g.
lactase g.
Lep g.
leptin receptor g.
lipoprotein lipase g.
malic enzyme g.
MEN1 g.
menin g.
multiexonic g.
murine g.
n-myc g.
ob g.
g. overexpression
P21 g.
p53 g.
P450arom g.
PAX3 g.
PDGF g.
PDS g.
Pendred syndrome g.
PER g.
period g.
peroxisome proliferator-activated receptor g.
phosphoenolpyruvate carboxykinase g.
Pit-1 g.
p57KIP2 g.
platelet-derived growth factor g.
pleiotropic g.
polypeptide hormone g.
POMC 8-kb g.
potassium inwardly-rectifying channel, subfamily J, member 1 g.
Pou1F1 g.
preproglucagone g.
preproinsulin g.
preproPTH g.
preprotachykinin A g.
procollagen g.
proenkephalin g.
proopiomelanocortin g.
Prop1 g.
p53 tumor-suppressor g.
$p21^{WAF1}$ tumor-suppressor g.
putative tumor-suppressor g.
Rad g.
Rb g.
Regl alpha g.
g. regulatory protein
reporter g.
retinoblastoma g. (Rb)
sex-determining region Y g. (SRY)
SLC12A1 g.
SLC12A3 g.
sodium/iodine cotransporter g.
somatostatin g.
SRY g.
sulfonylurea receptor g.
SV40 large T-antigen g.
Tabby g.
g. therapy
thyroid hormone target g.
TIM g.
tissue nonspecific alkaline phosphatase g.
g. transfer

TSH-R g.
tumor g.
tumor necrosis factor g.
tumor-suppressor g. (TSG)
ubiquitin fusion degradation 1 g.
VHL tumor suppressor g.
von Hippel-Lindau tumor-suppressor g.
v-*sis* transforming g.
wild-type K-ras g.
Wilms tumor 1 g.
WTI g.
Xist g.
Zeitgeber g.
ZFP g.
zinc finger Y g.
gene-activating sequence (GAS)
Genebs
Genentech biosynthetic human growth hormone
generalized
g. hyperpigmentation
g. resistance to thyroid hormone (GRTH)
g. thyroid hormone resistance (GTHR)
generation
malonaldehyde g.
thrombin g.
generator
pulse g.
genetic
g. counseling
g. hormone resistance syndrome
g. marker
g. obesity
g. polymorphism
genetically predisposing factor
gene transfer
Gen-Glybe
geniculohypothalamic tract (GHT)
genistein
Genistin
genital atrophy
genitalia
ambiguous g.
virilized external g.
genitogram
genitourinary autonomic neuropathy
Gen-Minoxidil
Genny holder
genome
haploid g.
g. scan
simian sarcoma virus g.
genomic imprinting
Genora
G. 0.5/35
G. 1/35
G. 1/50
Genotropin
G. 5.8-mg Intra-Mix
G. Mixer
G. Pen 5
G. Pen 5 growth hormone delivery device
G. Peri 12
G. powder
G. system
G. two-chamber cartridge
genotype
apo E g.
genotype-phenotype relationship
genotyping
Kell antigen g.
platelet antigen g.
Rh C, D, E g.
Genpril
Geref
geriatric
g. hypogonadism
g. hypoparathyroidism
germ-cell
g.-c. neoplasm
g.-c. tumor
germinal
g. arrest
g. cell aplasia
g. center
g. epithelium
germinoma
suprasellar g.
germline
g. amplification
g. deletion
g. PTEN mutation
g. putative protein-tyrosine phosphatase mutation
g. TP53 mutation
gestagen treatment
gestational
g. diabetes
g. diabetes mellitus (GDM)

NOTES

gestational *(continued)*
g. goitrogenesis
g. transient thyrotoxicosis (GTT)
g. trophoblastic disease
g. trophoblastic neoplasm (GTN)
gestodene
gestrinone
Gevrabon
G_q family
GFR
glomerular filtration rate
GG
Slo-Phyllin GG
GG-Cen
GG/DM
Kolephrin GG/DM
GH
growth hormone
GH cell adenoma
GH insulin
pentameric GH
placental GH
GH-1
GH-1 gene
GH-2
GH-2 gene
GHB
gamma-hydroxybutyrate
GHb
glycosylated hemoglobin
GHBP
growth hormone-binding protein
GHIH
growth hormone-inhibiting hormone
growth hormone inhibitory hormone
GH-N
growth hormone (normal)
ghost
g. cell
g. nucleus
GH-releasing
G.-r. factor (GRF)
G.-r. hormone
G.-r. hormone receptor (GHRH-R)
G.-r. hormone receptor gene
G.-r. peptide (GHRP)
G.-r. peptide receptor
GHRH
growth hormone-releasing hormone
GHRH-GH-IGF axis
GHRH-secreting tumor
GHRH-mRNA transcript
GHRH-R
GH-releasing hormone receptor
GHRH-R gene
GHRP
GH-releasing peptide
growth hormone-releasing peptide
GHRP receptor
GHRP-5
GHS
growth hormone secretagogue
GH-secreting pituitary adenoma
GHSR
growth hormone secretagogue receptor
GHT
geniculohypothalamic tract
GH-V
growth hormone (variant)
GI
gastrointestinal
giant
g. carotid aneurysm
g. cell carcinoma
g. cell thyroiditis
g. cell tumor
g. invasive pituitary adenoma
g. invasive prolactinoma
g. prolactinoma
giant-cell
g.-c. arteritis
g.-c. granuloma
g.-c. granulomatous hypophysitis
giardiasis
Gierke disease
GIF
glycosylation-inhibiting factor
GIFT
gamete intrafallopian transfer
gigantism
cerebral g.
pituitary g.
Gigli saw
GIP
gastric inhibitory peptide
gastric inhibitory polypeptide
GIT
glutathione-insulin transhydrogenase
Gitelman syndrome
GK
glucokinase
GLA
gamma-carboxyglutamic acid
gamma-linolenic acid
Gla
gamma-carboxyglutamic acid
Gla protein
gland
abnormal parathyroid g.
acinar g.
adenomatous adrenal g.
adrenal g.
anterior pituitary g.
apocrine sweat g.
autonomous nodular hyperplastic g.

Bartholin g.
Bowman g.
Brunner g.
bulbourethral g.
Cowper g.
eccrine sweat g.
endocrine g.
endometrial g.
exocrine g.
greater vestibular g.
great vestibular g.
high-lying thyroid g.
hyperplastic adrenal g.
hyperplastic parathyroid g.
hypoplastic g.
inferior parathyroid g.
lacrimal g.
lingual thyroid g.
lymphoepithelial endocrine g.
mammary g.
merocrine g.
neurosecretory g.
parathyroid g.
parotid g.
percutaneous alcohol ablation of the parathyroid g. (PAAP)
pineal g.
pituitary g.
posterior pituitary g.
preputial g.
prostate g.
radiation-damaged thyroid g.
salivary g.
sebaceous sweat g.
Skene paraurethral g.
Skene periurethral g.
somatotroph adenoma of pituitary g.
superior parathyroid g.
thymus g.
thyroid g.
tubuloalveolar salivary g.
ultimobranchial g.
urethral g.
uterine g.

glandular
g. acini
g. hypophysis
g. kallikrein
g. lesion
g. pattern

glandulocavernosal shunt

glans
g. clitoridis
g. penis

Glanzmann disease

glargine
insulin g.

glaucoma
low-tension g.

GlcNAc
N-acetylglucosamine
GlcNAc receptor

glia
g. maturation factor (GMF)

glia-activating factor (GAF)

glial
g. cell
g. cell line-derived neurotrophic factor (GDNF)
g. envelope
g. reaction
g. tumor

glibenclamide

glicentin

glicentin-related pancreatic polypeptide (GRPP)

gliclazide

glimepiride

glioblastoma
g. multiforme

glioma
benign optic g.
chiasmal g.
hypothalamic g.
hypothalamic/chiasmic g.
optic g.
optic apparatus g.
opticochiasmatic g.

glioneural tumor

gliosis
fibrillary g.

gliotic brain

glipizide
g. GITS

glitazone

globe subluxation

globoid cell leukodystrophy

globulin
antihemophilic g. (AHG)
antithymocyte g.
corticosteroid-binding g. (CBG)
cortisol-binding g. (CBG)
intramuscular immune g.

NOTES

G

globulin *(continued)*
lymphocyte immune g.
plasma sex hormone-binding g.
retinol-binding g. (RBG)
serum thyroxine-binding g.
sex-binding g.
sex hormone-binding g. (SHBG)
sex steroid-binding g. (SSBG)
testosterone-binding g. (TeBG)
testosterone estradiol-binding g.
thyroid-binding g. (TBG)
thyroid hormone-binding g. (TBG)
thyroxine-binding g. (TBG)
vitamin D-binding g.
globulin-vitamin D binding protein
globus pallidus
glomangioma
glomerular
g. disease
g. filtration rate (GFR)
glomerulitis
focal g.
glomerulonephritis
glomerulopressin
glomerulosa
adrenal zona g.
zona g.
glomerulosclerosis
focal segmental g. (FSGS)
glomerulotubular balance
glomerulus
glomus jugulare tumor
glossitis
glove-and-stocking distribution
GLP
glucagon-like peptide
GLP-1
glucagon-like peptide-1
glubionate
calcium g.
GlucaGen
glucagon
insulin-induced suppression of g.
g. receptor
g. stimulation test
g. storage disease
glucagon-like
g.-l. peptide (GLP)
g.-l. peptide-1 (GLP-1)
glucagonoma
g. syndrome
glucagon-producing tumor
glucagon-secreting tumor
glucoamylase
glucocerebrosidase deficiency
Glucocheck Pocketlab II blood glucose system
glucocorticoid
g. action
g. excess
exogenous g.
g. hormone
g. insensitivity
g. receptor (GR)
g. receptor deficiency
g. receptor dimer
g. receptor-interacting protein 1 (GRIP 1)
g. receptor-interacting protein 1 coactivator
g. remediable hypertension
g. replacement
g. replacement therapy
g. resistance
g. response element (GRE)
synthetic g.
glucocorticoid-free immunosuppressive regimen
glucocorticoid-induced
g.-i. growth failure
g.-i. osteoporosis
glucocorticoid-regulated gluconeogenesis
glucocorticoid-remediable
g.-r. aldosteronism (GRA)
g.-r. hyperaldosteronism (GRH)
g.-r. hyperandrogenism
glucocorticoid-remedial hyperaldosteronism
glucocorticoid-resistant depressive disorder
glucocorticoid-responsive element (GRE)
glucocorticoid-suppressible
g.-s. aldosteronism
g.-s. hyperaldosteronism
g.-s. mineralocorticoid excess
glucogenesis
glucoheptonate
calcium g.
glucokinase (GK)
enzyme g.
g. gene
Glucometer
G. DEX blood glucose monitor
G. DEX diabetes care system
G. Elite R meter
G. II
G. II home glucose monitoring system
gluconate
calcium g.
ferrous g.
gluconeogenesis
glucocorticoid-regulated g.
hepatic g.
renal g.

GlucoNIR glucose sensor
GluControl GC300
Glucophage
Gluco-Protein
G.-P. OTC self-test
G.-P. over-the-counter self-test
glucoregulatory neural reflex
glucosamine sulfate
glucose
B-D G.
blood g. (bG)
g. clamp method
g. concentration
g. counterregulatory hormone (GCRH)
fasting blood g. (FBG)
fasting plasma g. (FPG)
g. homeostasis
impaired fasting g. (IFG)
g. infusion rate
instant g.
insulin-induced g.
g. intolerance
g. measurement
g. metabolism
g. oxidase inhibitor
g. oxidase-platin
g. oxidation
g. phosphatase
g. phosphate
g. polymer
portohepatic g.
postprandial g. (PG)
g. receptor
g. response
g. sensing
g. tolerance
g. tolerance impairment
g. tolerance test (GTT)
g. toxicity
g. toxicity hypothesis
g. transporter (GLUT)
g. transporter translocation
uridine diphosphate g.
glucose-fatty acid cycle
glucose-induced insulin secretion
glucosensor
amperometric g.
glucose-6-phosphatase (G6Pase)
g.-p. deficiency
glucose-1-phosphate
glucose-6-phosphate (G6P)
g.-p. dehydrogenase (G6PD, G6PDH)
glucose-stimulated insulin secretion (GSIS)
glucose-transport
g.-t. protein 1 (GLUT-1)
g.-t. protein 2 (GLUT-2)
g.-t. protein 3 (GLUT-3)
g.-t. protein 4 (GLUT-4)
g.-t. protein 5 (GLUT-5)
g.-t. protein 6 (GLUT-6)
g.-t. protein 7 (GLUT-7)
g.-t. protein 6 pseudogene
glucosidase inhibitor
glucoside
cyanogenic g.
glucostatic hypothesis
glucosuria
glucosyltransferase
glucotoxicity
Glucotrol
G. XL
Glucovance
GlucoWatch
G. Biographer meter
G. Biographer transdermal sensor
G. glucose monitor
G. glucose monitoring device
glucuronic acid
glucuronidation
glucuronide
5-alpha-androstane-3-alpha,17-beta-diol g.
androstanediol g.
androsterone g. (AoG)
g. conjugate
glue
fibrin g.
Glukor
GLUT
glucose transporter
GLUT-1
glucose-transport protein 1
GLUT-2
glucose-transport protein 2
GLUT-3
glucose-transport protein 3
GLUT-4
glucose-transport protein 4
GLUT-5
glucose-transport protein 5

G

NOTES

GLUT-6
glucose-transport protein 6
GLUT-6 pseudogene
GLUT-7
glucose-transport protein 7
glutahione compound
glutamate
glutamate-cysteine ligase
glutamatergic fiber
glutamic
g. acid
g. acid codon (GAA)
g. acid decarboxylase (GAD)
glutamine
glutamyl transferase
glutaric
g. acidemia type II
g. aciduria type II
glutathione
g. peroxidase
reduced g. (GSH)
g. reductase
glutathione-insulin transhydrogenase (GIT)
glutathione-S-transferase (GST)
glutethimide
Glutose
Glu-X-Tyr
Glyate
glyburide
Albert G.
glycan
glycated
g. hemoglobin
g. hemoglobin A_{1c}
glycation
g. end product
nonenzymatic protein g.
glycemia
basal g.
glycemic
g. control
g. index
glyceraldehyde-3-phosphate dehydrogenase
glycerol
g. administration
iodinated g.
g. kinase
g. kinase deficiency
glycerol-3-phosphate dehydrogenase
Glycerol-T
glycerophosphate
glycine
g. cleavage complex
glycine-rich RNA-binding protein (GRP)
glycinuria
glycitein
glycobiology
glycocalyx
glycogen
g. phosphorylase
g. storage disease, types I/la, II, III, IV, V, VI, VII, VIII
g. store
g. synthase
g. synthase kinase-3 (GSK3)
g. synthesis
glycogenesis
glycogenic precursor
glycogenization
glycogenolysis
hepatic g.
glycogen synthesis
glycohemoglobin
glycol
ethylene g.
salicylic acid and propylene g.
glycolipid
glycolysis
glycolytic enzyme
glycopeptide hormone
glycoprotein
$alpha_1$ acid g. (AGP)
carbohydrate-deficient g. (CDG)
g. crystal growth inhibitor (CGI)
g. crystal growth-inhibitor protein
heterodimeric g.
homodimeric g.
g. hormone
g. hormone receptor
g. IIb and IIIb blocker
g. neuraminidase deficiency
zona pellucida receptor for g. 3
glycoproteinosis
glycoprotein-producing adenoma
glycoprotein-secreting pituitary tumor
glycopyrrolate
Glycosal diabetes test
glycosaminoglycan (GAG)
g. deposition
polysulfated g.
g. synthesis
glycosuria
overt g.
glycosylasparaginase deficiency
glycosylated
g. hemoglobin (GHb)
g. serum protein
glycosylation
g. consensus motif
N-linked g.
glycosylation-inhibiting factor (GIF)
glycosylphosphatidylinositol-anchored heparan sulfate proteoglycan (HSPG)
glycosyltransferase

glycotropic hormone
glycyrrhetinic acid
glycyrrhizin
glycyrrhizinic acid
glydiazinamide
Glynase PresTab
glypican-1
Glyset
Glytuss
GM1 gangliosidosis
GM-CFU
granulocyte-macrophage colony-forming unit
GM-CSF
G&M colony-stimulating factor
granulocyte-macrophage colony-stimulating factor
GMF
glia maturation factor
GMP
guanosine monophosphate
cyclic GMP
GNAS1
G. gene
G. locus
GNAS gene
GnRH
gonadotropin-releasing hormone
GnRH agonist
GnRH analog
GnRH mRNA
GnRH receptor
GnRHa
gonadotropin-releasing hormone agonist
GnRH-associated peptide (GAP)
GnRH-R
gonadotropin-releasing hormone receptor
GNRP
guanine nucleotide regulatory protein
GO
Graves ophthalmopathy
goal
serum phosphorus g.
goblet cell
goiter
adenomatous g.
amyloid g.
benign nodular g.
cervical g.
colloid g.
diffuse toxic g.
dyshormonogenetic g.
g. endemia
endemic colloid g.
endemic iodine-deficiency g.
enzootic g.
euthyroid diffuse g.
euthyroid nodular g.
exophthalmic g.
firm g.
Himalayan g.
hypothyroid g.
idiopathic colloid g.
intrathoracic g.
iodide g.
iodine-deficiency g.
iodine-deficient g.
lobulated g.
multinodular euthyroid g.
neonatal g.
nodular g.
nonautoimmune nontoxic diffuse g.
nontoxic multinodular g.
nontoxic nodular g.
nontoxic sporadic g.
ovarian g.
g. plongeont
g. reduction
g. regrowth
retrosternal g.
sequestered g.
simple nonendemic g.
small g.
sporadic g.
substernal g.
toxic diffuse g.
toxic multinodal g.
toxic multinodular g. (TMG)
toxic nodular g. (TNG)
uninodular g.
g. volume
goiter-deafness syndrome
goitrin
goitrogen
goitrogenesis
gestational g.
goitrogenic
g. agent
g. substance
goitrous
g. chronic autoimmune thyroiditis
g. cretinism
g. Hashimoto thyroiditis

NOTES

goitrous *(continued)*
g. hyperthyroidism
g. tissue
gold-198
colloidal g.
g. radioactive isotope
Goldberg-Hogness box
Goldman-Hodgkin-Katz equation
Goldmann
G. perimetry
G. visual field
gold thyroglucase
Golgi
G. apparatus
G. complex
G. network
G. phase
G. stack
Goltz syndrome
Gomori
G. chromalum-hematoxylin
G. staining method
gonad
dysgenetic g.
indifferent g.
streak g.
gonadal
g. axis
g. dysfunction
g. dysgenesis
g. failure
g. mosaicism
g. peptide
g. ridge
g. steroid
g. steroid level
g. steroidogenesis
g. steroid replacement
g. suppression
g. suppression treatment
45,X g. dysgenesis
46,XX g. dysgenesis
46,XY g. dysgenesis
gonadarche
gonadectomy
g. cell
gonadoblastoma
gonadorelin
gonadotoxicity
gonadotrope
g. adenoma
gonadotroph
g. cell
g. cell adenoma
g. cell hyperplasia
g. cell origin
g. hormone (GTH)
g. pituitary adenoma
gonadotropic adenoma
gonadotropin
alpha-human chorionic g. (alpha-hCG)
asialo-human chorionic g. (asialo-hCG)
beta-human chorionic g. (β-hCG)
g. bioinactivity
chorionic g. (CG)
g. deficiency
exogenous g.
g. gene
human chorionic g. (hCG)
human menopausal g. (HMG, hMG)
human pituitary g. (hPG)
g. hypersecretion
idiopathic g.
luteinizing hormone/human chorionic g. (LH/CG, LH/hCG)
g. receptor
g. secretion
sialylated human chorionic g.
gonadotropin-associated peptide
gonadotropinoma
gonadotropin-producing pituitary adenoma
gonadotropin-releasing
g.-r. hormone (GnRH)
g.-r. hormone activation
g.-r. hormone agonist (GnRH agonist, GnRHa)
g.-r. hormone-agonist therapy
g.-r. hormone analog
g.-r. hormone deficiency
g.-r. hormone pulse frequency
g.-r. hormone receptor (GnRH-R)
g.-r. hormone test
gonadotropin-secreting
g.-s. adenoma
g.-s. tumor
Gonal-F
gonarche
gondii
Toxoplasma g.
Gonic
gonorrhea
gonorrhoeae
Neisseria g.
Goodpasture syndrome
Goody's Headache Powders
Gordon syndrome
Gorham massive osteolysis
Gorlin syndrome
Gormel Creme
goserelin
gossypol
gourd-shaped sella

gout
G6P
glucose-6-phosphate
G6Pase
glucose-6-phosphatase
GPCR
G protein-coupled receptor
GPCR mutation
G6PD
glucose-6-phosphate dehydrogenase
G6PDH
glucose-6-phosphate dehydrogenase
G-protein
heterotrimeric G.-p.
G.-p. intermediary
G.-p. signaling pathway
G.-p. trimer
G.-p. trimeric complex
GR
glucocorticoid receptor
GRA
glucocorticoid-remediable aldosteronism
graafian follicle
gracile
grade
Ki67 g.
PAHO g. 0, 1, 2
Pan American Health Organization g. (0–2)
gradient
calcium g.
chemical g.
corticomedullary osmotic g.
corticopupillary osmolality g.
electrical g.
electrochemical g.
hydrostatic pressure g.
negative arterial-portal glucose g.
Percoll g.
g. pressure garment
voltage g.
gradient-echo sequence
gradient-recalled
spoiled g.-r. (SPGR)
Graefenberg spot
Graefe sign
graft
g. versus host (GVH)
g. versus host reaction
granidinium thiocyanate
granin
granular
g. cell tumor
g. chromophil cell
granulated cell
granule
beta cell secretory g.
Birbeck g.
calcium bilirubinate g.
chromaffin g.
g. extrusion
keratohyaline g.
neurosecretory g. (NSG)
secretory g.
Snaplets-FR G.
zymogen g.
granulocyte
g. colony-stimulating factor (G-CSF)
granulocyte-macrophage
g.-m. colony-forming unit (GM-CFU)
g.-m. colony-stimulating factor (GM-CSF)
granulocytopenia
iatrogenic g.
granulocytosis
granuloma
g. annulare
caseating g.
giant-cell g.
noncaseating g.
reparative g.
sperm g.
granulomatosa
struma g.
granulomatosis
bronchocentric g.
Wegener g.
granulomatous
g. disease
g. hypophysitis
g. inflammation
g. sarcoidosis
g. thyroiditis
granulosa
g. cell death
g. cell defect
g. cell tumor
g. cell tumor of the ovary
g. lutein
g. lutein cell

G

NOTES

granulosus
Echinococcus g.
granzyme
Graves
G. disease
G. ophthalmopathy (GO)
gravidarum
chloasma g.
thyrotoxicosis of hyperemesis g.
gravis
gravity
specific g.
gray (Gy)
gray patch
Grb-2 protein
GRE
glucocorticoid response element
glucocorticoid-responsive element
greater vestibular gland
great vestibular gland
Greenberg
G. bar
G. retractor mounting system
green birefringent amyloid protein
Grey Turner sign
GRF
GH-releasing factor
growth hormone-releasing factor
GRH
glucocorticoid-remediable hyperaldosteronism
growth-releasing hormone
Grimelius stain technique
GRIP 1
glucocorticoid receptor-interacting protein 1
GRIP 1 coactivator
Grocott stain
groove
Harrison g.
hydrophobic g.
g. pancreatitis
ground substance
group
5-amino g.
arylmethyl g.
g. A *Streptococcus*
g. B coxsackievirus
5-cyano g.
high mobility g. (HMG)
International Diabetes Immunotherapy G.
iodophenoxyl g.
keto g.
National Diabetes Data G. (NDDG)
perikaryal g.
thioureylene g.
group-specific component (Gc)
growth
appositional g.
bone g.
chondrocytic g.
g. curve
g. differentiation factor (GDF)
g. differentiation factor-9 (GDF-9)
g. disorder
epitaxial g.
excess acral g.
g. factor expression
g. factor-inducible chemokine (FIC)
g. factor therapy
g. hormone (GH)
g. hormone axis
g. hormone-binding protein (GHBP)
g. hormone cell
g. hormone cell adenoma (GH cell adenoma)
g. hormone cell hyperplasia
g. hormone deficiency
g. hormone-deficient adult
g. hormone-deficient child
g. hormone dose
g. hormone dose-response curve
g. hormone-expressing cell
g. hormone-1 gene
g. hormone-2 gene
g. hormone-inhibiting hormone (GHIH)
g. hormone inhibitory hormone (GHIH)
g. hormone insensitivity
g. hormone insulin
g. hormone/insulin-like growth factor axis
g. hormone (normal) (GH-N)
g. hormone-producing giant invasive adenoma
g. hormone-producing tumor
g. hormone-prolactin cell
g. hormone-prolactin cell adenoma
g. hormone protein-sparing effect
g. hormone release-inhibiting hormone
g. hormone-releasing factor (GRF)
g. hormone-releasing hormone (GHRH)
g. hormone-releasing hormone-growth hormone-insulin-like growth hormone axis
g. hormone-releasing hormone-secreting tumor
g. hormone-releasing peptide (GHRP)
g. hormone replacement
g. hormone resistance
g. hormone resistance syndrome

g. hormone response
g. hormone secretagogue (GHS)
g. hormone secretagogue receptor (GHSR)
g. hormone-secreting pituitary adenoma (GH-secreting pituitary adenoma)
g. hormone-secreting pituitary tumor
g. hormone secretion
g. hormone synthesis
g. hormone therapy
g. hormone (variant) (GH-V)
hypothalamic hamartomatous g.
longitudinal g.
pituitary tumor cell g.
prolactinoma g.
g. retardation
g. spurt
g. velocity (GV)

growth-blocking antibody
growth-releasing hormone (GRH)
growth-stimulating antibody
GrowTrak Plus
GRP
gastrin-releasing peptide
glycine-rich RNA-binding protein
GRPP
glicentin-related pancreatic polypeptide
GRTH
generalized resistance to thyroid hormone
Gs-cAMP pathway
GSH
reduced glutathione
GSIS
glucose-stimulated insulin secretion
GSK3
glycogen synthase kinase-3
gsp-positive somatotroph tumor
GST
glutathione-S-transferase
G-stimulating protein (G_s)
GTH
gonadotroph hormone
GTHR
generalized thyroid hormone resistance
GTN
gestational trophoblastic neoplasm
GTP
guanosine triphosphate
guanosine 5′ triphosphate
GTP-binding protein
GTP-dependent regulatory protein complex
GTPase
guanosine triphosphatase
GTPase-activating protein (GAP)
GTT
gestational transient thyrotoxicosis
glucose tolerance test
Guaituss AC
guanabenz
guanethidine
guanine
g. nucleotide binding protein
g. nucleotide regulatory protein (GNRP)
guanosine
g. 5′ diphosphate (GDP)
g. diphosphate-binding
g. monophosphate (GMP)
g. triphosphatase (GTPase)
g. triphosphate (GTP)
g. 5′ triphosphate (GTP)
g. triphosphate-activating protein (GAP)
g. triphosphate binding protein
g. triphosphate-dependent regulatory protein complex
g. trophosphate
guanylate
g. cyclase
g. cyclase enzyme
guanylin
guanyl nucleotide
guanylyl
g. cyclase
g. cyclase-linked receptor
guar gum
gubernaculum
guidelines
American Diabetes Association g.
California Diabetes and Pregnancy Sweet Success G.
National Cholesterol Education g.
Guillain-Barré syndrome
Gull disease
gum
guar g.
Nicorette G.
Nicorette DS G.
gumma, pl. **gummata**
syphilitic g.
gummata of the thyroid

NOTES

gummatous lesion
gustatory
g. neurosensory process
g. sweating
gut-associated lymphoid tissue (GALT)
gut-brain peptide
gut peptide
gut-peptide hypothesis
guttering
GV
growth velocity
GVH
graft versus host
GVH disease
GVH reaction
Gy
gray
gynandroblastoma
gynecoid obesity
gynecomastia
late-onset g.
Gynogen L.A. Injection
gynoid fat distribution
gyrata
cutis verticis g.
gyrate atrophy
gyrus
cingulate g.
paraterminal g.
parolfactory g.

H
carboxypeptidase H
cathepsin H
Margesic H
H_2
prostaglandin H. (PGH_2)
H19 gene
habenular commissure
Habitrol Patch
habitus
eunuchoid body h.
marfanoid h.
Haemolance lancet
Hagedorn
neutral protamine H. (NPH)
Hageman factor
hair
axillary h.
h. effect
h. follicle
parallel development of axillary h.
parallel development of pubic h.
pubic h.
terminal h.
vellus h.
HAIRAN
hyperandrogenism, insulin resistance, acanthosis nigricans
HAIRAN syndrome
hairless woman syndrome
hairpin loop
Haldrone
half-life
biologic h.-l.
effective h.-l.
physical h.-l.
Halfprin
hallucination
formed visual h.
unformed visual h.
visual h.
hallux
plantar surface of h.
halo
hypoechoic band
sonographic halo
halofenate
haloperidol
Halotestin
Haltran
HAM
hypoparathyroidism, adrenal insufficiency, mucocutaneous candidiasis
hamartoblastoma
hypothalamic h.
hamartoma
cutaneous h.
gastrointestinal h.
hypothalamic neuronal h.
neuronal h.
oral h.
retinal h.
tuber cinereum h.
h. of tuber cinereum
hamartomatous nodule
hamburger thyrotoxicosis
hamster oocyte penetration test (HOPT)
hand
h. enlargement
h. grip strength
Hand-Schüller-Christian disease
Hansen disease
haploid
h. genome
haploinsufficiency
haplotype
diabetogenic h.
h. linkage
Hardy
H. classification of pituitary tumor
H. ring curette
H. spoon dissector
Hardy-Weinberg law
Harris-Benedict equation
Harrison groove
Hartnup syndrome
Harvey-Ras oncogene
Hashimoto
atrophic H. thyroiditis
H. disease
H. encephalopathy
H. thyroiditis
hashitoxicosis
Hassall corpuscle
HAT
histone acetyltransferase
H^+-ATPase
hydrogen adenosine triphosphatase
haversian
h. canal
h. system
Hb
hemoglobin
HbA1c
hemoglobin A_{1c}
HBD
hormone-binding domain

HBGF-2
heparin-binding growth factor-2
HBP
helix-bundle peptide
HC
Bancap HC
HCB
hexachlorobenzene
HCF
high-carbohydrate high-fiber
HCF diet
hCG
human chorionic gonadotropin
hCG pregnancy test
sialylated hCG
β-hCG
beta-human chorionic gonadotropin
hCG-modulated thyroid activity
hCG-secreting hepatoblastoma
HCl
pioglitazone H.
HCMA
hyperchloremic metabolic acidosis
Hcrtr1 receptor
Hcrtr2 receptor
hCS
human chorionic somatomammotropin
HDE
humanitarian device exemption
H-dexamethasone
HDL
high-density lipoprotein
HDL-C
high-density lipoprotein C
headache
frontotemporal h.
headlight
fiberoptic h.
head of pancreas
healing
poor wound h.
wound h.
Health
National Institutes of H. (NIH)
Heart
H. and Estrogen/Progestin Replacement Study (HERS)
H. Outcome Prevention Evaluation (HOPE)
heat
h. intolerance
h. shock protein (HSP, Hsp)
h. shock protein autoantibody
heating
radiofrequency capacitive h.
heat-stable protein
heatstroke
heavy metal poisoning
Hectorol
H. Injection
hedgehog
Indian h.
heel-to-pubis measurement
Heidenhain pouch
height
h. loss
midparental h. (MPH)
helical
h. computed tomography
h. CT
helicine artery
Helicobacter pylori
helix-bundle peptide (HBP)
helix-loop-helix
basic h.-l.-h. (bHLH)
h.-l.-h. family
h.-l.-h. structure
HELLP
hemolysis, elevated liver enzymes, and low platelets
HELLP syndrome
helper/inducer T-lymphocyte
helper T cell
hemachromatosis
hereditary h. (HH)
hemadsorption
hemangioblastoma
retinal h.
hemangioblastomatosis
cerebelloretinal h.
retinal cerebellar h.
hemangioendothelioma
malignant h.
hemangioma
cavernous h.
hemangiopericytoma
Hematinic
Theragran H.
hematocrit
hematogenous
hematopoiesis
extramedullary h. (EMH)
hematopoiesis-supporting stroma
hematopoietic
h. cell growth factor
h. compartment
h. stem cell precursor
h. system
hematoxylin
lead h.
h. stain
heme-binding protein
hemiagenesis
hemianopia
bitemporal h.

hemianopic
h. defect
h. scotoma
hemianopsia
bilateral h.
bitemporal h.
hemicastration
hemichoreoathetosis
hemifield slide phenomenon
hemigastrectomy
hemihypophysectomy
blind h.
hemithyroidectomy
hemizona
h. assay
h. assay index (HZI)
hemizygosity
hemizygous
hemochorial
h. placenta
hemochromatosis
h. gene
hemoconcentration
hemocrine
h. action
HemoCue blood glucose system
Hemocyte
hemocytoblastoma
hemodialysis
chronic h.
h. membrane bioincompatibility
h. therapy
hemodilution
hemofiltration
hemoglobin (Hb)
h. A
h. A_{1b}
h. A_{1c} (HbA1c)
h. A_0
h. A_1a
h. A_1b
h. C
h. E
glycated h.
glycosylated h. (GHb)
h. Raleigh
h. Russ
h. S
hemoglobinopathy
hemoglobinuria
paroxysmal nocturnal h.
hemolysis
h., elevated liver enzymes, and low platelets (HELLP)
h., elevated liver enzymes, and low platelets syndrome
hemolytic anemia
hemolyticus
Streptococcus h.
hemoperfusion
charcoal h.
resin h.
hemoperitoneum
hemophilia A
hemopoietin
hemoprotein
cytochrome P450 h.
hemorrhage
active variceal h.
adrenal h.
apoplectic h.
vitreous h.
hemorrhagic
h. diathesis
h. nodule
hemorrhagicum
corpus h.
hemosiderin
hemosiderosis
thyroid h.
hemostasis
metabolic h.
osmotic h.
Henderson-Hasselbalch equation
Henle
loop of H.
H. loop
medullary thick ascending limb of H.
hentermine
heparan
h. sulfate
h. sulfate proteoglycan
heparin-binding
h.-b. EGF
h.-b. epidermal growth factor
h.-b. growth factor-2 (HBGF-2)
heparin-bound growth factor
hepatectomy
hepatic
h. artery
h. artery embolization
h. disease

NOTES

hepatic *(continued)*
h. effect
h. failure
h. fibrogenic activity
h. free fatty acid uptake
h. gluconeogenesis
h. glucose efflux
h. glucose output (HGO)
h. glucose production (HGP)
h. glycogenolysis
h. glycogen synthesis
h. hydroxymethylglutaryl coenzyme A reductase inhibitor
h. insufficiency
h. insulin sensitivity
h. lipase
h. lipase activity
h. lipase deficiency
h. necrosis
h. neoplasm
h. somatomedin
h. steatosis
h. tumor
h. vein
hepatis
peliosis h.
hepatitis
h. A
acute infectious h.
h. A virus
h. B
h. C
h. C-associated osteosclerosis
cholestatic h.
chronic active h.
h. E
h. F
hepatoblastoma
hCG-secreting h.
human chorionic gonadotropin-secreting h.
hepatocellular
h. enzyme
h. tumor
hepatocyte
h. growth factor (HGF)
h. nuclear factor (HNF)
h. nuclear factor-3 (HNF3)
h. nuclear factor-4 (HNF4)
h. nuclear factor-4a (HNF-4a)
h. transcription factor-1
hepatofugal flow
hepatoma
h. cell insulin receptor
hepatomegaly
hepatopetal flow
hepatotoxicity
Heptavax-B vaccine
hereditary
h. angioneurotic edema
h. ataxia
h. end-organ resistance
h. fructose intolerance
h. hemachromatosis (HH)
h. hemorrhagic telangiectasia
h. nephrogenic diabetes insipidus
h. neuropathy with liability to pressure palsy (HNPP)
h. nonpolyposis colon cancer (HNPCC)
h. nonpolyposis colon cancer/ovarian cancer syndrome
h. pancreatitis (HP)
h. panhypopituitarism
h. pseudovitamin D deficiency rickets
h. thyrotoxicosis
h. vitamin D resistance
heredofamilial disorder
heregulin
heritable
Hermansky-Pudlak syndrome
hermaphrodite
hermaphroditism
true h.
herpes
h. simplex virus thymidine kinase (HSV-TK)
h. zoster
herpetiformis
dermatitis h.
Herring body
HERS
Heart and Estrogen/Progestin Replacement Study
Hertel
H. exophthalmometer
HESX1
homeobox gene expressed in ES cells
Hesx1
factor H.
HETE
hydroxyeicosatetraenoic acid
12-HETE
12-hydroxyeicosatetraenoic acid
heterochromatic nucleus
heterochromatin
constitutive h.
facultative h.
heterochromia iridium
heterodimer
cFos-cJun h.
RelA-p50 h.
thyroid hormone receptor-retinoid X receptor h.
TR-RXR h.

heterodimeric
h. glycoprotein
h. luteinizing hormone (hLH)
h. structure
heterodimerization
heterodimerize
heterodisomic chromosome
heterogeneity
heterogenicity
osteoblast h.
heterologous
heterooligomer
heterophilic antibody
heteroplasty
heterosexual precocity
heterotetramer
hybrid h.
heterotetrameric molecule
heterotrimer
type I collagen h.
heterotrimeric
h. G-protein
h. protein
heterozygosity
compound h.
loss of h. (LOH)
heterozygote
heterozygous
h. cystathione beta synthase deficiency
heuristic
hexachlorobenzene (HCB)
Hexadrol
hexameric domain
hexarelin
hexokinase
h. B gene
h. enzyme
h. II gene
h. IV
HFA
Proventil HFA
hFGF
Kaposi sarcoma human growth factor
HGF
hepatocyte growth factor
hGH
human growth hormone
somatotropin
HGO
hepatic glucose output
HGP
hepatic glucose production
H-graft
portacaval H-g.
HH
hereditary hemachromatosis
H_1 histone
HHM
humoral hypercalcemia of malignancy
HHPS
hypothalamohypophysial portal system
HHRH
syndrome of hereditary hypophosphatemic rickets with hypercalciuria
HHS
hyperglycemic hyperosmolar syndrome
5-HIAA
5-hydroxyindoleacetic acid
hibernoma
hidrosis
HIF-1alpha
hypoxia-inducible factor-1-alpha
high
h. circulating parathyroid hormone
h. glycemic index diet
h. jugular vein sampling
h. mobility group (HMG)
h. mobility group box
high-arched palate
high-attenuation iodinated contrast media
high-calcium dialysate
high-carbohydrate
h.-c. high-fiber (HCF)
h.-c. high-fiber diet
high-density
h.-d. lipoprotein (HDL)
h.-d. lipoprotein C (HDL-C)
high-dose
h.-d. corticosteroid
h.-d. dexamethasone suppression test
h.-d. intraperitoneal aprotinin
h.-d. statin treatment
high-fiber
high-carbohydrate h.-f. (HCF)
high-impact activity
high-$K_M$isoenzyme
high-lying thyroid gland

NOTES

H

high-mannose
h.-m. oligosaccharide
h.-m. precursor
high-performance liquid chromatography (HPLC)
high-phosphorus diet
high-pressure baroreceptor
high-resolution coronal axis imaging
high-salt diet
high-speed microsurgical drill
hilar cell
hilus cell
Himalayan goiter
Himbin
Dayto H.
^{3}H-imipramine binding
hindgut
HIOMT
hydroxyindole-*O*-methyltransferase
Hippel-Lindau
von H.-L. (VHL)
hippocampal
h. formation
h. neuron
hippocampus
hippurate
Hirschsprung disease
hirsute
hirsutism
androgen-type h.
facial h.
Ferriman scale of h.
idiopathic h. (IH)
lagunal h.
hirsutism-anovulation syndrome
His-Pro-DKP
histidyl-proline-diketopiperazine
histamine
h. (H_2) antagonist
histamine-N-methyltransferase
histaminergic
h. afferent
Histerone Injection
histidase
histidine
histidinemia
ocular h.
histidine-rich calcium-binding protein (HRC)
histidyl-proline-diketopiperazine (His-Pro-DKP)
histiocyte
Langerhans cell h.
histiocytic neoplasm
histiocytosis, histocytosis
granulomatous h.
Langerhans cell h.
malignant h.
h. X
histochemistry
hybridization h.
histocompatibility
h. class I
h. complex gene
h. locus antigen (HLA)
major h.
histocytosis (*var. of* histiocytosis)
histofluorescence
histology
bone h.
mineralized bone h.
histomorphic feature
histomorphometric
h. assessment
h. examination
h. study
h. technique
histomorphometry
dynamic h.
quantitative bone h.
histone
h. acetylation
h. acetyltransferase (HAT)
h. deacetylase activity
h. deacetylation
H_1 h.
Histoplasma capsulatum
histoplasmosis
histrelin
HIV
human immunodeficiency virus
Hi-Vegi-Lip
hKGK1
human kidney glandular kallikrein-1 gene
hKGK1 gene
HLA
histocompatibility locus antigen
human leukocyte antigen
HLA allele
HLA DR antigen association
HLA restricted
HLA-A antigen
HLA allele
HLA-B35
HLA-B8 antigen
HLA-B antigen
HLA-C antigen
HLA-D antigen
HLA-DP antigen
HLA-DQ
H.-D. antigen
HLA-DQα501
HLA-DR
H.-D. antigen
HLA-DR3 antigen

HLA-DR4 antigen
HLA-DR5 antigen
HLA-Dw3 antigen
^{3}H-leucine
hLH
heterodimeric luteinizing hormone
HMG
high mobility group
human menopausal gonadotropin
HMG box
hMG
human menopausal gonadotropin
HMG-CoA
beta-hydroxy-beta-methylglutaryl-coenzyme A
HMG-CoA reductase inhibitor
HNF
hepatocyte nuclear factor
HNF3
hepatocyte nuclear factor-3
HNF3 transcription factor
HNF4
hepatocyte nuclear factor-4
HNF4 transcription factor
HNF-4a
hepatocyte nuclear factor-4a
HNK-1 antigen
HNP-4
human neutrophil peptide-4
HNPCC
hereditary nonpolyposis colon cancer
HNPP
hereditary neuropathy with liability to pressure palsy
H_2O_2 amperometric electrode
13-HODE
13-hydroxyoctadecadienoic acid
Hodgkin disease
Hofbauer cell
Hoffmann syndrome
Hofmeister
anion of the H. series
hOKT3g1
hOKT3y1
Hold
holder
Bra Pocket pump h.
Genny h.
Leg Thing pump h.
Pump-N-Shorts pump h.
Thigh Thing pump h.
Waist It pump h.
hole zone
Holmes-Adie syndrome
holoenzyme
Hologic QDR 4500 DXA bone densitometer
holoprosencephaly
homatropine
homeobox
h. gene expressed in ES cells (HESX1)
homeodomain factor
homeostasis
calcium h.
fetal mineral h.
fuel h.
glucose h.
intracellular h.
mineral h.
osmotic h.
phosphorus h.
potassium h.
skeletal h.
sleep-wake h.
sodium h.
water h.
homeotherm
homeothermia
homeotic
paired box h. 3 (PAX3)
paired box h. 8 (PAX8)
hominis
Mycoplasma h.
homocarnosinase
homocarnosine
homocarnosinosis
homocysteine
h. level
homocystinemia
methylmalonic acidemia with h.
homocystinuria
homodimer
catalytic h.
regulatory h.
thyroid hormone receptor h.
TR h.
homodimeric glycoprotein
homodimerization
homogenate
xanthoma h.
homogentisic acid
homologous
h. pseudogene

NOTES

H

homologous *(continued)*
h. recombination
h. thyroid antigen
homologue
TNF-weak h. (TWEAK)
homology
homonymous
homoplasty
homotetramer
homovanillic acid (HVA)
homozygote
homozygous
h. cystinuric
h. missense mutation
Honvol
HOPE
Heart Outcome Prevention Evaluation
HOPE trial
HOPT
hamster oocyte penetration test
hormogenesis
hormonal
h. add-back therapy
h. hyperfunction
h. milieu
h. regulator
h. signal
h. study
hormone
activational h.
adenohypophysial h.
adipokinetic h.
adrenal androgen-stimulating h. (AASH)
adrenal medullary h.
adrenocortical h.
adrenocorticotrophin h. (ACTH)
adrenocorticotropic h. (ACTH)
adrenomedullin h.
aldosterone-stimulating h. (ASH)
alpha-melanocyte-stimulating h.
alpha-melanocyte-stimulating h.
alpha-MSH h.
altered degradation of parathyroid h.
amino acid-peptide h.
angiotensin II antidiuretic h.
antidiuretic h. (ADH)
anti-müllerian h. (AMH)
antithyroid-stimulating h. (anti-TSH)
atrial natriuretic h. (ANH)
beta-melanocyte-stimulating h.
beta-thyroid-stimulating h. (beta-TSH)
bioactive parathyroid h.
h. biosynthesis
bound h.
bovine parathyroid h. (bPTH)
brain h.
calciotropic peptide h.
calcitonin gene-related h. (CGRH)
calcitropic h.
calcium-lowering h.
calcium-regulating h.
contrainsulin h.
cortical androgen-stimulating h. (CASH)
corticotropin-releasing h. (CRH)
corticotropin-releasing h. 1R (CRH1R)
corticotropin-releasing h.-R1 (CRH-R1)
corticotropin-releasing h. 2R (CRH2R)
counterregulatory h.
C-terminal assay for parathyroid h.
h. degradation
dexamethasone-suppressed ovine corticotropin-releasing h.
diabetogenic h.
eclosion h.
endogenous gonadal h.
endogenous growth h.
exogenous thyroid h.
fasting growth h.
follicle-stimulating h. (FSH)
follicle-stimulating hormone-releasing h. (FSH-RH)
follicular stimulating h. (FSH)
free h.
gamma-melanocyte-stimulating h. (gamma-MSH)
gastrointestinal h.
Genentech biosynthetic human growth h.
generalized resistance to thyroid h. (GRTH)
GH-releasing h.
glucocorticoid h.
glucose counterregulatory h. (GCRH)
glycopeptide h.
glycoprotein h.
glycotropic h.
gonadotroph h. (GTH)
gonadotropin-releasing h. (GnRH)
growth h. (GH)
growth hormone-inhibiting h. (GHIH)
growth hormone inhibitory h. (GHIH)
growth hormone release-inhibiting h.
growth hormone-releasing h. (GHRH)
growth h. (normal) (GH-N)

growth-releasing h. (GRH)
growth h. (variant) (GH-V)
heterodimeric luteinizing h. (hLH)
high circulating parathyroid h.
human corticotropin-releasing h.
human growth h. (hGH)
human parathyroid h. (hPTH)
human placental uterotropic h. (hPUTH)
hydrophilic h.
hydrophobic h.
hyperglycemic h.
hypocalcemic h.
hypophyseotropic h.
hypothalamic h.
hypothalamic inhibitory h.
hypothalamic-releasing h.
immunoradiometric assay of circulating parathyroid h.
immunoreactive parathyroid h. (iPTH)
inappropriate secretion of thyroid-stimulating h.
indole h.
inhibin h.
inhibitory h.
intact parathyroid h.
interstitial cell-stimulating h. (ICSH)
lactogenic h.
lactotropic h.
LH-releasing h. (LHRH, LH-RH, LRH)
lipophilic h.
"little" h.
luteinizing h.-beta (LH-β)
luteinizing hormone-releasing h. (LHRH, LH-RH, LRH)
luteotropic h.
magnocellular h.
melanin-concentrating h. (MCH)
melanocyte-concentrating h.
melanocyte-inhibiting h.
melanocyte-releasing h. (MRH)
melanocyte-stimulating h. (MSH)
mineralocorticoid h.
mini h.
müllerian-inhibiting h. (MIH)
müllerian inhibitory h. (MIH)
myotropic h.
natriuretic h.
neurohypophysial h.
neurotrophic h.
nuclear accessory h.
ouabain-like h.
ovine corticotropin-releasing h.
paraneoplastic growth h.
parathyroid h. (PTH)
parotid h.
pentameric growth h.
peptide-amino acid h.
peripheral tissue resistance to thyroid h. (PTRTH)
pituitary glycoprotein h.
pituitary growth h.
pituitary resistance to thyroid h. (PRTH)
polypeptide h.
posterior lobe h.
primary adrenal medullary h.
prolactin-inhibiting h. (PIH)
prolactin inhibitory h. (PIH)
prolactin release-inhibiting h. (PIH)
prolactin-releasing h. (PRH)
ProLease encapsulated sustained-release growth h.
prothoracotropic h. (PTTH)
h. receptor
h. receptor-ligand complex
h. receptor-mediated response
h. receptor-negative tumor
h. receptor-positive tumor
recombinant human growth h. (RHGH, rhGH)
recombinant human thyroid-stimulating h. (rhTSH)
release-inhibiting h.
releasing h.
h. replacement therapy (HRT)
h. resistance
resistance to thyroid h. (RTH)
h. response element (HRE)
h. response unit (HRU)
h. rhythm
SciTojet needle-free injector for human growth h.
h. secretion
secretory burst of growth h.
selective peripheral resistance to thyroid h.
selective pituitary resistance to thyroid h. (PRTH)
h. sensitive lipase
h. serum level
sex steroid h.

NOTES

H

hormone *(continued)*
sine qua nonsuppressed thyroid-stimulating h.
somatomammotropic h.
somatotroph h. (STH)
somatotropic h.
somatotropin release-inhibiting h. (SRIH)
steroid h.
sterol h.
stress h.
syndrome of bioinactive growth h.
syndrome of inappropriate secretion of antidiuretic h. (SIADH)
syndrome of inappropriate thyroid-stimulating h.
synthetic corticotropin-releasing h.
thyroid h.
thyroid-stimulating h. (TSH)
thyroid-stimulating hormone-releasing h.
thyrotropin-releasing h. (TRH)
thyrotropin-stimulating h. (TSH)
total h.
trophic h.
tropic anterior pituitary h.
urinary follicle-stimulating h.
water-soluble h.
Y h.
hormone-binding
h.-b. domain (HBD)
h.-b. negative
h.-b. protein
hormone-dependency effect
hormone-fuel interrelationship
hormone-resistant
h.-r. breast cancer
h.-r. state
hormone-responsive
h.-r. epithelium
hormone-secreting
h.-s. adrenal tumor
h.-s. cell
h.-s. pituitary tumor
hormone-sensitive adenylate cyclase system
hormone-specific neurophysin
hormonogenesis
thyroid h.
horn
temporal h.
Horner syndrome
horny cell
hospital-acquired hyponatremia
hospital gangrene
host
h. cell
graft versus h. (GVH)
HOT
Hypertensive Optimal Treatment Trial
hot
h. flashes
h. nodule
h. spot
Hour
Acutrim 16 H.
24-hour
24-h. fractionated metanephrine
24-h. urinary aldosterone excretion
24-h. urinary fractionated metanephrine
24-h. urine collection
24-h. urine free cortisol
hourglass constriction
housekeeping gene
Houssay phenomenon
Howell aspiration needle
Hoxa3 homeobox gene
HP
hereditary pancreatitis
Ku-Zyme HP
Profasi HP
HPA
hypothalamic-pituitary-adrenal
hypothalamopituitary adrenal
HPA axis
HPA axis suppression
HPA function
H.P. Acthar Gel
hPASP
human pancreas-specific protein
5-HPETE
5-hydroperoxyeicosatetraenoic acid
12-HPETE
12-hydroperoxyeicosatetraenoic acid
HPG
hypothalamic-pituitary-gonadal
HPG axis
hPG
human pituitary gonadotropin
hPL
human placental lactogen
HPLC
high-performance liquid chromatography
HPRT
hypoxanthine-guanine phosphoribosyltransferase
HPRT deficiency
HPT
hyperparathyroidism
HPT axis
hPTH
human parathyroid hormone
hPUTH
human placental uterotropic hormone

H-*ras*

HRC
histidine-rich calcium-binding protein

HRE
hormone response element

HRT
hormone replacement therapy

HRU
hormone response unit

H.S.
Estratest H.S.

hs-CRP

HSD
hydroxysteroid dehydrogenase

HSG
hysterosalpingogram

HSP
heat shock protein

Hsp
heat shock protein

HSPG
glycosylphosphatidylinositol-anchored heparan sulfate proteoglycan

hst-1
human stomach cancer-transforming factor-1

hst-2
human stomach cancer-transforming factor-2

HSV-TK
herpes simplex virus thymidine kinase

5-HT
monoamine serotonin

5HT
5-hydroxytryptamine

HTA
hypophysiotropic area

hTg
human thyroglobulin

HTLV-1
human T-cell leukemia virus type I

5HTP
5-hydroxy-L-tryptophan

hTR
human thyroid hormone receptor

$5HT_2$ receptor antagonist

H-TRON plus V100 insulin infusion pump

huang
ma h.

Humalog
H. Mix 50/50
H. Mix 75/25
H. Pen

human
h. calcitonin
h. chorionic gonadotropin (hCG)
h. chorionic gonadotropin-modulated thyroid activity (hCG-modulated thyroid activity)
h. chorionic gonadotropin-secreting hepatoblastoma
h. chorionic somatomammotropin (hCS)
h. chorionic thyrotropin
h. corticotropin-releasing hormone
h. demineralized bone matrix
H. Genome Project
h. growth hormone (hGH)
h. growth hormone gene
h. immunodeficiency virus (HIV)
h. insulin
h. kidney glandular kallikrein-1
h. kidney glandular kallikrein-1 gene (hKGK1)
h. leukocyte antigen (HLA)
h. leukocyte antigen allele (HLA allele)
h. leukocyte antigen DR antigen association
h. leukocyte antigen restricted
h. malignant osteopetrosis
h. menopausal gonadotropin (HMG, hMG)
h. neutrophil peptide-4 (HNP-4)
h. pancreas-specific protein (hPASP)
h. parathyroid hormone (hPTH)
h. pituitary gonadotropin (hPG)
h. placental lactogen (hPL)
h. placental uterotropic hormone (hPUTH)
h. pluripotent stem cell
h. proCHR gene
h. prokaryotic chromosome gene
h. stomach cancer-transforming factor-1 (hst-1)
h. stomach cancer-transforming factor-2 (hst-2)
h. T-cell leukemia virus type I (HTLV-1)
h. thyroglobulin (hTg)
h. thyroid hormone receptor (hTR)

NOTES

human *(continued)*
h. X chromosome, gene 1
h. zona pellucide binding test
humanitarian device exemption (HDE)
Humatrope
HumatroPen
Humegon
Humibid
H. L.A.
H. Sprinkle
humor
aqueous h.
humoral
h. factor
h. hypercalcemia of malignancy (HHM)
h. immune response
h. immunity
h. signal
h. symptom
hump
buffalo h.
dowager h.
Humphrey visual field
Humulin
H. 50/50
H. 70/30
H. L
H. Mix 75/25 Pen
H. N
H. 70/30 pen
H. R
H. R pen
H. U
hunger
bone h.
hungry
h. bone
h. bone syndrome
Hunter syndrome
Huntington
H. chorea
H. disease
Hurler-Scheie syndrome
Hurler syndrome
Hürthle
H. cell
H. cell adenoma
H. cell neoplasm
H. cell tumor
Hutchinson-Gilford syndrome
HVA
homovanillic acid
hyaline
h. body
h. cartilage
h. membrane disease
hyalinization
afferent arteriole h.
Crooke h.
hyalinizing
h. trabecular adenoma
h. trabecular neoplasm
hyaluronan
hyaluronic acid
hyaluronidase
H-Y antigen
Hybolin
H. Decanoate
H. Improved Injection
hybrid
h. heterotetramer
h. steroid
hybridization
allele-specific oligonucleotide h.
fluorescence in situ h. (FISH)
h. histochemistry
h. histochemistry probe
molecular probe h.
in situ h.
hybridoma
h. cell
Hycodan
hydatidiform mole
hydoxylase
hydradenitis
suppurative h.
hydramnios
hydrate
H. Injection
terpin h.
hydremia
hydrocarbon
polyaromatic h.
hydrocele
hydrocephalus
X-linked h.
Hydrocet
hydrochloride
clonidine h.
cyproheptadine h.
desipramine h.
eflornithine h.
fluoxetine h.
hydromorphone h.
metformin h.
metoclopramide h.
oxymetazoline h.
ranitidine h.
hydrochlorothiazide
hydrocortisone
h. replacement therapy
h. sodium succinate
Hydrocortone
H. Acetate Injection

H. Oral
H. Phosphate Injection
HydroDIURIL
hydroflumethiazide
hydrogen
h. adenosine triphosphatase (H^+-ATPase)
h. breath test
h. ion
h. ion buffering
h. peroxide
hydrogenase
3-hydroxysteroid h.
hydrogen-bonding effect
Hydrogesic
hydrolase
cholesterol ester h.
maleylacetoacetate h.
hydrolink gel electrophoresis
hydrolysate
aluminum-contaminated casein h.
casein h.
hydrolysis
phosphoinositide h.
thyroglobulin h.
hydrolyzed lithostathine fibril
Hydromet
hydrometry
hydromorphone
h. hydrochloride
hydronephrosis
Hydro-Par
hydropathy
Kyte-Doolittle h. analysis
hydroperiodide
tetraglycine h.
hydroperoxyeicosatetraenoic
5-h. acid (5-HPETE)
12-h. acid (12-HPETE)
Hydrophed
hydrophilic
h. hormone
h. macromolecule
hydrophobic
h. amino acid
h. groove
h. hormone
h. protein
hydrophobicity
hydrostatic
h. pressure
h. pressure gradient
hydroxide
aluminum h.
magnesium h.
4-hydroxyandrostenedione
11-hydroxyandrostenedione
hydroxyapatite crystal
hydroxyapatite/tricalcium phosphate particle
hydroxychloroquine
hydroxycorticoid
hydroxycorticosteroid
17-hydroxycorticosteroid (17-OHCS)
urinary 17-h.
18-hydroxycorticosterone
18-hydroxydeoxycorticosterone
hydroxyeicosatetraenoic
h. acid (HETE)
5-h. acid
12-h. acid (12-HETE)
15-h. acid
11-C-hydroxyephedrine scintigraphy
2-hydroxyestrone
4-hydroxyestrone
2-hydroxyglutaric acid
5-hydroxyindoleacetic acid (5-HIAA)
hydroxyindole-*O*-methyltransferase (HIOMT)
3-hydroxyisovalerate
hydroxyisovaleric acid
hydroxylase (Ohase)
h. deficiency
steroid h.
tryptophan h.
tyrosine h.
11-hydroxylase
11-h. deficiency
11-h. enzyme
17-hydroxylase
17-h. deficiency
18-hydroxylase
21-hydroxylase
21-h. deficiency
21-h. gene
24-hydroxylase
vitamin D 24-h. (24-OHase)
hydroxylation
17-hydroxylation
25-hydroxylation
hydroxyl radical
hydroxylysine (OHL)
6-hydroxymelatonin
hydroxymethylglutarate

NOTES

H

3-hydroxy-3-methylglutaryl-CoA carboxylase deficiency
hydroxymethylglutaryl-coenzyme A carboxylase
13-hydroxyoctadecadienoic acid (13-HODE)
4-hydroxyphenylpyruvate dioxygenase
17-hydroxypregnenolone
hydroxyprogesterone
h. caproate
17-hydroxyprogesterone (17-OHP, 17-OPH)
hydroxyproline
h. oxidase
urinary h.
hydroxypropyl-β-cyclodextrin
hydroxysteroid
h. dehydrogenase (HSD)
11-h. dehydrogenase
3-hydroxysteroid hydrogenase
6α-hydroxytetrahydro-11-deoxycortisol
5-hydroxytryptamine (5HT)
-h. subtype 2 receptor antagonist
5-hydroxytryptophan
5-hydroxy-L-tryptophan (5HTP)
hydroxyvitamin D
25-hydroxyvitamin D (25OH-VitD)
25-hydroxy-vitamin D 1α-hydroxylase (1-alpha-OHase)
hydroxyzine
hygroma
cystic h.
Hygroton
Hylutin
hyoid bone
hyoscyamine
Hyosophen
hypadrenia
Hy-Pam Oral
hypatocyte
hyperabsorptive hypercalciuric stone disease
hyperaldosteronism
bilateral idiopathic h.
dexamethasone-suppressible h.
familial h.
glucocorticoid-remediable h. (GRH)
glucocorticoid-remedial h.
glucocorticoid-suppressible h.
idiopathic h. (IHA)
secondary h.
syndrome of primary h.
tertiary h.
hyperalimentation
hyperaminoacidemia
hyperammonemia
hyperamylasemia
hyperandrogenemia
cryptic h.
hyperandrogenesis
ovarian h.
hyperandrogenic
h. anovulation
h. state
hyperandrogenism
early pubertal h.
functional ovarian h.
glucocorticoid-remediable h.
h., insulin resistance, acanthosis nigricans (HAIRAN)
ovarian h.
hyperandrogen state
hyperapobetalipoproteinemia
hyperargininemia
hyperation
intracranial h.
hyperbaric
h. boot
h. chamber
h. oxygen
h. oxygen treatment
hyper-beta-alaninemia
hyperbilirubinemia
hyperbradykininism
hypercalcemia
benign hypocalciuric h.
calcitriol-mediated h.
familial hypocalciuric h. (FHH)
Fanconi-type idiopathic h.
immobilization-related h.
infantile h.
malignancy-associated h.
theophylline-induced h.
hypercalcemic
hypercalcinemia
hypercalcitonemia
hypercalciuria
absorptive h.
benign familial h.
idiopathic h.
normocalcemic h.
syndrome of hereditary hypophosphatemic rickets with h. (HHRH)
hypercalciuric
h. hypophosphatemic rickets
h. hypophosphatemic state
hypercapnia
hypercarnosinuria
hypercarotenemia
hyperchloremia
hyperchloremic metabolic acidosis (HCMA)

hypercholesterolemia
familial h. (FH)
polygenic h.
hyperchylomicronemic syndrome
hypercontractile state
hypercortisolemia
pathologic h.
hypercortisolism
chronic h.
endogenous h.
exogenous h.
food-related h.
iatrogenic h.
metyrapone-induced h.
hypercytokinemia
hyperdeviation
hyperdibasicaminoaciduria
hyperechogenicity
hyperechoic
hyperestrinism
hyperestrogenic
h. state
hyperestrogenism
hypereuthroid
hyperextensibility
joint h.
hyperfibrinogenemia
hyperfractionated radiotherapy
hyperfunction
autoimmune thyroid h.
autonomous h.
endocrine h.
hormonal h.
primary adrenal h.
secondary adrenal h.
hyperfunctioning
h. tissue
hypergastrinemia
hyperglycemia
fasting h.
hypoinsulinemic h.
postprandial h.
rebound h.
hyperglycemic
h. coma
h. glucose clamp
h. hormone
h. hyperosmolar syndrome (HHS)
hyperglycinemia
nonketotic h.
hypergonadotrophic hypogonadism
hypergonadotropic
h. hypogonadism
h. state
hyperhidrosis
central h.
hyperhomocystinemia
resistant h.
hyperhomocyteinemia
hyperhydroxyprolinemia
hyperimidodipeptiduria
hyperinsulinemia
exogenous h.
islet beta-cell h.
maternal hyperglycemia-induced fetal h.
hyperinsulinemic
h. hypoglycemia
h. hypoglycemia marker
h. polycystic ovary syndrome
hyperinsulinemic-euglycemic clamp technique
hyperinsulinism
congenital h.
familial h.
hyperinsulinoma
hyperintense
hyperirritability
hyperkalemia
familial h.
hyperkeratosis
hyperkinesia
hyperlactemia
hyperleucine-isoleucinemia
hyperlipasemia
hyperlipidemia
combined h.
familial combined h. (FCH)
type IV h.
hyperlipoproteinemia
type 3 h.
hyperlysinemia
hypermagnesemia
hypermelatoninism
hypermenorrhea
hypermethioninemia
hypermethylation
hypermineralocorticoidism
licorice-induced h.
renin-independent h.
hypernatremia
essential h.
hypernatremic

NOTES

H

hyperoral behavior
hyperornithinemia
hyperosmolality
hyperosmolar nonketotic coma
hyperosmotic
hyperostosis
h. corticalis
diaphyseal cortical h.
diffuse idiopathic skeletal h. (DISH)
endosteal h.
h. frontalis interna
infantile cortical h.
hyperoxaluria
enteric h.
hyperoxia
hyperparathyroid bone disease
hyperparathyroidism (HPT)
acute primary h.
h. axis
compensatory h.
familial isolated primary h. (FIHP, FIPH)
neonatal severe h. (NSHPT)
normocalcemic primary h.
persistent h.
phosphorus-induced h.
primary h. (PHPT)
secondary h.
tertiary h.
hyperphagia
hyperphenylalaninemia
hyperphosphatasemia
familial h.
idiopathic h.
hyperphosphatasia
osteoectasia with h.
hyperphosphatemia
hyperphosphaturia
hyperpigmentation
cutaneous h.
generalized h.
hyperpigmented skin
hyperpituitarism
hyperplasia
ACTH-independent bilateral macronodular h. (AIBH)
adenomatous h.
adrenal medullary h.
adrenomedullary h.
autonomous adrenal h.
autosomal dominant toxic thyroid h.
beta cell h.
bilateral macronodular h.
C cell h.
chronic lobular h.
congenital adrenal h. (CAH)
congenital lipoid adrenal h.
congenital virilizing adrenal h.
corticotroph h.
corticotroph cell h.
cystic h.
ECL cell h.
enterochromaffin-like cell h.
epidermal h.
erythroid h.
familial C-cell h.
focal epithelial h.
gonadotroph cell h.
growth hormone cell h.
intraductal mucinous h.
Kupffer cell h.
lactotroph h.
Leydig cell h.
lipoid adrenal h.
lymphoid h.
macronodular adrenal h.
massive macronodular h.
micronodular h.
neointimal h.
nonsalt-wasting congenital adrenal h.
paraadenomatous corticotroph h.
parathyroid gland h.
pineal h.
pituitary h.
primary macronodular h.
prolactin cell h.
stromal h.
thecal h.
thymic h.
thyroid h.
thyrotroph cell h.
type I congenital adrenal h.
type II congenital adrenal h.
type IV congenital adrenal h.
type V congenital adrenal h.
hyperplastic
h. adrenal gland
h. parathyroid gland
hyperpneumatization
hyperproinsulinemia
hyperprolactinemia
idiopathic h.
radiation-induced h.
secondary h.
hyperprolactinemic
h. disorder
h. endocrinopathy
hyperprolinemia
hyperprostaglandin E syndrome
hyperreactio luteinalis
hyperreflexia
hyperreninemia
hyperreninemic hypoaldosteronism

hyperreninism
hyperrespond
hypersarcosinemia
hypersecretion
ACTH h.
adrenocorticotrophic hormone h.
adrenocorticotropic hormone h.
gonadotropin h.
pituitary h.
hypersensitivity response
hypersexuality
paroxysmal h.
hypersomnia
hypertelorism
hypertension
benign intracranial h.
endocrine h.
essential h.
glucocorticoid remediable h.
idiopathic intracranial h.
intracranial h. (IH)
licorice-induced h.
low-renin essential h.
pregnancy-induced h. (PIH)
renovascular h.
systemic arterial h.
Hypertensive Optimal Treatment Trial (HOT)
hyperthecosis
follicular h.
ovarian h.
stromal h.
hyperthermia
cyclic h.
fulminant h.
malignant h.
microwave h.
paroxysmal h.
thyroid storm h.
hyperthyroid
clinically h.
h. periodic paralysis
hyperthyroidism
apathetic h.
autoimmune h.
congenital h.
factitious h.
familial nonautoimmune h.
fetal h.
goitrous h.
iatrogenic h.
iodine-induced h. (IIH)
masked h.
monosymptomatic h.
monosystemic h.
neonatal Graves h.
nonautoimmune familial h.
non-Graves disease h.
painless h.
postpartum h.
primary h.
secondary h.
subacute h.
subclinical h.
hyperthyrotropinemia
hyperthyroxinemia
complex h.
dysalbuminemic h.
euthyroid h.
familial dysalbuminemic h. (FDH)
prealbumin-associated h. (PAH)
hypertonic
h. encephalopathy
h. syndrome
h. volume depletion
hypertonicity
impaired medullary h.
plasma h.
hypertrichosis
villous h.
hypertriglyceridemia
carbohydrate-induced h.
familial h.
hypertriiodothyroninemia
familial dysalbuminemic h.
hypertrophic
h. cardiomyopathy
h. lichen planus
h. osteoarthropathy
h. state
hypertrophied
h. corneal nerve
h. thyroglossal duct remnant
hypertrophy
benign prostatic h.
compensatory h.
fiber h.
periosteal h.
thymus h.
hyperuricemia
hyperuricosuria
hypervalinemia

NOTES

hypervitaminosis
h. A
h. D
hypervolemia
hypha, pl. **hyphae**
aseptate h.
thick-walled h.
Hy-Phen
hypnosedation
hypoactivity
hypoadrenalism
central h.
primary h.
secondary h.
hypoadrenocorticism
hypoalbuminemia
hypoaldosteronism
congenital h.
hyperreninemic h.
hyporeninemic h.
syndrome of hyporeninemic h. (SHH)
hypoalphalipoproteinemia
familial h.
hypoaminoacidemia
hypoandrogenic milieu
hypoandrogenism
ovarian h.
hypoatremia
hypobetalipoproteinemia
hypocalcemia
autosomal dominant h.
early h.
late h.
neonatal h.
optic h.
phosphorus-induced h.
symptomatic h.
hypocalcemic
h. emergency
h. hormone
h. tetany
hypocalciuria
hypocalciuric-hypomagnesemic variant
hypocaloric diet
hypocellular
h. bone surface
h. marrow without fibrosis
hypochlorhydria
hypochondroplasia
hypochromic microcytic red blood cell
hypocitraturia
primary h.
secondary h.
hypocorticotropic state
hypocortisolemia
hypocortisolism
postadenomectomy h.
hypocretin
hypodipsia
hypodipsic disorder
hypoechogenicity
hypoechoic
h. band (halo)
hypoestrogenemia
hypoestrogenic
hypoestrogenism
hypofunction
autoimmune polyglandular h.
pituitary hormone h.
hypofunctioning
hypogammaglobulinemia
hypogeusia
hypoglossal nerve
hypoglycemia
alimentary h.
artifactual h.
h. crisis
ethanol h.
factitial h.
factitious h.
fasting h.
functional h.
hyperinsulinemic h.
idiopathic reactive h.
insulin factitial h.
insulin-induced systemic h.
ketotic h.
late h.
nadir h.
nocturnal h.
noninsulinoma pancreatogenous h.
nonislet-cell tumor-induced h.
postabsorptive h.
postprandial h.
reactive h.
h. unawareness
h. unresponsiveness
hypoglycemia-associated autonomic failure
hypoglycemic
h. coma
h. shock
hypoglycin
hypoglycorrhachia
hypogonadal hypogonadism
hypogonadism
acquired hypogonadotropic h.
central h.
central h. types IIA, III
functional hypothalamic h.
geriatric h.
hypergonadotrophic h.
hypergonadotropic h.
hypogonadal h.
hypogonadotrophic h.
hypothalamic hypogonadotropic h.

idiopathic hypogonadotropic h. (IHH)
neurogenic h.
primary h.
secondary h.
tertiary h.

hypogonadotrophic
h. hypogonadism

hypoinsulinemia
relative h.

hypoinsulinemic hyperglycemia

hypokalemia
licorice-induced h.
spontaneous h.

hypokalemic
h. metabolic alkalosis
h. periodic paralysis

hypoleptinemia

hypolipidemic agent

hypomagnesemia

hypomagnesiuria

hypomelatoninism

hypomenorrhea

hypometabolic

hypomineralization

hyponatremia
asymptomatic h.
hospital-acquired h.
iatrogenic h.
symptomatic h.

hyponatremic encephalopathy

hypoosmolality

hypoparathyroidism
autoimmune h.
autosomal dominant h.
familial h.
geriatric h.
idiopathic h.
permanent h.
postsurgical h.
primary h.
secondary h.
transient h.

hypoparathyroidism, adrenal insufficiency, mucocutaneous candidiasis (HAM)

hypophosphatasia

hypophosphatemia
congenital h.
fasting h.
X-linked h. (XLH)

hypophosphatemic
h. bone disease
h. osteomalacia
h. rickets

hypophyseal (*var. of* hypophysial)

hypophysectomized

hypophysectomy
endoscopic transsphenoidal h.
stereotactic h.
transsphenoidal h.

hypophyseotropic hormone

hypophysial, hypophyseal
h. artery
h. cleft
h. lesion
h. portal system
h. stalk
h. stalk circulation

hypophysial-hypothalamic portal system

hypophysial-portal circulation

hypophysiotropic
h. area (HTA)
h. factor
h. hormonal function
h. neuron
h. system

hypophysis
chromophilic h.
glandular h.
pharyngeal h.

hypophysitis
autoimmune h.
chronic lymphocytic h.
giant-cell granulomatous h.
granulomatous h.
idiopathic granulomatous h.
lymphocytic h.
purulent h.

hypopituitarism
complete h.
idiopathic h.
isolated h.
partial h.
postpartum h.
radiotherapy-induced h.
selective h.

hypopituitary adult

hypoplasia
congenital lipoid adrenal h.
cytomegalic-type congenital adrenal h.
focal dermal h.

NOTES

hypoplasia *(continued)*
- Leydig cell h.
- miniature-type congenital adrenal h.
- h. of nipples
- pituitary h.
- somatotroph h.

hypoplastic
- h. gland
- h. mandible
- h. nail
- h. vulva
- h. zygoma

hypoprolactinemia
hypoproliferative anemia
hypoproteinemia
hypoprothrombinemia
hyporeflexia
hyporeninemic hypoaldosteronism
hyporesponsiveness
- partial thyroid-stimulating hormone h.
- partial TSH h.

hyposmia
hyposmotic
hyposomatotropism
- obesity-related h.

hypospadias
- familial h.
- penoscrotal h.
- perineoscrotal h.

hypospermatogenesis
hyposthenuria
hypotension
- idiopathic orthostatic h.
- orthostatic h.
- postural h.
- primary orthostatic h.
- secondary orthostatic h.

hypothalamic
- h. acromegaly
- h. amenorrhea
- h. anovulation
- h. center
- h. diabetes insipidus
- h. dysregulation
- h. eunuchism
- h. glioma
- h. gonadotropin-releasing hormone deficiency
- h. hamartoblastoma
- h. hamartomatous growth
- h. hormone
- h. hypogonadotropic hypogonadism
- h. hypothyroidism
- h. inhibitory hormone
- h. neuroendocrine regulation
- h. neuronal hamartoma
- h. obesity
- h. opioidergic tone
- h. paraventricular nucleus
- h. regulatory mechanism
- h. sulcus
- h. tumor
- h. zone

hypothalamic/chiasmic glioma
hypothalamic-hypophyseal
- h.-h. portal vessel

hypothalamic-midbrain junction
hypothalamic-pituitary
- h.-p. axis
- h.-p. control
- h.-p. disease
- h.-p. disorder
- h.-p. response

hypothalamic-pituitary-adrenal (HPA)
- h.-p.-a. axis
- h.-p.-a. axis suppression
- h.-p.-a. function

hypothalamic-pituitary-gonadal (HPG)
- h.-p.-g. axis

hypothalamic-pituitary-ovarian axis
hypothalamic-pituitary-thyroid axis
hypothalamic-releasing
- h.-r. factor
- h.-r. hormone

hypothalamohypophyseal complex
hypothalamohypophysial
- h. nerve tract
- h. portal system (HHPS)

hypothalamoneurohypophysial tract
hypothalamopituitary adrenal (HPA)
hypothalamopituitary-adrenocortical axis
hypothalamus
- arcuate nucleus of the h. (ARC)
- dorsomedial nucleus of the h.
- lateral h.
- medial basal h.
- paraventricular nucleus of the h.
- preoptic area of the h. (POA)
- PVN of the h.
- rostral h.
- SCN of the h.
- suprachiasmatic nucleus of the h.
- supraoptic nucleus of the h. (SON)
- ventromedial nucleus of the h. (VMN)

hypothalmo-neurohypophyseal neuron
hypothermia
- cyclic h.
- paroxysmal h.

hypothermic cold adaptation
hypothesis
- estrone h.
- glucose toxicity h.
- glucostatic h.
- gut-peptide h.

lipostatic h.
Lyon h.
null h.
overworked B-cell h.
Pedersen h.
single gateway h.
SNARE h.
somatomedin h.
Somogyi h.
thermostatic h.
thrifty genotype h.

hypothyroid
h. goiter
h. mononeuropathy
h. myopathy
h. polyneuropathy
h. rhabdomyolysis

hypothyroidism
amiodarone-induced h.
biochemical h.
central h.
childhood h.
clinical h.
congenital h.
fetal h.
hypothalamic h.
hypothyrotropic h.
idiopathic hypothalamic h.
iodine-induced h.
juvenile h.
lithium-induced h.
maternal h.
minimally symptomatic h. (MSH)
neonatal h.
pituitary h.
postablative h.
post-therapeutic h.
preclinical h.
primary thyroidal h.
secondary h.
spontaneous primary h.
sporadic congenital h.
subclinical h.
tertiary h.
thyroidal h.
transient neonatal h.
transient postradioiodine h.

hypothyrotropic
h. hypothyroidism

hypothyroxinemia
fetal h.
maternal h.
h. of prematurity

hypotonia

hypotonic
h. duodenography
h. saline
h. syndrome
h. urine

hypotriglyceridemic action

hypouricemia

hypovascular islet cell tumor

hypoventilation

hypovolemia

hypovolemic
h. shock

hypoxanthine
h. phosphoribosyltransferase

hypoxanthine-guanine
h.-g. phosphoribosyltransferase (HPRT)
h.-g. phosphoribosyltransferase deficiency

hypoxemia
fetal h.

hypoxia

hypoxia-inducible factor-1-alpha (HIF-1alpha)

hypoxic
h. brain injury
h. encephalopathy

Hyprogest 250

hysterectomy

hystericus
syndrome of globus h.

hysterosalpingogram (HSG)

hysterosalpingography

hystidyl-methionine-27
peptide h.-m. (PHM-27)

Hytakerol

Hytinic

Hytuss

Hytuss-2X

Hyzine-50 Injection

HZI
hemizona assay index

NOTES

^{123}I
iodine-123
^{125}I
iodine-125
^{127}I
iodine-127
^{131}I
iodine-131
radioactive iodine
^{131}I isotope
^{131}I therapy
thyroid ablation with ^{131}I
I_2
prostaglandin I. (PGI_2)
IA
central hypogonadism type IA
Ia
fumarylacetoacetate hydrolase type Ia
pseudohypoparathyroidism type Ia
IAA
insulin autoantibody
IAEA
International Atomic Energy Agency
IAPP
islet amyloid polypeptide
iatrogenic
i. Cushing syndrome
i. granulocytopenia
i. hypercortisolism
i. hyperthyroidism
i. hyponatremia
i. thyrotoxicosis
IB
central hypogonadism type IB
Excedrin IB
isolated growth hormone deficiency type IB (IGHD-IB)
Midol IB
Motrin IB
Pamprin IB
Ib
maleylacetoacetate hydrolase, type Ib
pseudohypoparathyroidism type Ib
Iberet-Folic-500
Iberet-Liquid
Ibuprin
ibuprofen
Ibuprohm
Ibu-Tab
ICA
islet cell antigen
ICAM
intercellular adhesion molecule
ICAM-1
intercellular adhesion molecule-1
Icaps
ICARUS
Islet Cell Antibody Registry of Users Study
ICCIDD
International Council for Control of Iodine Deficiency Disorder
I-cell disease
ICER
inducible cAMP early repressor
inducible cyclic adenosine monophosphate early repressor
ICF
intracellular fluid
ichthyosis
congenital i.
X-linked i.
ICMA
immunochemiluminescence assay
immunochemiluminescent assay
immunochemiluminometric assay
ICSA
islet cell surface antibody
ICSH
interstitial cell-stimulating hormone
ICSI
intracytoplasmic sperm injection
ICTP
carboxyterminal cross-linked telopeptide of type I collagen
IDC
invasive ductal carcinoma
IDD
insulin-dependent diabetes
iodine-deficiency disorder
IDDM
insulin-dependent diabetes mellitus
IDE
insulin-degrading enzyme
ideation
identity
gender i.
idiogenic osmole
idiopathic
i. Addison disease
i. adrenal insufficiency
i. aldosteronism
i. colloid goiter
i. complete precocious puberty
i. diabetes
i. diabetes insipidus
i. exophthalmos
i. galactorrhea

idiopathic *(continued)*
i. gonadotropin
i. granulomatous hypophysitis
i. hirsutism (IH)
i. hyperaldosteronism (IHA)
i. hypercalcemia of infancy
i. hypercalciuria
i. hyperphosphatasemia
i. hyperprolactinemia
i. hypogonadotropic hypogonadism (IHH)
i. hypoparathyroidism
i. hypopituitarism
i. hypothalamic hypothyroidism
i. intracranial hypertension
i. ischemic necrosis
i. juvenile osteoporosis
i. myxedema
i. orthostatic hypotension
i. osteolysis
i. osteoporosis in men
i. pancreatitis
i. parkinsonism
i. paroxysmal myoglobinuria
i. postprandial syndrome
i. reactive hypoglycemia
i. sexual precocity
i. short stature (ISS)
i. thrombocytopenic purpura (ITP)
i. true precocious puberty

idioventricular pacemaker

IDL
intermediate-density lipoprotein

IDO
indoleamine 2,3-dioxygenase

Idox

idoxifene

IDUS
intraductal ultrasound

IFG
impaired fasting glucose

IFN
interferon

IFN-α
interferon-alpha

IFN-β
interferon-beta

IFN-ε
interferon-epsilon

IFN-γ
interferon-gamma

IFN-ω
interferon-omega

IFN-α_1
interferon-alpha_1

Ig
immunoglobulin
Ig gene

IgA
immunoglobulin A

IgD
immunoglobulin D

IgE
immunoglobulin E

IGF
insulinlike growth factor

IGF1
insulinlike growth factor-1

IGF2
insulinlike growth factor-2
IGF2 gene

IGF-binding protein (IGFBP)

IGF-binding protein-1

IGFBP
IGF-binding protein
insulinlike growth factor-binding protein

IGFBP-1
insulinlike growth factor-binding protein-1

IGFBP-2
insulinlike growth factor-binding protein-2

IGFBP-3
insulinlike growth factor-binding protein-3

IGFBP-4
insulinlike growth factor-binding protein-4

IGFBP-5
insulinlike growth factor-binding protein-5

IGFBP-6
insulinlike growth factor-binding protein-6

IGF-I
insulinlike growth factor-I
interleukin growth factor I

IGF-II
IGF-II gene

IGF-IIR
insulinlike growth factor-II receptor
IGF-IIR gene

IgG
immunoglobulin G
aggregated human IgG (AHuG)

IGHD
isolated growth hormone deficiency

IGHD-IB
isolated growth hormone deficiency type IB

IGHD-II
isolated growth hormone deficiency type II

IGHD-III
isolated growth hormone deficiency type III

I

IgM
immunoglobulin M
IGT
impaired glucose tolerance
IH
idiopathic hirsutism
intracranial hypertension
IHA
idiopathic hyperaldosteronism
bilateral IHA
IHC
immunohistochemical
IHC stain
IHH
idiopathic hypogonadotropic hypogonadism
IIH
iodine-induced hyperthyroidism
^{131}I-19-iodocholesterol scintigraphy
I–IV
urotensin I–IV
IJV
internal jugular vein
IJV sampling
IL
interleukin
IL-1
interleukin-1
IL-2
interleukin-2
IL-3
interleukin-3
IL-4
interleukin-4
IL-5
interleukin-5
IL-6
interleukin-6
IL-7
interleukin-7
IL-8
interleukin-8
IL-9
interleukin-9
IL-10
interleukin-10
IL-11
interleukin-11
IL-12
interleukin-12
IL-13
interleukin-13
IL-14
interleukin-14
IL-16
interleukin-16
IL-17
interleukin-17
IL-18
interleukin-18
ILA
insulinlike activity
^{131}I-labeled
^{131}I-l. iodocholesterol
^{131}I-l. metaiodobenzylguanidine (^{131}I-labeled MIBG)
^{131}I-l. MIBG
IL-1-alpha
interleukin-1-alpha
IL-1-beta
interleukin-1-beta
ileal-brake effect
Iletin
I. I
Lente I. (I, II)
Pork Regular I. (II)
ileus
myxedema i.
paralytic i.
iliac
i. artery
i. crest bone biopsy
ill-defined nodule
illicit hormone receptor
illness
affective i.
nonthyroidal i. (NTI)
Ilozyme
IL-1RA
interleukin-1 receptor antagonist
IMA
immunometric assay
image
i. intensifier
midsagittal i.
T1-weighted i.
T2-weighted spin-echo i.
imaging
diagnostic i.
endorectal magnetic resonance i.
fluorescence i.
high-resolution coronal axis i.
magnetic resonance i. (MRI)
radioiodine thyroid i.

NOTES

imaging *(continued)*
radionuclide i.
i. technique
i. thermography
thyroid magnetic resonance i.
IMD
immune-mediated diabetes
^{131}I-MIBG
iodine 131-metaiodobenzylguanidine
^{131}I-MIBG scan
imidazole
i. derivative
i. dioxolone
imidodipeptide
imiglucerase
imipramine
immitis
Coccidioides i.
immobilization-related hypercalcemia
immune
i. amyloid
i. cell-mediated cytotoxicity
i. complex
i. response antigen
i. system
immune-mediated diabetes (IMD)
immunity
acquired i.
active i.
cell-mediated i.
cellular i.
humoral i.
maternal i.
passive i.
immunoassay
chemiluminescent i. (CLIA)
Crosslaps i.
enzyme i. (EIA)
enzyme-linked i.
Pyrilinks-D i.
sandwich i.
two-site sandwich i.
immunobead test
immunoblastic lymphoma
immunoblotting
immunochemiluminescence assay (ICMA)
immunochemiluminescent assay (ICMA)
immunochemiluminometric assay (ICMA)
immunocompetence
immunocytochemical
i. analysis
i. staining
immunocytochemistry
neuropeptide i.
immunocytology
immunodeficiency
combined i.
secondary i.
severe combined i.
immunodominant serologic determinant
immunoelectrophoresis
immunogenetics
immunogenic glucose oxidase
immunoglobulin (Ig)
i. A (IgA)
i. D (IgD)
i. E (IgE)
i. G (IgG)
i. G gene
intravenous i. (IVIg)
iodothyronine-binding i.
i. M (IgM)
stimulatory i.
i. synthesis
thyroid growth i. (TGI)
thyroid growth-blocking i. (TGBI)
thyroid-stimulating i. (TSI)
thyroid-stimulating hormone-binding inhibitor i. (TBII)
thyroid-stimulating hormone-binding inhibitor immunoglobulin i.
thyrotropin-binding inhibitory i. (TBII)
TSH-binding inhibitory i. (TBII)
i. V gene
immunogold-labeling technique
immunogold staining
immunoheterogeneity
immunohistochemical (IHC)
i. analysis
i. stain
i. staining
i. staining technique
immunohistochemistry
i. technique
immunoliposome
immunometric assay (IMA)
immunomodulator
immunomodulatory
immunoneuropeptide
immunoneutralization
immunopathogenesis
immunoperoxidase
i. technique
immunophilin
immunoprecipitation
i. assay
immunoradiometric
i. assay (IRMA)
i. assay of circulating calcium
i. assay of circulating parathyroid hormone
immunoradiometric assay (IRMA)

immunoreactive
- i. insulin
- i. parathyroid hormone (iPTH)

immunoreactivity
- insulinlike i.

immunoregulation

immunoregulatory effect

immunoscreening

immunosenescence

immunostain

immunostaining
- endothelin i.

immunosuppression

immunotherapy

impaired
- i. downgaze
- i. fasting glucose (IFG)
- i. glucose counterregulation
- i. glucose tolerance (IGT)
- i. medial gaze
- i. medullary hypertonicity
- i. thirst

impairment
- beta-cell i.
- erectile i.
- glucose tolerance i.
- mineralization i.

impedance
- bioelectrical i.

imperfecta
- amelogenesis i.
- dentinogenesis i.
- fibrogenesis i.
- osteogenesis i. (OI)
- osteogenesis i. types I, II, III, IV

implant
- breast silicone i.
- endometriotic i.
- islet cell i.
- testosterone i.
- Zoladex I.

implantable
- i. biosensor
- i. glucose sensor
- i. intraperitoneal pump
- i. programmable insulin infusion pump

impotence
- erectile i.
- functional i.
- psychogenic i.
- stuttering i.

impression
- frank basilar i.

imprinting
- genomic i.

Imuran

in
- I. Charge Diabetes Control System
- i. situ hybridization
- i. vitro
- i. vitro bioassay
- i. vitro collagen invasion assay
- i. vitro fertilization (IVF)
- i. vivo
- i. vivo assessment
- i. vivo bioassay

In-111 octreotide

inactivating mutation

inactivation
- X chromosome i.

inactive
- i. agent
- i. renin concentration

inanition

inappropriate
- i. dieting
- i. hormone receptor
- i. secretion of thyroid-stimulating hormone
- i. secretion of TSH

Inapsine

incerta
- zona i.
- zone i.

incidental adrenal mass

incidentaloma
- adrenal i.
- pituitary i.

incisura
- tentorial i.

inclusion cell disease

incomplete
- i. androgen resistance
- i. cell basement membrane
- i. isosexual precocity
- i. precocious puberty
- i. testicular feminization
- i. XY gonadal dysgenesis

incompletely pneumatized sphenoid sinus

incontinence

increased
- i. adenyl cyclase activity

NOTES

increased *(continued)*
i. aldosterone excretion
i. fibrinolysis
incretin
i. effect
incubation
chase i.
pulse i.
indapamide
indentation
clival i.
Inderal
I. LA
index
baseline body mass i.
body mass i. (BMI)
cardiac i.
free T_4 i. (FT_4I)
free thyroxine i. (FTI, FT4I, FT_4I, FT4i)
glycemic i.
hemizona assay i. (HZI)
karyopyknotic i. (KPI)
Ki67 i.
maturation i. (MI)
penile brachial i.
ponderal i.
Psychological Well Being I.
quantitative insulin sensitivity check i. (QUICKI)
Indian hedgehog
indifferent gonad
indium-111
i. octreotide imaging
i. pentetreotide
Indocin
I. I.V. Injection
I. SR Oral
Indocollyre
indole
i. hormone
indoleamine
i. 2,3-dioxygenase (IDO)
indomethacin
Indotec
indoxyl sulfate
induced hypermetabolic state
inducer T lymphocyte
inducible
i. cAMP early repressor (ICER)
i. cyclic adenosine monophosphate early repressor (ICER)
induction
ovulation i.
infancy
diencephalic syndrome of i.
idiopathic hypercalcemia of i.
minipuberty of i.
persistent hyperinsulinemic hypoglycemia of i. (PHHI)
infantile
i. agranulocytosis
i. cortical hyperostosis
i. cystinosis
i. embryonic carcinoma
i. hypercalcemia
i. osteopetrosis
infantilism
sexual i.
infantility
sexual i.
infarction
diabetic myocardial i.
pituitary i.
postpartum pituitary i.
infected pancreatic necrosis
infection
congenital cytomegalovirus i.
cryptococcal i.
Diabetes Mellitus Insulin-Glucose Infusion in Acute Myocardial I. (DIGAMI)
filarial i.
mycotic i.
sexually transmitted i. (STI)
i. stone
viral i.
infectious
i. adrenalitis
i. mononucleosis
i. thyroiditis
InFeD
inferior
i. pancreaticoduodenal artery
i. parathyroid artery
i. parathyroid gland
i. petrosal sinus
i. petrosal sinus sampling (IPSS)
i. phrenic artery
i. thyroid artery
infertile
i. male
i. male syndrome
infertility
anovulatory i.
cervical factor i.
eugonadal i.
female i.
male i.
primary i.
secondary i.
infiltrate
exuberant neutrophilic i.
inflammatory cell i.

I

infiltrating
i. ductal carcinoma
i. lobular carcinoma
infiltration
lymphocytic i.
infiltrative
i. dermopathy
i. disorder
i. eye sign
i. ophthalmopathy
i. orbitopathy
inflammation
granulomatous i.
sarcoidlike noncaseating granulomatous i.
inflammatory
i. cell
i. cell infiltrate
i. cytokine
i. lesion
influence
inotropic i.
influenzae
influx
iodide i.
net calcium i.
infra
vide i.
infraclavicular fat pad
infradian rhythm
infrahyoid
i. muscle
infundibular
i. eminence
i. pouch
i. process
i. recess
i. stalk
infundibularis
pars i.
infundibulohypophysial region
infundibulum
i. eminence
pars i.
infuser
button i.
infusion
bombesin i.
continuous regional arterial i. (CRAI)
continuous subcutaneous insulin i. (CSII)
intracarotid artery i.
somatostatin i.
inhaled insulin
inheritance
Mendelian i.
sex-linked i.
X-linked i.
inherited hormone resistance syndrome
inhibin
i. A
i. B
i. hormone
inhibition
aromatase i.
feedback i.
oligonucleotide i.
short-loop i.
inhibitor
aldose reductase i. (ARI)
allosteric i.
alpha-glucosidase i.
angiotensin-converting enzyme i.
aromatase i.
calcineurin i.
carbonic anhydrase i.
gamma-aminobutyric acid transaminase i.
glucose oxidase i.
glucosidase i.
glycoprotein crystal growth i. (CGI)
hepatic hydroxymethylglutaryl coenzyme A reductase i.
HMG-CoA reductase i.
luteinization i.
mammary-derived growth i. (MGDI)
monoamine oxidase i.
nonergot long-acting prolactin i.
oocyte meiotic i.
phosphodiesterase i.
plasminogen activator i. (PAI)
postreceptor i.
prereceptor i.
selective serotonin reuptake i. (SSRI)
serine protease i. (SERPIN)
vascular endothelial cell growth i. (VEGI)
wheat amylase i. (WAI)
inhibitor-1
plasminogen activator i. (PAI-1)

NOTES

inhibitor-2
inhibitory
i. factor
i. guanine nucleotide binding regulatory protein
i. hormone
i. receptor (R_i)
i. response element (IRE)
i. transmitter
inhomogeneity
inhomogeneous
i. texture
injectable multiple vitamin
injection
Adlone I.
A-hydroCort I.
Amcort I.
A-methaPred I.
Andro-L.A. I.
Andropository I.
AquaMEPHYTON I.
Aristocort Forte I.
Aristocort Intralesional I.
Aristospan Intraarticular I.
Aristospan Intralesional I.
Astramorph PF I.
Ben-Allergin-50 I.
Celestone Phosphate I.
Cel-U-Jec I.
Cleocin Phosphate I.
Decadron I.
Delatestryl I.
depAndro I.
depGynogen I.
depMedalone I.
Depo-Estradiol I.
Depogen I.
Depoject I.
Depo-Medrol I.
Depopred I.
Depo-Provera I.
Depotest I.
Depo-Testosterone I.
Dihyrex I.
Dilaudid I.
Dilaudid-HP I.
Dinate I.
Dioval I.
D-Med I.
Dramilin I.
Duralone I.
Duramorph I.
Duratest I.
Durathate I.
Dymenate I.
Estra-L I.
Estro-Cyp I.
Everone I.
Gynogen L.A. I.
Hectorol I.
Histerone I.
Hybolin Improved I.
Hydrate I.
Hydrocortone Acetate I.
Hydrocortone Phosphate I.
Hyzine-50 I.
Indocin I.V. I.
intracavernosal i.
intracytoplasmic sperm i. (ICSI)
Kenaject I.
Kenalog I.
Key-Pred I.
Key-Pred-SP I.
Konakion I.
Lyphocin I.
Marmine I.
Medralone I.
M-Prednisol I.
Neucalm-50 I.
Orinase Diagnostic I.
Osmitrol I.
paricalcitol i.
pegvisomant for i.
percutaneous bone marrow i.
percutaneous fine-needle ethanol i. (PFNEI)
Phenazine I.
Phenergan I.
Prednisol TBA I.
Prorex I.
Quiess I.
i. site
i. site rotation
Solu-Cortef I.
Solu-Medrol I.
Sublimaze I.
Tac-3 I.
Tac-40 I.
Tesamone I.
Triam-A I.
Triam Forte I.
Triamonide I.
Tri-Kort I.
Trilog I.
Trilone I.
Triostat I.
Trisoject I.
Ureaphil I.
Vancocin I.
Vancoled I.
Vistacon-50 I.
Vistaquel I.
Vistaril I.
Vistazine I.
zoledronic acid for i.

I

injector
jet i.
injury
demyelination i.
hypoxic brain i.
osmotic cell i.
parenchymal brain i.
pituitary-hypothalamic i.
radiation i.
thermal i.
vascular i.
innervate
innervated
innervation
somatostatinergic i.
innominate vein
Innovar
inorganic
i. iodide
i. orthophosphate (P_i)
i. phosphate
i. pyrophosphate
inositol
i. diphosphate
i. phosphate pathway
i. triphosphate (IP3)
i. 1,4,5-triphosphate (IP3)
inositophosphoglycan
inotropic
i. bipyridine
i. glutamate receptor antagonist
i. influence
^{111}In-pentetreotide
input
excitatory i.
insecticide
organochlorine i.
insemination
intrauterine i. (IUI)
therapeutic donor i. (TDI)
insensate feet
insensitivity
congenital androgen i.
glucocorticoid i.
growth hormone i.
partial androgen i.
insert
Estring vaginal i.
insidious proptosis
insipidus
acquired diabetes i.
central diabetes i. (CDI)
cranial diabetes i.
diabetes i.
dipsogenic diabetes i.
familial central diabetes i.
familial nephrogenic diabetes i.
hereditary nephrogenic diabetes i.
hypothalamic diabetes i.
idiopathic diabetes i.
nephrogenic diabetes i. (NDI)
neurogenic diabetes i.
neurohypophysial diabetes i.
peripheral diabetes i.
permanent diabetes i.
prolonged diabetes i.
renal form of diabetes i.
transient diabetes i.
triphasic diabetes i.
X-linked diabetes i.
insole
Plastazote i.
instability
microsatellite i.
Insta-Glucose
instant glucose
InstantPlus
Accu-Chek I.
instrumentation
antegrade i.
retrograde i.
insufficiency
adrenal i.
central adrenocortical i.
chronic renal i. (CRI)
corpus luteum i. (CLI)
exocrine pancreatic i. (EPI)
hepatic i.
idiopathic adrenal i.
Leydig cell i.
luteal phase i.
panadrenal i.
pancreatis i.
parathyroid i.
primary adrenocortical i.
pseudocorpus luteum i.
renal i.
tertiary adrenal i.
Insuflon
insular
i. carcinoma
i. pattern
insulin
i. absorption

NOTES

insulin *(continued)*
i. action
i. allergy
i. analog
i. antagonism
i. antagonist
aspart i.
autoantibodies against i.
i. autoantibody (IAA)
bedtime i.
beef i.
i. binding
i. binding affinity
biosynthetic human i.
bovine i.
i. clearance
i. concentration
i. deficiency
endogenous i.
i. factitial hypoglycemia
fast-acting i.
i. gene
i. gene transcription factor
i. gene transfer
GH i.
i. glargine
i. growth factor
i. growth factor-binding protein
i. growth factor-binding protein type 1–6
growth hormone i.
human i.
immunoreactive i.
i. infusion rate
i. infusion specialist
inhaled i.
intermediate-acting i.
intranasal i.
intraperitoneal i.
isophane i.
i. lack
Lente I.
i. level
i. lipoatrophy
i. lipodystrophy
Lispro I.
i. lispro
long-acting i.
long-lasting i.
nasal i.
neutral protamine Hagedorn i.
NPH i.
Omnican Piston syringe for i.
ophthalmic administration of i.
oral administration of i.
i. pen
i. phosphorylation cascade
plasma i.
porcine i.
pork i.
premixed i.
i. preparation
i. preprohormone
i. promoter factor-1 (IPF-1)
protamine zinc i.
i. protease
i. pump therapy
purified pork i. (PPI)
i. receptor (IR)
i. receptor antibody
i. receptor gene
i. receptor knockout (IRKO)
i. receptor-related receptor (IRR)
i. receptor substrate (IRS)
i. receptor substrate-1 (IRS-1)
i. receptor substrate-2 (IRS-2)
i. receptor substrate protein (IRS-protein)
recombinant human i.
rectal administration of i.
Regular I.
Regular Purified Pork I.
i. resistance
i. secretagogue
i. secretion
i. secretory defect
i. secretory response (ISR)
semisynthetic i.
i. sensitivity
i. sensitizer
i. shock
short-acting i.
i. signaling pathway
i. surrogate
i. surrogate value
synthetic human i.
i. target tissue
i. tolerance test (ITT)
Ultralente i.
Velosulin BR i.

insulinase
insulin-autoimmune syndrome
insulin-combination regimen
insulin/C-peptide molar ratio
insulin-degrading enzyme (IDE)
insulin-dependent diabetes (IDD)
insulin-dependent diabetes mellitus (IDDM)
insulinemia
Insulin-Free World Foundation
insulin-induced
i.-i. glucose
i.-i. receptor downregulation
i.-i. suppression of glucagon
i.-i. systemic hypoglycemia

insulinlike
i. activity (ILA)
i. growth factor (IGF)
i. growth factor-1 (IGF1)
i. growth factor-2 (IGF2)
i. growth factor-binding protein (IGFBP)
i. growth factor-binding protein-1 (IGFBP-1)
i. growth factor-binding protein-2 (IGFBP-2)
i. growth factor-binding protein-3 (IGFBP-3)
i. growth factor-binding protein-4 (IGFBP-4)
i. growth factor-binding protein-5 (IGFBP-5)
i. growth factor-binding protein-6 (IGFBP-6)
i. growth factor-binding protein protease
i. growth factor-I (IGF-I)
i. growth factor-II
i. growth factor-II gene
i. growth factor-II receptor (IGF-IIR)
i. growth factor-II receptor gene
i. immunoreactivity
insulin-mediated glucose uptake
insulinogenesis
insulinoma
calcified malignant i.
i. cell
malignant i.
Whipple trial of i.
insulinomimetic effect
insulinopathy
insulinopenia
insulinopenic
i. diabetes mellitus
i. impaired glucose tolerance
insulinotropininsulin resistance syndrome
insulin-producing cell
insulin-receptor
i.-r. autoantibody
insulin-resistance syndrome
insulin-resistant syndrome X
insulin-sensitive enzyme
insulin-stimulated
i.-s. autophosphorylation
i.-s. glucose transport
insulitis
int2
integration gene 2
intact
i. parathyroid hormone
i. thirst mechanism
intake
caloric i.
dietary calcium i.
fluid i.
Intal
integration gene 2 (int2)
integrative model of seasonality
integrin
i. alpha v beta 3
alpha v beta 3 vitronectin receptor i.
intense thirst
intensifier
image i.
intensive
i. insulin administration
i. therapy
intention tremor
interaction
agonist-receptor i.
cell-bone matrix i.
ligand-receptor i.
sperm-cervical mucus i.
interassay
intercalated
i. cell
i. lamella
intercellular
i. adhesion molecule (ICAM)
i. adhesion molecule-1 (ICAM-1)
interception
interconversion
intercostal nerve
interdental spacing
interdigitate
interferon (IFN)
i. therapy
interferon-alpha (IFN-α)
recombinant i.-a. (rIFN-α)
interferon-alpha$_1$ (IFN-α_1)
interferon-alpha-induced thyroiditis
interferon-beta (IFN-β)
interferon-epsilon (IFN-ε)
interferon-gamma (IFN-γ)
interferon-omega (IFN-ω)
interfollicular stroma

NOTES

interieur
milieu i.
interleukin (IL)
i. growth factor I (IGF-I)
i. type 2 receptor
interleukin-1 (IL-1)
i. receptor antagonist (IL-1RA)
interleukin-2 (IL-2)
interleukin-3 (IL-3)
interleukin-4 (IL-4)
interleukin-5 (IL-5)
interleukin-6 (IL-6)
interleukin-7 (IL-7)
interleukin-8 (IL-8)
interleukin-9 (IL-9)
interleukin-10 (IL-10)
interleukin-11 (IL-11)
interleukin-12 (IL-12)
interleukin-13 (IL-13)
interleukin-14 (IL-14)
interleukin-16 (IL-16)
interleukin-17 (IL-17)
interleukin-18 (IL-18)
interleukin-1-alpha (IL-1-alpha)
interleukin-1-beta (IL-1-beta)
interlobular fibrosis
intermedia
massa i.
pars i.
intermediary
G-protein i.
intermediate
i. lymphocytic lymphoma
i. nucleus
phosphorylated glycolytic i.
i. pituitary lobe
postreceptor signaling i.
i. trophoblast
intermediate-acting insulin
intermediate-density lipoprotein (IDL)
intermediolateral
i. cell column
i. gray column
intermolecular dityrosine bridge
interna
hyperostosis frontalis i.
theca i.
internal
i. capsule
i. intraperitoneal insulin infusion pump
i. jugular vein (IJV)
i. jugular vein sampling
i. milieu
i. ophthalmoplegia
i. urethra
international
I. Atomic Energy Agency (IAEA)
I. Council for Control of Iodine Deficiency Disorder (ICCIDD)
I. Diabetes Federation
I. Diabetes Immunotherapy Group
i. unit (IU)
interosseous atrophy
interpeduncular
i. chiasmatic cistern
i. fossa
interphase
Interpore
interposition method
interpositum
velum i.
interrelationship
hormone-fuel i.
interstitial
i. cell-stimulating hormone (ICSH)
i. edema
i. fluid (ISF)
i. fluid compartment
i. hyperthermic technique
i. osmolality
i. urea
interstitium
renal medullary i.
intertrabecular space
intertrigo
interval
QKd i.
QT i.
intervening peptide (IP)
intervillous space
intestinal
i. bypass
i. fistula
i. lymphectasia
intolerance
alcohol i.
carbohydrate i.
fructose i.
galactose i.
glucose i.
heat i.
hereditary fructose i.
lysinuric protein i.
intorsion
intoxication
acute water i.
aluminum i.
chronic water i.
syndrome of water i.
vitamin A i.
vitamin D i.
water i.
intoxification
metal i.

I

intraabdominal
i. adiposity
i. testis
intraadrenal pressure
intraamniotic
intracarotid artery infusion
intracavernosal injection
intracavernous venous connection
intracellular
i. calcium
i. cAMP level
i. cyclic adenosine monophosphate level
i. effector enzyme
i. fluid (ICF)
i. function
i. homeostasis
i. killing
i. lysosomal membrane
i. messenger
i. metabolic process
i. receptor
i. solute
i. store
intracellulare
Mycobacterium i.
intracranial
i. hyperation
i. hypertension (IH)
intracrine
i. action
intractable vomiting
intracystic
i. radiation therapy
i. radiotherapy
intracytoplasmic
i. oncocytic change
i. sperm injection (ICSI)
intraductal
i. mucinous hyperplasia
i. oncocytic papillary neoplasm (IOPN)
i. pancreatic adenoma
i. papillary mucinous neoplasm (IPNM)
i. papilloma
i. ultrasound (IDUS)
intragastric balloon
intraglandular
i. fibrous septa
i. lymphatic network
intrahepatic
i. bile duct
i. cholestasis
intrahistocompatibility locus antigen recombination
intra-HLA recombination
intrahypophyseal
i. portal vessel
i. pressure
intralesional fluorinated steroid
intralobular
i. duct
i. fibrosis
intramembranous
i. bone
i. ossification
intramitochondrial compartment
Intra-Mix
Genotropin 5.8-mg I.-M.
intramural uterine part
intramuscular
i. immune globulin
i. testosterone
intranasal
i. desmopressin
i. insulin
intraocular pressure
intraoperative
i. radiotherapy
i. ultrasound (IOUS)
intraovarian
i. regulator
i. rest
intrapancreatic calculus
intrapenile nitric oxide
intraperitoneal
i. insulin
i. lavage
i. reinfusion
intrapituitary
i. adenoma
intrasellar
i. adenohypophyseal neuronal choristoma
i. adenoma
i. cavity
i. cystic lesion
i. gangliocytoma
i. hydatid cyst
i. pressure
i. tuberculoma
intratesticular adrenal rest

NOTES

intrathoracic
i. goiter
i. goitrous component
intrathyroglobulin iodotyrosine coupling reaction
intrathyroidal primary
intrathyroid iodide concentration
intraurethral alprostadil
intrauterine
i. device (IUD)
i. growth retardation (IUGR)
i. insemination (IUI)
intravaginal
i. dose
i. estrogen
intravascular
i. compartment
i. volume
intravenous
i. glucose tolerance test (IVGTT)
i. immunoglobulin (IVIg)
i. pamidronate
i. pyelogram
i. urography
intraviral microscopy
intrinsic
i. gut neuron
i. response
intron
invasion
basophilic cell i.
i. suppressive factor
invasive
i. ductal carcinoma (IDC)
i. fibrous thyroiditis
i. hormonally active pituitary adenoma
i. hormonally inactive pituitary adenoma
i. macroprolactinoma
i. prolactinoma
Inventory
Minnesota Multiphasic Personality I. (MMPI)
inversus
situs i.
involute
involution
lymph node i.
splenic i.
thymic i.
involutional osteoporosis
inward-directed voltage-gated Ca^{2+} channel
inward-rectifying K^+-channel 6.2 (K_{ir}6.2)
iodide
i. channel
i. deficiency
i. efflux
fluorescent i.
i. goiter
i. influx
inorganic i.
potassium i.
i. pump
saturated solution of potassium i. (SSKI)
supersaturated potassium i. (SSKI)
i. symporter
i. transport
i. transport defect
i. trap
i. trapping
i. trapping function
iodide-127
iodinase enzyme
iodinated
i. contrast dye
i. contrast media
i. glycerol
iodination
thyroglobulin i.
iodine
butanol-extractable i.
i. deficiency
i. 131-metaiodobenzylguanidine (^{131}I-MIBG)
i. organification defect
polyvinylpyrrolidone i.
radioactive i. (^{131}I, RAI)
i. release
i. tincture
iodine-123 (^{123}I)
iodine-125 (^{125}I)
iodine-127 (^{127}I)
iodine-131 (^{131}I)
i. isotope
i. therapy
i. total body scan (^{131}I-TBS)
iodine-deficiency
i.-d. disorder (IDD)
i.-d. goiter
iodine-deficient goiter
iodine-induced
i.-i. hyperthyroidism (IIH)
i.-i. hypothyroidism
i.-i. thyrotoxicosis
iodine-perchlorate discharge test
iodine-replete goitrous population
iodine-trapping defect
iodism
iodization
universal salt i. (USI)
iodized oil
iodoacetate
iodoalbumin

iodoamino acid
iodocholesterol
^{131}I-labeled i.
i. scan
iodoglibenclamide
iodolipid compound
Iodo-Niacin
Iodopen
iodopeptid
iodophenoxyl group
iodoprotein
iodothyronine
i. coupling
i. deiodinase
i. metabolism
i. ring
iodothyronine-binding immunoglobulin
iodothyronine metabolism
iodotyrosine
i. coupling
i. coupling defect
i. dehalogenase
i. dehalogenase defect
radioiodinated i.
iodotyrosine-specific deiodinase
iodotyrosyl
ion
calcium i.
carbonate i.
i. channel
citrate i.
divalent i.
i. exchange chromatography
hydrogen i.
isocitrate i.
phosphate i.
potassium i. (K^+)
Ionamin
ion-exchange resin
ionic
i. calcium
i. strength
i. transport
ionized
i. calcium concentration
i. calcium level
ionizing radiation
ionomycin
ionophore
calcium i.
ion-selective electrode
iontophoretic sampling procedure
iopanoate
iopanoic
i. acid
Iophen
IOPN
intraductal oncocytic papillary neoplasm
IOUS
intraoperative ultrasound
IP
intervening peptide
IP3
inositol triphosphate
inositol 1,4,5-triphosphate
IPF-1
insulin promoter factor-1
IPNM
intraductal papillary mucinous neoplasm
ipodate
sodium i.
ipratropium
i. and albuterol
ipriflavone
ipsilateral
i. contraction
i. paramesonephric duct
IPSS
inferior petrosal sinus sampling
iPTH
immunoreactive parathyroid hormone
IR
insulin receptor
Ircon
IRE
inhibitory response element
irides
bicolored i.
iridium
heterochromia i.
IRKO
insulin receptor knockout
IRMA
immunoradiometric assay
iron (Fe)
i. clearance
i. deposition
i. dextran complex
i. overload
Prussian blue stain for i.
i. storage disease
i. turnover
iron-binding protein

NOTES

IRR
insulin receptor-related receptor
irradiation
childhood head and neck i.
cranial i.
fractionated linear accelerator-based i.
pituitary i.
irrigation
therapeutic i.
IRS
insulin receptor substrate
IRS-1
insulin receptor substrate-1
IRS-2
insulin receptor substrate-2
IRS-protein
insulin receptor substrate protein
ISAtx247
ischemia
diffuse renal i.
skeletal muscle i.
ischemic necrosis
ischiocavernosus
i. muscle
ISF
interstitial fluid
Ishikawa cytodiagnostic technique
islet
i. alpha-cell
i. amyloid polypeptide (IAPP)
i. autoantigen
i. autoimmunity
i. beta-cell
i. beta-cell hyperinsulinemia
capsule of i.
i. cell
i. cell adenoma
i. cell adenomatosis
I. Cell Antibody Registry of Users Study (ICARUS)
i. cell antigen (ICA)
i. cell carcinoma
i. cell implant
i. cell surface antibody (ICSA)
i. cell transplant
i. cell transplantation
i. cell tumor
i. of Langerhans
mantle i.
pseudoatrophic i.
i. transplantation
i. xenograft
Isletest
I. ICA kit
isletitis
Ismotic
isoandrosterone
isobologram analysis
iso-B prolactin
isobutyric acid
isocalorically substituted diet
isocaproate
isochromosome
isocitrate ion
isodisomic chromosome
isoechoic
isoelectric focusing
isoenzyme
brain i.
carbonic anhydrase II i.
4-galactosyltransferase i. II
Galtose i. II
isoetharine
Arm-a-Med i.
Dey-Lute i.
isoflavone
soy i.
isoform
fibronectin peptide i.
melanocortin receptor i.
thyroid hormone nuclear receptor i.
isoform-specific thyroid hormone receptor
isohormone
isointense
isokinetic dynamometer
isolated
i. familial somatotropinoma
i. gonadotropin deficiency
i. growth hormone deficiency (IGHD)
i. growth hormone deficiency type IB (IGHD-IB)
i. growth hormone deficiency type II (IGHD-II)
i. growth hormone deficiency type III (IGHD-III)
i. hypopituitarism
isoleucine
peptide histidine i. (PHI)
i. transaminase
isomerase
i. dehydrogenase deficiency
disulfide i.
protein disulfide i. (PDI)
triose isomerase (TIM)
isometric knee extensor strength
isoniazid
isoosmolar semielemental formula
isopeptide
endothelin i.
isophane insulin
isoprenoid

isoproterenol
Arm-a-Med i.
Dey-Dose i.
Isoptin
isosexual
i. precocious puberty
i. precocity
i. pubertal development
isosmotic
isosorbide
isothiocyanate
4,4′-di-isothiocyanatostilbene-2,2′-disulfonic acid (DIDS)
isotonic
isotonicity
isotope
i. dilution
gold-198 radioactive i.
^{131}I i.
iodine-131 i.
i. scanning
yttrium-90 radioactive i.
isotretinoin
isovaleric
i. acid
i. acidemia
isovaleryl-CoA dehydrogenase
isovalerylglycine
isoxsuprine
isozyme
ISR
insulin secretory response
ISS
idiopathic short stature
isthmectomy
isthmus
thyroid i.
i. uteri
Isuprel
^{131}I-TBS
iodine-131 total body scan
ITP
idiopathic thrombocytopenic purpura
itraconazole
I-Tropine
ITT
insulin tolerance test
IU
international unit
IUD
intrauterine device
Progestasert IUD
IUGR
intrauterine growth retardation
IUI
intrauterine insemination
IVF
in vitro fertilization
IVGTT
intravenous glucose tolerance test
IVIg
intravenous immunoglobulin

NOTES

isotope *(continued)*
i. scanning
yttrium-90 radioactive i.
isotretinoin
isovaleric
i. acid
i. acidemia
isovaleryl-CoA dehydrogenase
isovalerylglycine
isoxsuprine
isozyme
ISR
insulin secretory response
ISS
idiopathic short stature
isthmectomy
isthmus
thyroid i.
i. uteri
Isuprel
^{131}I-TBS
iodine-131 total body scan
ITP
idiopathic thrombocytopenic purpura
itraconazole
I-Tropine
ITT
insulin tolerance test
IU
international unit
IUD
intrauterine device
Progestasert IUD
IUGR
intrauterine growth retardation
IUI
intrauterine insemination
IV
hexokinase IV
osteogenesis imperfecta types I, II, III, IV
Sillence type I, II, III, IV
IVF
in vitro fertilization
IVGTT
intravenous glucose tolerance test
IVIg
intravenous immunoglobulin
IX
factor IX

Jaa-Prednisone
Jackson-Weiss syndrome
Jadelle
Jak
Janus kinase
Jak1
Janus kinase 1
Jak1 kinase
Jak2
Janus kinase 2
Jak2 kinase
Jannetta
bayoneted J. microdissector
45-degree angled J. microdissector
Jansen metaphyseal chondrodysplasia (JMC)
Janus
J. kinase (Jak)
J. kinase 1 (Jak1)
J. kinase 2 (Jak2)
Jarcho cannula
jaundice
cholestatic j.
JDF
Juvenile Diabetes Foundation
jejunocolic anastomosis
jejunoileal bypass
jejunostomy
needle catheter j.
jejunum
jelly
Wharton j.
Jenest-28
Jerusalem syndrome
jet injector
Jew
Ashkenazi J.
JG
juxtaglomerular
JG cell
JGA
juxtaglomerular apparatus
JMC
Jansen metaphyseal chondrodysplasia
JNK
Jun kinase
JOD
juvenile-onset diabetes
Jod-Basedow, jodbasedow
J.-B. disease
J.-B. effect
J.-B. mechanism
J.-B. phenomenon
Joffroy sign
Johanson-Blizzard syndrome
joint
apophyseal j.
Charcot j.
cricothyroid j.
j. hyperextensibility
Joslin Diabetes Center
Jost model
Jr.
Caltrate J.
J-shaped sella
J-type diabetes
jugular
j. bulb
j. chain
juice
pancreatic j.
pure pancreatic j. (PPJ)
junction
adherens j.
gap j.
hypothalamic-midbrain j.
mesodiencephalic j.
ribosome-membrane j.
tight j.
ureteropelvic j.
ureterovesical j.
junctional
j. arrhythmia
j. scotoma
Junior Strength Motrin
Jun kinase (JNK)
Jurkat cell
juvenile
j. Austin-type sulfatidosis
j. cystinosis
J. Diabetes Foundation (JDF)
j. hypothyroidism
j. papillomatosis
j. pilocytic astrocytoma
juvenile-onset
j.-o. diabetes (JOD)
j.-o. diabetes mellitus
juxtacrine
j. factor
juxtaglomerular (JG)
j. afferent arteriole
j. apparatus (JGA)
j. cell
j. function
j. stretch receptor
juxtamembrane
juxtathyroidal tissue
juxtathyroid node

K
potassium
cathepsin K
neuromedin K
Pen-Vee K
substance K
K^+
potassium ion
K_1
vitamin K_1
K_2
vitamin K_2
K_7
vitamin K_7
K_5
vitamin K_5
K_6
vitamin K_6
K_d
equilibrium dissociation constant
K_a
equilibrium association constant
K_{ir}6.2
inward-rectifying K^+-channel 6.2
Kabi International Growth Study (KIGS)
Kahn syndrome
kainate receptor channel
KAL gene
Kalgutkar
KALIG-1
Kallmann syndrome interval gene 1
kaliuresis
kaliuretic stimulus
kallidin
desArg k.
kallikrein
k. activator
glandular k.
human kidney glandular k.-1
plasma k.
k. protease
tissue k.
kallikrein-kinin system
Kallmann
K. syndrome
K. syndrome interval gene 1 (KALIG-1)
kansasii
Mycobacterium k.
kaolin
Kaposi
K. sarcoma
K. sarcoma human growth factor (hFGF)
Kapseals
Thera-Combex H-P K.
kaput
circadian locomotor output cycles k. (CLOCK)
Kartagener syndrome
Karydakis
K. flap
K. operation
K. technique
karyopyknotic index (KPI)
karyotype
classical XO k.
karyotyping
katacalcin (KC)
Kaybovite-1000
Kayexalate
kb
kilobase
KC
katacalcin
Kcal
kilocalorie
KCNJ1
potassium inwardly-rectifying channel, subfamily J, member 1
KCNJ1 gene
^{40}K counting
9-kDA
calbindin 9-k.
kDa
kilodalton
8-kDa protein
37-kDa protein
150-kDa ternary complex
Kearns-Sayre
K.-S. disease
K.-S. syndrome
K_m effect
Keflex
Keftab
Kell antigen genotyping
Kelly clamp
keloid formation
Kenacort Oral
Kenaject Injection
Kenalog Injection
Kennedy
K. disease
K. syndrome
Kenney-Caffey syndrome
keratan sulfate
keratin
acellular desquamated k.

keratin *(continued)*
k. content
wet k.
keratinization
keratinocyte
k. growth factor (KGF)
keratitis
exposure k.
keratoconjunctivitis
keratography
keratohyaline granule
keratopathy
band k.
keratosis
palmar k.
palmoplantar k.
k. pilaris
plantar k.
Kerrison rongeur
Kestrone
ketamine adduct
ketoacid disorder
ketoacidosis
alcoholic k.
diabetic k. (DKA)
ketoaciduria
branch chain k.
ketoconazole
3-keto-desogestrel
ketogenesis
ketogenic
k. steroid
17-k. steroid
keto group
ketone
k. body
ketonemia
ketonuria
ketoprofen
17-ketoreductase
ketorolac tromethamine
ketosis
KetoSite test
ketosteroid
17-ketosteroid
17-k. reductase (17-KR)
17-k. reductase deficiency
urinary 17-k.
3-ketothiolase deficiency
ketotic hypoglycemia
keyhole
MacCarty k.
Key-Pred Injection
Key-Pred-SP Injection
kg
kilogram
KGF
keratinocyte growth factor
Ki
antibody Ki
Ki67
K. grade
K. index
kidney
pancreas after k. (PAK)
simultaneous pancreas-k. (SPK)
KIGS
Kabi International Growth Study
killer
lymphokine-activated k. (LAK)
natural k. (NK)
killing
bactericidal k.
intracellular k.
kilobase (kb)
kilocalorie (Kcal)
kilodalton (kDa)
kilogram (kg)
osmoles per k. (Osm/kg)
Kimmelstiel-Wilson nodule
kinase
activinlike receptor k.
AMP-activated protein k. (AMPK)
beta-adrenergic receptor k. (βARK)
Bruton tyrosine k. (BTK)
casein K. I, II
calcium-dependent protein k.
calmodulin-dependent protein k. (CaM-kinase)
carboxyl k.
cGMP-dependent protein k.
conserved helix-loop-helix ubiquitous k. (CHUK)
creatine k. (CK)
cyclic guanosine 3′,5′-monophosphate-dependent protein k.
cyclin-dependent k. (CDK, Cdk)
cytokinin-regulated k. (Crk)
cytokinin-regulated k. II (CrkII)
cytokinin-regulated k. L (CrkL)
extracellularly regulated k. (ERK)
extracellular-regulated k.
extracellular signal-regulated k. (ERK)
extracellular signal related k.
glycerol k.
herpes simplex virus thymidine k. (HSV-TK)
Jak1 k.
Jak2 k.
Janus k. (Jak)
Janus k. 1 (Jak1)
Janus k. 2 (Jak2)
Jun k. (JNK)
MAP k.
MAP/ERK k. (MEK)

MEK k. (MEKK)
mitogen-activated protein k. (MAPK)
MLC k. (MLCK)
myosin light chain k. (MLCK)
NAD k.
periodically fluctuating protein k. (PFK)
phosphoglycerate k. (PGK)
3-phosphoinositide-dependent protein k. (PDK)
phosphorylase b k.
protein 70-kDa S6 ribosomal subunit k. (p70S6k)
protein tyrosine k. (PTK)
pyruvate k.
receptor tyrosine k. (RTK)
rhodopsin k.
tyrosine k.
tyrosine k.-2 (Tyk-2)

3′-kinase
phosphatidylinositol 3′-k. (PI3-K)

kinase-3
glycogen synthase k. (GSK3)

kinase-deficient activin receptor

Kindred
Bercu patient of K. S

kindreds
Canadian-Dutch Mennonite k.

kinematics
sperm k.

kinin

kininase
k. I
k. II

kininogen

kit
Isletest ICA k.
One Touch Fast Take meter k.

***kit* oncogene**

Klebsiella pneumoniae

Kleine-Levin syndrome

Klenow fragment

Klimodien

Klinefelter syndrome

Klippel-Trenaunay-Weber syndrome

Klüver-Bucy syndrome

Kmuna trial

Kniest dysplasia

Kniest-Stickle dysplasia

Knife
Gamma K.
Leksell Gamma K.
model U Gamma K.

knockout
insulin receptor k. (IRKO)

knot
cystine k.

Knudson
K. model of tumor suppression gene
K. two-hit model of tumorigenesis

Kobberling-Dunnigan syndrome

Kocher-Debré-Sémélaigne syndrome

Kolephrin GG/DM

Kombu

Konakion Injection

Kornchenzellen cell

Korotkoff sound

Kozak consensus translation initiation sequence

K-Phos Neutral tablet

KPI
karyopyknotic index

17-KR
17-ketosteroid reductase

Krabbe disease

Krebs-Ringer solution

Krev-1 gene

kringle domain

KT
Orudis KT

Kulchitsky cell

Kumetrix microneedle technology

Kupffer
K. cell
K. cell hyperplasia

kuru

Ku-Zyme HP

Kveim test

kwashiorkor
k. disease
k. syndrome

Kwelcof

kyphoscoliosis

kyphosis

Kyrle disease

kystis

Kyte-Doolittle hydropathy analysis

NOTES

L
liter
cathepsin L
L cell
Humulin L
27L
30L
40L
L_1
vitamin L_1
L_2
vitamin L_2
LA
laparoscopic adrenalectomy
Dexone LA
Inderal LA
L.A.
Dexasone L.A.
Humibid L.A.
Solurex L.A.
Theoclear L.A.
label
luminescent l.
labeling
tetracycline l.
labetalol
labial fusion agglutination
labile previtamin D_3
lack
insulin l.
lacrimal
l. gland
l. nucleus
l. system
lactacidosis
lactalbumin
lactase gene
lactate
calcium l.
l. dehydrogenase (LDH)
sodium l.
lactation
l. optic neuritis
lactational amenorrhea
lactic
l. acid
l. acidosis
l. dehydrogenase
lactiferous
l. duct
l. sinus
lactobacillus
l. acidophilus
l. bifidus
lactoferrin
lactogen
human placental l. (hPL)
placental l. (PL)
lactogenesis
lactogenic hormone
lactoglandin
lactogogue
lactose synthase
lactotrope
lactotroph
l. adenoma
l. hyperplasia
l. tumor
lactotropic hormone
lacuna
osteoclastic resorption l.
resorption l.
LADA
latent autoimmune diabetes of adults
laeve
chorion l.
laevis
Xenopus l.
lag
lid l.
lagophthalmos
lagunal hirsutism
LAK
lymphokine-activated killer
LAK cell
L-alpha-aminomethyl-encyclopropylproprionic acid
lambdoidal suture
lamella
circumferential l.
intercalated l.
lamellar bone
lamina
basal l.
dental l.
l. dura
l. propria
l. terminalis
laminated calcification
laminin (LN)
l. B1 element
l. enzyme
laminography
lampbrush state
Lanacaps
Ferralyn L.
Lanaphilic Topical
lancet
Haemolance l.
Techlite l.

L

Langerhans
L. cell
L. cell histiocyte
L. cell histiocytosis
islet of L.
Langhans cytotrophoblast
lanosterol
lanreotide
slow-release l.
lansoprazole
lanthanum-containing compound
Lantus
LAP
latency-associated peptide
liver-enriched activating protein
LAP-1
Los Angeles preservation solution 1
laparoscopic adrenalectomy (LA)
laparoscopy
lateral transabdominal l.
LAR
long-acting release
octreotide LAR
Parlodel LAR
Sandostatin LAR
large
l. fiber neuropathy
l. for gestational age (LGA)
large-needle aspiration biopsy (LNAB)
large-volume paracentesis (LVP)
L-arginine:nitric oxide pathway
Larodopa
Laron
L. disease
L. dwarfism
L. syndrome
Laron-type dwarfism (LTD)
laryngeal nerve
laryngomalacia
laryngospasm
laser
Altea MicroPor l.
argon l.
l. Doppler flowmetry
l. prostatectomy
Lasette
L. laser lancing device
Personal L.
Lasix
lasofoxifene
last menstrual period (LMP)
late
l. distal tubule
l. dumping syndrome (LDS)
l. hypocalcemia
l. hypoglycemia
l. luteal phase
l. luteal phase disorder
l. onset hydroxylase deficiency
latency-associated peptide (LAP)
latent
l. autoimmune diabetes of adults (LADA)
l. tetany
late-onset
l.-o. gynecomastia
l.-o. idiopathic chronic pancreatitis
lateral
l. aberrant thyroid
l. aberrant thyroid tissue
l. anlage
l. cricoarytenoid
l. hypothalamus
l. rectus palsy
l. retrochiasmatic area
l. thyroid anlage
l. transabdominal laparoscopy
l. zone
lateralization
pituitary tumor l.
LATS
long-acting thyroid stimulator
LATS protector
LATS-P
long-acting thyroid stimulator-protector
Laurence-Moon-Biedl syndrome
Laurence-Moon syndrome
LAV
lymphadenopathy-associated virus
lavage
bronchial l.
intraperitoneal l.
law
Hardy-Weinberg l.
Lawrence syndrome
layer
endothelial l.
Nitabuch l.
LBA_4
leukotriene B_4
LBM
lean body mass
LBW
low birth weight
LCAD
long chain acyl-CoA dehydrogenase
LCAD deficiency
LCAT
lecithin-cholesterol acyltransferase
LCAT deficiency
LCED
liquid chromatography with electrochemical detection
LCFA-CoA
long chain fatty acyl-CoA

LCHAD
long chain 3-hydroxyacyl-CoA dehydrogenase
LCHAD deficiency
LDB
ligand-binding domain
LDH
lactate dehydrogenase
LDL
low-density lipoprotein
LDL deficiency
dense LDL
LDL direct test
LDL receptor-related protein (LRP)
L-dopa test
LDS
late dumping syndrome
LDSST
low-dose short synacthen test
LE
leucine enkephalin
leader
aminoterminal l.
lead hematoxylin
leafy chorion
leaking endometrioma
lean
l. body mass (LBM)
l. mass
l. physique
l. tissue
Leber hereditary optic neuropathy
lecithin
lecithin-cholesterol acyltransferase (LCAT)
lecithin/sphingomyelin (L/S)
l. ratio
Lederplex
left
l. anterior mediastinal adenoma
l. internal mammary arteriogram
l. temporal projection
leg
bow l.
***Legionella pneumophila* pneumonia**
Leg Thing pump holder
Leiden mutation
Leigh disease
leiomyoma
early-onset uterine l.
spermatic cord l.
uterine l.
leiomyosarcoma
gastric epithelioid l.
Leishmania major
Leksell
L. Gamma Knife
L. model G stereotactic frame
Lemmel syndrome
length
erect penile l.
flaccid penile l.
penile l.
stretched penile l.
lens opacity
Lente
L. Iletin I
L. Iletin II
L. Insulin
lentiginosis syndrome
lentis
ectopia l.
Lenz-Majewski syndrome
Lep gene
leprae
Mycobacterium l.
leprechaunism
l. syndrome
leptin
l. concentration
l. deficiency
l. deficiency/resistance
l. receptor gene
leptomeninges
LES
lower esophageal sphincter
Lesch-Nyhan
L.-N. disease
L.-N. syndrome
lesion
adynamic bone l.
aplastic bone l.
benign cystic l.
blade-of-grass l.
blueberry l.
café au lait l.
chest wall l.
cortisol secreting l.
cystic bone l.
extraglandular l.
glandular l.
gummatous l.
hypophysial l.
inflammatory l.

NOTES

lesion *(continued)*
intrasellar cystic l.
low-turnover bone l.
mixed bone l.
neoplastic pathologic l.
nonneoplastic pathologic l.
osteolytic l.
pagetic bone l.
polyostotic l.
polypoid l.
rachitic-like l.
radial scar breast l.
strawberry l.
suprasellar cystic l.
trophoblastic l.
letdown
lethal
l. paroxysm
letrozole
Letterer-Siwe disease
leu-7
l. antigen
leucine
l. enkephalin (LE)
l. rich repeat (LRR)
l. zipper gene family
leucine-zipper domain
leucovorin
leucyl-beta-naphthylaminidase
leu-enkephalin
leukemia
acute lymphoblastic l.
acute lymphocytic l. (ALL)
acute myelogenous l.
adult T-cell l. (ATL)
chronic granulocytic l. (CGL)
chronic myelogenous l. (CLL)
l.-inhibiting factor (LIF)
l. inhibitory factor (LIF)
human T-cell l. type I (HTLV-1)
radiation-induced l.
leukemoid reaction
leukocyte
l. common antigen
leukocytosis
polymorphonuclear l.
leukodystrophy
globoid cell l.
metachromatic l. (MLD)
sudanophilic l.
leukoencephalitis
leukoerythroblastic anemia
leukoma
acromegaly, cutis verticis, l. (ACL)
corneal l.
leukopenia
leukorrhea
leukosis
leukotriene (LT)
l. A_4 (LTA_4)
l. B_4 (LBA_4)
l. C_4 (LTC_4)
l. D_4 (LTD_4)
l. E_4 (LTE_4)
leukovirus
leuprolide
l. acetate
levalbuterol
levamisole
levator
l. aponeurosis
l. palpebrae superioris muscle
Levbid
LeVeen shunt
level
albumin-bound testosterone l.
aldolase l.
aluminum bone l.
antithrombin III l.
antithyroperoxidase l.
basal l.
basal aluminum l.
basal plasma GH l.
basal plasma growth hormone l.
basal serum prolactin l.
bioavailable testosterone l.
cerebrospinal fluid ACE l.
cerebrospinal fluid angiotensin-converting enzyme l.
circulating estrogen l.
complement l.
C-peptide l.
cryoglobulin l.
elastase-1 l.
endothelin l.
free testosterone l.
gonadal steroid l.
homocysteine l.
hormone serum l.
insulin l.
intracellular cAMP l.
intracellular cyclic adenosine monophosphate l.
ionized calcium l.
normal gonadal steroid l.
Osteocalcin l.
plasma ACTH l.
plasma aluminum l.
plasma endothelin l.
plasma galanin l.
plasma growth hormone-releasing hormone l.
plasma homocysteine l.
plasma hormone l.
plasma insulin l.

plasma ketone l.
plasma testosterone l.
postchallenge glucose l.
preinfusion l.
procollagen l.
proinsulin l.
P-selectin l.
random cortisol l.
salivary cortisol l.
serum C-peptide l.
serum dehydroepiandrosterone sulfate l.
serum fructosamine l.
serum growth hormone l.
serum parathyroid hormone l.
sex steroid l.
somatomedin l.
somatomedin C l.
supranormal gonadal steroid l.
thyroglobulin l.
urine glucose l.
urine hydroxyproline l.

Levi-Lorain dwarf
Levlen
Levlite
levodopa
l. and carbidopa
Levo-Dromoran
levonorgesterol-releasing intrauterine device
levonorgestrel
ethinyl estradiol and l.
levonorgestrel-releasing intrauterine device
Levoprome
Levora
levormeloxifene
levorphanol
Levo-T
Levothroid
levothyroxine
free l.
l. sodium
l. suppression therapy
Levoxyl
Levsin
Levsinex
Levsin/SL
Lewis
axon response of L.
triple response of L.
LewisA
sialyl L.
Leydig
L. cell
L. cell agenesis
L. cell aplasia
L. cell hyperplasia
L. cell hypoplasia
L. cell insufficiency
L. cells of the testis
L. cell tumor
LFA-1
lymphocyte function-associated antigen-1
LGA
large for gestational age
LH
lutropin
LH-β
luteinizing hormone-beta
LH/CG
luteinizing hormone/human chorionic gonadotropin
LH-dependent androgen excess
Lhermitte-Duclos disease
LH/hCG
luteinizing hormone/human chorionic gonadotropin
LH-releasing hormone (LHRH, LH-RH, LRH)
LHRH, LH-RH, LRH
LH-releasing hormone
luteinizing hormone-releasing hormone
LHRH deficiency
libido
decreased l.
libitum
ad l.
Librax
lichen
l. myxedematosus
l. sclerosus
lichenified dermatitis
licorice-induced
l.-i. hypermineralocorticoidism
l.-i. hypertension
l.-i. hypokalemia
lid
l. fissure
l. lag
Liddle
L. syndrome
L. test

NOTES

LIF
leukemia-inhibiting factor
leukemia inhibitory factor
LifeGuide
L. glucose meter
L. System
lifestyle
sedentary l.
life-years
quality-adjusted l.-y. (QALYs)
Li-Fraumeni syndrome
ligament
Berry l.
broad l.
falciform l.
gastrohepatic l.
ovarian l.
round l.
ligamentum
l. arteriosum
l. flavum
ligand
A proliferation-inducing l. (APRIL)
4-1BB l. (4-1BBL)
l. binding determinant
CD 27 l. (CD 27L)
CD 30 l. (CD 30L)
CD 40 l. (CD 40L)
c-*mpl* l.
erb B2/HER2 l.
E-selectin l.
Fas l. (Fas-L)
osteoprotegerin l. (OPGL)
OX40 l. (OX40L)
polypeptide l.
PPAR l.
radioactive l.
TNF-related apoptosis inducing l. (TRAIL)
ligand-binding domain (LDB)
ligand-dependent action of thyroid hormone receptor
ligand-gated channel
ligand-independent
l.-i. action of thyroid hormone receptor
l.-i. stimulation
ligand-receptor
l.-r. complex
l.-r. interaction
ligase
glutamate-cysteine l.
lignan
lignin
Liliequist membrane
limb
adrenal gland l.
l. ataxia
thick ascending l. (TAL)
thickened adrenal l.
limbic
l. lobe
l. system
limbus
nasal l.
limitans
sulcus l.
limited
l. fragment proteolysis
l. joint mobility (LJM)
Limitrol-DM
linamarin
lindane
line
AtT20 pituitary cell l.
canthomeatal l.
cement l.
l. of Farré
Fischer rat thyroid l.-5 (FRTL-5)
milk l.
Muercke l.
multiple myeloma cell l.
nasotuberculum l.
pituitary cell l.
thyroid T-cell l. (TCL)
Lineac particle beam radiotherapy
lineage
chondrocytic l.
linear nevus sebaceous syndrome
linguae
foramen caecum l.
lingual
l. thyroid
l. thyroid gland
linkage
diphenyl ether l.
haplotype l.
phosphodiester l.
X-chromosome l.
linoleic acid
linomide
liothyronine
l. sodium
liotrix
LIP
liver-enriched inhibiting protein
lipase
hepatic l.
hormone sensitive l.
lipoprotein l. (LPL)
preduodenal l.
lipectomy
lipemia
postprandial l.
l. retinalis

lipid
l. cholesterol
l. myopathy
l. peroxidation
l. peroxide
l. phosphorus
l. profile
l. tumor
lipid-containing tumor
lipid-laden
l.-l. clear cell
l.-l. homogeneous adrenocortical carcinoma
l.-l. lysosome
lipid-lowering
l.-l. agent
l.-l. therapy
lipidosis
Lipitor
lipoatrophic diabetes
lipoatrophy
diabetic l.
insulin l.
lipoblast
lipocalin protein
lipocortin
lipocortin-1
lipodystrophy
insulin l.
l. syndrome
lipofuscin
lipogenesis
lipogenic enzyme
lipogranulomatosis
lipohypertrophy
diabetic l.
lipoid
l. adrenal hyperplasia
l. cell
l. cell tumor
lipolysis
lipoma
lipomatosis
retroperitoneal l.
lipophilic
l. drug
l. hormone
l. molecule
lipopolysaccharide (LPS)
lipoprotein
l. (a)
high-density l. (HDL)
high-density l. C (HDL-C)
intermediate-density l. (IDL)
l. lipase (LPL)
l. lipase deficiency
l. lipase gene
low-density l. (LDL)
l. remnant
very low density l. (VLDL)
lipoprotein(a) (Lp(a))
liposarcoma
liposomal amphotericin B
lipostatic hypothesis
lipostat mechanism
liposuction
lipotrophic diabetes
lipotropin (LPH)
Lipovite
lipoxin
lipoxygenase
l. pathway
5-lipoxygenase
5-l. activating protein (FLAP)
12-lipoxygenase
lips
bumpy l.
Liquibid
Liqui-Caps
liquid
l. chromatography with electrochemical detection (LCED)
L. Pred
Liqui-E
Liquiprin
liquor folliculi
Lisofylline (LSF)
Lispro
L. Insulin
insulin L.
lissencephaly
Listeria
listeriosis
liter (L)
osmoles per l. (Osm/L)
lithiasis
renal l.
lithium
l. carbonate
lithium-associated thyrotoxicosis
lithium-induced hypothyroidism
litholysis
lithostathine assay

NOTES

lithotripsy
shock wave l.
"little" hormone
livedo reticularis
liver
l. cancer
l. disease
l. enzyme
l. failure
fatty l.
l. phosphorylase
l. volume
liver-enriched
l.-e. activating protein (LAP)
l.-e. inhibiting protein (LIP)
living segmental donor pancreas transplantation
LJM
limited joint mobility
LKV-Drops
l-lysine
LMP
last menstrual period
LN
laminin
LNAB
large-needle aspiration biopsy
L-nitro-L-arginine methyl ester
load
phenytoin l.
phosphate l.
loading
aluminum l.
calcium l.
salt l.
lobe
anterior pituitary l.
conical l.
contralateral l.
intermediate pituitary l.
limbic l.
neural l.
pyramidal l.
lobectomy
unilateral l.
lobulated goiter
lobule
breast l.
localized myxedema
local symptom
lochia
red l.
l. rubra
Locilex
L. pexiganan acetate cream 1%
L. topical cream
locus, pl. **loci**
adenosine deaminase l.
l. ceruleus
class II HLA l.
class II human leukocyte antigen l.
diabetogenic l.
GNAS1 l.
quantitative trait l. (QTL)
Lodine
L. XL
Loestrin
L. 1.5/30
L. 1/20
logarithm
l. of odds
log dose-response relationship
LOH
loss of heterozygosity
lomefloxacin
long
l. bone
l. chain acyl-CoA dehydrogenase (LCAD)
l. chain acyl-CoA dehydrogenase deficiency
l. chain fatty acyl-CoA (LCFA-CoA)
l. chain 3-hydroxyacyl-CoA dehydrogenase (LCHAD)
l. chain 3-hydroxyacyl-CoA dehydrogenase deficiency
long-acting
l.-a. insulin
l.-a. release (LAR)
l.-a. thyroid stimulator (LATS)
l.-a. thyroid stimulator-protector (LATS-P)
longitudinal
l. growth
l. relaxation time
long-lasting insulin
long-loop
l.-l. feedback
l.-l. feedback signal
loop
advanced insulin infusion with a control l. (ADICOL)
disulfide l.
l. diuretic
feedback l.
Galen l.
hairpin l.
Henle l.
l. of Henle
negative feedback l.
neuroendocrine control l.
Looser
L. fissure
L. pseudofracture
L. zone

Lo/Ovral
loperamide
Lorcet
L. 10/650
L. Plus
Lorcet-HD
Lortab
L. ASA
Los Angeles preservation solution 1 (LAP-1)
loss
distal motor axonal l.
height l.
l. of heterozygosity (LOH)
male pattern hair l.
postimplantation embryofetal l.
receptor l.
sensorineural hearing l.
visual l.
weight l.
loss-of-function mutation
Louis-Bar and Nijmegen breakage syndrome
lovastatin
low
l. birth weight (LBW)
l. bone density
l. glycemic index diet
low-bone-turnover syndrome
low-calcium dialysate
low-density
l.-d. lipoprotein (LDL)
l.-d. lipoprotein deficiency
l.-d. lipoprotein receptor
l.-d. lipoprotein receptor-related protein (LRP)
low-dose
l.-d. dexamethasone test
l.-d. short synacthen test (LDSST)
l.-d. vaginal estrogen
Lowe
L. disease
L. syndrome
lower esophageal sphincter (LES)
low-grade astrocytoma
low-phosphorus diet
low-pressure baroreceptor
low-renin essential hypertension
low-tension glaucoma
low-triiodothyronine syndrome
low-T_3 syndrome
low-turnover
l.-t. bone lesion
l.-t. disease
l.-t. osteoporosis
Lozol
Lp(a)
lipoprotein(a)
LPH
lipotropin
LPL
lipoprotein lipase
LPS
lipopolysaccharide
LRH (*var. of* LHRH)
LRP
LDL receptor-related protein
low-density lipoprotein receptor-related protein
LRR
leucine rich repeat
L/S
lecithin/sphingomyelin
L/S ratio
LSF
Lisofylline
LT
leukotriene
LT_4
l-thyroxine
LTA_4
leukotriene A_4
LTC_4
leukotriene C_4
LTD
Laron-type dwarfism
LTD_4
leukotriene D_4
LTE_4
leukotriene E_4
l-thyroxine (LT_4)
L-triiodothyronine uptake
L-type calcium channel
lucent zone
luciferase
firefly l.
Luedde exophthalmometer
LUFS
luteinized unruptured follicle syndrome
Lufyllin
lumbar
l. cerebrospinal fluid catheter
l. spine bone density

NOTES

lumen
follicular l.
residual l.
luminal
l. brush-border membrane
l. compartment
l. endothelium
l. surface
luminescent
l. label
l. paint
lumisterol
lumone
Lunelle
lung
Wilms l.
Lupron
L. Depot
L. Depot-3 Month
L. Depot-4 Month
L. Depot-Ped
lupus
cutaneous l.
drug-induced l.
l. erythematosus
Luschka
foramina of Magendie and L.
luteal
l. cyst
l. dysfunction
l. phase
l. phase defect
l. phase deficiency
l. phase insufficiency
luteectomy
lutein
l. cell
granulosa l.
luteinalis
hyperreactio l.
luteinization
l. inhibitor
premature l.
l. stimulant
luteinization-inhibiting factor
luteinized
l. theca cell
l. unruptured follicle syndrome (LUFS)
luteinizing
l. hormone-beta (LH-β)
l. hormone beta core fragment
l. hormone/chorionic gonadotropin (LH/CG) receptor
l. hormone/human chorionic gonadotropin (LH/CG, LH/hCG)
l. hormone receptor
l. hormone-releasing hormone (LHRH, LH-RH, LRH)
l. hormone-releasing hormone deficiency
l. hormone-secreting tumor
luteinizing hormone-dependent androgen excess
luteogenesis
luteolysis
luteoma
l. of pregnancy
luteotropic hormone
luteum
corpus l.
Lutrepulse
lutropin (LH)
Luveris
Luxol fast blue stain
LVP
large-volume paracentesis
lyase
argininosuccinate l.
peptidyl-alpha-hydroxyglycine alpha-amidating l. (PAL)
17,20-lyase
Lycolan Elixir
Lyme disease
lymph
l. node
l. node involution
l. node metastasis
lymphadenitis
lymphadenoma
lymphadenopathy-associated virus (LAV)
lymphangiectasis
lymphangioma
lymphangiosarcoma
lymphectasia
intestinal l.
lymphedema
congenital hereditary l.
lymphocutaneous sporotrichosis
lymphocyte
l. adenylate cyclase response
B l.
CD4 helper l.
CD8 suppressor l.
cytotoxic T l.
Epstein-Barr transformed l.
l. function-associated antigen-1 (LFA-1)
l. immune globulin
inducer T l.
peripheral blood l. (PBL)
regulatory l.
T l.
T-effector l.

thymic l.
T-suppresser l.
lymphocytic
l. hypophysitis
l. infiltration
l. thyroiditis
lymphocytopenia
lymphoepithelial
l. endocrine gland
lymphoid
l. cell
l. follicle
l. hyperplasia
lymphokine
secrete l.
lymphokine-activated
l.-a. killer (LAK)
l.-a. killer cell
lymphoma
aggressive hypothalamic l.
Burkitt l.
immunoblastic l.
intermediate lymphocytic l.
lymphoplasmacytoid l.
mantle zone l.
PCNS l.
primary central nervous system l.
primary thyroid l.
small cleaved l.
small noncleaved l.
T-cell l.
lymphomatosa
struma l.
lymphoplasmacytoid lymphoma
lymphoproliferative disorder
lymphoreticular neoplasm
lymphoscintigraphy
lymphotoxin
lymphotoxin-beta
Lynch syndrome
lynestrenol
Lynoral
Lyon
L. hypothesis
L. phenomenon
lyonization
Lyphocin Injection
lypressin
lysine
l. dehydrogenase
l. vasopressin
lysinuric protein intolerance
lysophosphatidylcholine
lysosomal
l. dense body
l. membrane
lysosome
lipid-laden l.
lysozyme
l. F_2 element
lysuride
lysyl-bradykinin
lysyl oxidase

L

NOTES

M
immunoglobulin M (IgM)
1/50M
Norethin 1/50M
MA
megestrol acetate
Maalox
M. Plus
MAb, Mab
monoclonal antibody
MacCarty keyhole
maceration of epithelium
MacFee extension
macroadenoma
pituitary growth hormone-secreting m.
pluripotent pituitary m.
prolactin-secreting pituitary m.
solitary unilateral m.
macroalbuminuria
macroalteration in muscle tissue
macroangiopathy
dysglycemic m.
macrocephaly
macrofollicular
m. adenoma
m. pattern
macroglossia
macrognathia
macrolipasemia
macromastia
macromolecule
hydrophilic m.
macronodular adrenal hyperplasia
macroorchidism
macrophage
m. colony-stimulating factor (M-CSF)
m. inflammatory protein-1-alpha (MIP-1-alpha)
m. inflammatory protein-1-beta (MIP-1-beta)
m. migration-inhibiting factor
m. migration inhibitory factor
macrophage-activating factor
macropinocytotic
macroprolactinemia
macroprolactinoma
invasive m.
macrosomia
fetal m.
macrovascular disease
macula
m. densa
m. densa cell
m. densa chemoreceptor
m. densa receptor
macular
m. degeneration
m. edema
macule
café au lait m.
mad cow disease
Madelung deformity
magaldrate
m. and simethicone
magnesium
m. ammonium phosphate
m. carbonate
m. deficiency
m. depletion
m. hydroxide
m. oxide
m. salt
m. sulfate
magnesium-lipid salt
magnetic
m. resonance cholangiography (MRC)
m. resonance cholangiopancreatography (MRCP)
m. resonance elastography (MRE)
m. resonance imaging (MRI)
m. resonance spectroscopy (MRS)
magnocellular
m. cholinergic neuron
m. hormone
m. hypothalamohypophyseal neuron
m. neurosecretory neuron
m. neurosecretory system
m. perikaryon
Magnum food scale
mahogany cofactor
ma huang
Maillard
M. product
M. reaction
M. site
main
m. d'accoucheur
m. pancreatic duct (MPD)
maintenance
bone mass m.
major
m. depression
m. depressive disorder (MDD)
m. gangrene
m. histocompatability complex (MHC)
m. histocompatibility

major *(continued)*
Leishmania m.
m. proglucagon fragment (MPF)
thalassemia m.
m. tranquilizer
majora
malabsorption
bile-salt m.
calcium m.
carbohydrate m.
maldescent
maldevelopment
maldigestion/malabsorption
fat m.
male
m. climacteric
infertile m.
m. infertility
m. orgasm
m. pattern baldness
m. pattern hair loss
m. phenotype
m. precocious puberty
m. pseudohermaphrodites
m. pseudohermaphroditism
m. sperm
m. Turner syndrome
undervirilized m.
maleate
rosiglitazone m.
male-limited familial precocious puberty
maleylacetoacetate
m. hydrolase
m. hydrolase, type Ib
malformation
arteriovenous m. (AVM)
malic
m. enzyme
m. enzyme gene
malignancy
humoral hypercalcemia of m. (HHM)
periampullary m.
secondary m.
malignancy-associated hypercalcemia
malignant
m. external otitis
m. hemangioendothelioma
m. histiocytosis
m. hyperthermia
m. insulinoma
m. islet cell tumor
Mallamint
malleable brain retractor
malnutrition
protein-calorie m.
protein-energy m. (PEM)
malnutrition-related diabetes mellitus
malonaldehyde generation
Maloney stain for aluminum
malonyl-CoA
MALT
marginal zone/mucosa-associated lymphoid tissue
mucosa-associated lymphoid tissue
maltase
mammalian
m. achaete-scute homologous protein-2 (Mash-2)
m. bombesin
m. target of rapamycin (mTOR)
mammary
m. crest
m. dysplasia
m. fibroadenoma
m. gland
m. ridge
m. tumor virus (MTV)
mammary-derived growth inhibitor (MGDI)
mammillary
m. body
m. fasciculus
m. peduncle
m. region
mammillotegmental fasciculus
mammillothalamic tract
mammography
ultrasound m.
mammosomatotroph
m. cell
m. cell adenoma
mammotrope
m. acidophil
mandible
hypoplastic m.
manifestation
morphologic m.
neuroophthalmologic m.
mannitol
m. administration
mannose
mannose-6-phosphate/IGF-2 receptor (M6P/IGF-2R)
manometry
sphincter of Oddi m.
Mansonella perstans
mantle
m. islet
m. zone lymphoma
MAO
monoamine oxidase
Maox
MAP
mean arterial pressure
mitogen-activated protein

MAP kinase
MAP kinase pathway
Mapap
MAP/ERK kinase (MEK)
MAPK
mitogen-activated protein kinase
MAPK cascade
MAPK pathway
maple syrup urine disease
mapping
c-*fos* m.
MAR
mineral apposition rate
Maranox
marasmus
m. syndrome
Marax
marble
m. bone disease
m. bone pattern
marcescens
Serratia m.
Marcillin
marfanoid habitus
Marfan syndrome
Margesic H
margin
adrenal gland m.
coast of California smooth m.
coast of Maine irregular m.
marginal zone/mucosa-associated lymphoid tissue (MALT)
Marine-Lenhart syndrome
marine vibrios
Marinol
marker
biochemical m.
genetic m.
hyperinsulinemic hypoglycemia m.
microsatellite m.
postreceptor m.
short tandem repeat m.
STR m.
variable number of tandem repeat m.'s
VNTR m.'s
Marmine
M. Injection
M. Oral
marrow
bone m.
m. cavity formation
m. cell vacuolization
m. hematopoietic stem cell
m. monocyte
red bone m.
yellow bone m.
marsupialization
Marthritic
MAS
McCune-Albright syndrome
masculinization
Mash-2
mammalian achaete-scute homologous protein-2
masked
m. hyperthyroidism
m. thyroid autonomy
mask sign
***mas* oncogene**
mass
body cell m.
bone m.
cold m.
decreased lean m.
density of the fat m. (d_{FF})
density of the fat-free m. (d_{FFM})
fat m. (FM)
fat-free m. (FFM)
incidental adrenal m.
m. isotopomer distribution analysis (MIDA)
lean m.
lean body m. (LBM)
musculoskeletal m.
peak adult bone m. (PABM)
protein m.
pseudoadrenal m.
red cell m.
skeletal m.
m. spectrometry
syncytiotrophoblast m.
T- and Z- scores of bone m.
massa intermedia
mass-forming pancreatitis
massive macronodular hyperplasia
Masson trichrome stain
mastalgia
mast cell
mastitis
chronic cystic m.
cystic m.
mastocytoma
mastocytosis

NOTES

mastoparan
maternal
m. antibody
m. deprivation syndrome
m. estradiol rhythm
m. hyperglycemia-induced fetal hyperinsulinemia
m. hypothyroidism
m. hypothyroxinemia
m. immunity
m. postpartum thyroid dysfunction
maternally inherited diabetes and deafness (MIDD)
maternotoxic effect
matrix
cellulose-derived m.
estradiol m.
extracellular m.
m. Gla protein (MGP)
human demineralized bone m.
mesangial m.
m. metalloprotease (MMP)
m. metalloproteinase (MMP)
m. metalloproteinase-12 (MMP-12)
m. mineralization
mineralized m.
mitochondrial m.
noncollagen bone m.
organic m.
osseous m.
porous collagen m.
m. transdermal system
m. vesicle
matrix-dissolution product
maturation
endochondral bone m.
epiphyseal m.
m. index (MI)
precocious m.
mature
m. follicle
m. teratoma
mature-onset diabetes of the young (MODY)
maturity-onset
m.-o. diabetes (MOD)
m.-o. diabetes mellitus
m.-o. diabetes in the young (MODY)
m.-o. diabetes of youth (MODY)
Maurie syndrome
maximal urinary flow rate
maximum
m. intensity projection (MIP)
M. Strength Dex-A-Diet
M. Strength Dexatrim
tubular transport m. (T_m)
Maxolon
May-Giemsa-Grünwald stain
Mayo scissors
Mazanor
mazindol
MB-35 peptide
MBH
medial basal hypothalamic region
MBP
myelin basic protein
MCAD
medium chain acyl-CoA dehydrogenase
MCAD deficiency
MCAR
melanocortin receptor type 4
McCabe nerve dissector
McCardle syndrome
McCune-Albright syndrome (MAS)
MCD
medullary collecting duct
MCH
melanin-concentrating hormone
MCP
membrane cofactor protein
MCP-1
monocyte chemotactic protein-1
MC2-R
melanocortin-2 receptor
MC3-R
melanocortin-3 receptor
MC4-R
melanocortin-4 receptor
M-CSF
macrophage colony-stimulating factor
MCT
medullary carcinoma of the thyroid
MDC
minimal detectable concentration
MDD
major depressive disorder
mDNA
mitochondrial deoxyribonucleic acid
MDR
multidrug resistance protein
MDRD
Modification of Diet in Renal Disease
ME
methionine enkephalin
MEA
multiple endocrine abnormalities
multiple endocrine adenopathies
meal timing
mean arterial pressure (MAP)
Means-Lerman
M.-L. scratch
M.-L. scratch murmur
measurement
gastric impedance m.
glucose m.

heel-to-pubis m.
pubis-to-crown m.
skin fold m.
transrectal ultrasound m.
TSH receptor antibody m.

Measurin

mechanism
autonomic cooling m.
cell-signaling m.
cis m.
counterregulation m.
hypothalamic regulatory m.
intact thirst m.
Jod-Basedow m.
lipostat m.
photoperiodic m.
prolactin inhibitory m.
Randle m.
thirst m.
trans m.
ubiquitin m.
urinary concentrating m.

mechanoreceptor

Meckel cartilage

meclofenamate

Meda
M. Cap
M. Tab

media
high-attenuation iodinated contrast m.
iodinated contrast m.
radiopaque iodinated radiographic contrast m.
tunica m.

medial
m. anlage
m. basal hypothalamic region (MBH)
m. basal hypothalamus
m. forebrain bundle
m. longitudinal fasciculus
m. zone

median
m. anlage
m. eminence

mediastinal
aberrant m. thyroid tissue
m. parathyroid adenoma

mediastinitis
sclerosing m.

mediastinum testis

mediator
bioactive m.

medicamentosa
rhinitis m.
thyrotoxicosis m.

Medicare Bone Mass Measurement Standardization Act

medication
aluminum-containing m.
antidiabetic m.
antithyroid m.

medicine
weight-loss m.

Medi-Glybe

Medihaler-Iso

Medi-Ject needle-free insulin injection system

Medi-Jector
M.-J. Choice
M.-J. Choice needle-free insulin injection system

mediobasal brain structure

Medipren

Medisense
M. Pen 2
M. Pen 2 self-blood glucose monitor

Medi-Tuss

medium
m. chain acyl-CoA dehydrogenase (MCAD)
m. chain acyl-CoA dehydrogenase deficiency
gadolinium-diethylenetriaminepentaacetic acid contrast m.

Medralone Injection

medrogestone

Medrol
M. Oral
M. Veriderm Cream

medroxyprogesterone
m. acetate (MPA)
depot m.
estrogen and m.

medulla
adrenal m.
m. oblongata
m. pons
rostral ventrolateral m.
ventrolateral m.

NOTES

M

medullary
- m. carcinoma of the thyroid (MCT)
- m. cavity
- m. cell
- m. collecting duct (MCD)
- m. thick ascending limb of Henle
- m. thyroid cancer (MTC)
- m. thyroid carcinoma (MTC)

mefenamic acid
Mega B
Megace
megakaryocyte
megalencephaly
megaloblastic anemia
Megaton
megestrol acetate (MA)
meglitinide
Meige disease
meiosis
meiotic
- m. division
- m. nondysjunction

MEK
MAP/ERK kinase
- MEK kinase (MEKK)

MEKK
MEK kinase

Mel1a melatonin receptor
Mel1b melatonin receptor
melancholia
- syndrome of m.

melanin
melanin-concentrating hormone (MCH)
melanoblastoma
melanocortin
- m. receptor isoform
- m. receptor type 4 (MCAR)

melanocortin-2 receptor (MC2-R)
melanocortin-3 receptor (MC3-R)
melanocortin-4 receptor (MC4-R)
melanocyte-concentrating hormone
melanocyte-inhibiting hormone
melanocyte-releasing hormone (MRH)
melanocyte-stimulating
- m.-s. factor (MRF)
- m.-s. hormone (MSH)
- m.-s. hormone sequence

melanocytoma
melanoma
- familial atypical multiple mole-m. (FAMMM)
- m. growth stimulatory activity (MGSA)

Melanotan II
melanotropic
- m. cell

MELAS
myopathy, encephalopathy, lactic acidosis, stroke-like episodes
- MELAS syndrome

melatonin (MLT)
- m. rhythm

Melfiat-105 Unicelles
meliloti
- *Rhizobium m.*

melitensis
- *Brucella m.*

mellitus
- adult-onset diabetes m.
- atypical diabetes m. (ADM)
- autoimmune diabetes m.
- autosomal dominant diabetes m.
- diabetes m.
- gestational diabetes m. (GDM)
- insulin-dependent diabetes m. (IDDM)
- insulinopenic diabetes m.
- juvenile-onset diabetes m.
- malnutrition-related diabetes m.
- maturity-onset diabetes m.
- noninsulin-dependent diabetes m. (NIDDM)
- obese type 2 noninsulin-dependent diabetes m.
- posttransplant diabetes m. (PTDM)
- tropical diabetes m.
- type 1 diabetes m.
- type 2 diabetes m.
- White classification of diabetes m.

melorheostosis
melphalan
memapsin 2
membrana
- m. granulosa cell
- m. limitans externa

membrane
- apical m.
- arachnoid m.
- basolateral plasma m.
- brush-border m. (BBM)
- cell basement m.
- m. cofactor protein (MCP)
- cricothyroid m.
- cuprophane dialysis m.
- dialysis m.
- endosteal m.
- m. excitability
- incomplete cell basement m.
- m. integral protein (MIP)
- intracellular lysosomal m.
- Liliequist m.
- luminal brush-border m.
- lysosomal m.
- nitrocellulose m.

parathyroid cell m.
periodontal m.
piarachnoid m.
postsynaptic m.
tubular dialysis m.
vasculosyncytial m.
membrane-associated estrogen receptor
membrane-bound
m.-b. receptor
m.-b. receptor molecule
membranous
m. bone
m. urethra
Memorial Sloan-Kettering Cancer Center
MEN
multiple endocrine neoplasia
MEN syndrome
MEN 1
multiple endocrine neoplasia type 1
MEN 2
multiple endocrine neoplasia type 2
MEN 3
multiple endocrine neoplasia type 3
men
idiopathic osteoporosis in m.
***MEN1* gene**
MEN 2A
multiple endocrine neoplasia type 2A
Menadol
menarche
MEN 2B
multiple endocrine neoplasia type 2B
Mendelian inheritance
Mendenhall syndrome
Menest
menin
m. gene
meningioma
parasellar m.
pituitary m.
meningitis
basilar m.
tuberculous m.
meningococcal sepsis
meningococcemia
meningoencephalitis
Menkes disease
menometrorrhagia
menopausal estrogen
menopause
precocious emotional m.
premature m.
surgical m.
menorrhagia
menotropin
menses
oligomenorrhea with anovulatory m.
menstrual cycle
menstruation
retrograde m.
MENT
7-alpha-methyl-19-nortestosterone
mental retardation
mepenzolate
Mepergan
meperidine
m. and promethazine
Mephyton Oral
meprednisone
6-mercaptopurine
Meridia
Merkel cell carcinoma
merocrine
m. gland
mesangial
m. cell
m. matrix
mesangiocapillary
mesangium
extraglomerular m.
mesencephalon
mesenchymal
m. progenitor
m. stem cell
m. tumor
mesenchyme
mesenteric artery
mesh
titanium m.
mesoderm
extraembryonic somatic m.
mesodermal cell
mesodiencephalic junction
mesomelic shortening
mesometric dysplasia
mesonephros
mesosalpinx
mesothelioma
mesovarium
messenger
chemical m.
first m.
intracellular m.

NOTES

messenger *(continued)*
m. ribonucleic acid (mRNA)
m. RNA (mRNA)
second m.
tertiary m.
mesterolone
mestranol
m. and norethindrone
mesylate
2-Br-alpha-ergocryptine m.
nafomostat m.
pergolide m.
metabolic
m. acidosis
m. alkalosis
m. bone disease
m. clearance rate
m. control
m. effect
m. hemostasis
m. signal
m. stone workup
m. stress episode
m. syndrome
m. web
metabolism
basal m.
bone mineral m.
calcium phosphorus m.
cobalamin m.
disordered water m.
estrogen m.
fuel m.
glucose m.
iodothyronine m.
peripheral thyroid hormone m.
phosphorus m.
prereceptor m.
protein m.
purine m.
selenoprotein m.
sterol m.
thyroid hormone m.
water m.
metabolite
calciferol m.
phosphatidylinositide m.
vitamin D m.
metachromatic leukodystrophy (MLD)
Metahydrin
metaiodobenzylguanidine (MIBG)
^{131}I-labeled m. (^{131}I-labeled MIBG)
^{131}I-m. scan
131-metaiodobenzylguanidine
iodine -m. (^{131}I-MIBG)
^{131}metaiodobenzylguanidine
metal
m. intoxification
paramagnetic m.
trace m.
metalloprotease
matrix m. (MMP)
metalloproteinase
matrix m. (MMP)
tissue inhibitor of m. (TIMP)
zinc m.
metalloproteinase-12
matrix m. (MMP-12)
metalloproteinases-1
tissue inhibitor of m. (TIMP-1)
metallothionein (MT)
metamyelocyte
Met and Leu enkephalin
Metandren
metanephrine
24-hour fractionated m.
24-hour urinary fractionated m.
metanephros
metaphyseal, metaphysial
m. dysplasia
m. exostosis
m. sclerosis
metaphyses
metaphysis
metaplasia
clear cell m.
myeloid m.
oxyphilic m.
Metaprel
metaproterenol
Arm-a-Med m.
Dey-Dose m.
metastasis
distant m.
lymph node m.
pituitary m.
prior distant m.
sellar m.
tumor m.
metastatic
m. deposit
m. extraosseal calcification
m. tumor
metatarsal-phalangeal flexion deformity
metenkephalin
meter
Accu-Chek Advantage glucose m.
Accu-Chek Instant glucose m.
Chemstrip MatchMaker blood glucose m.
ExacTech blood glucose m.
Glucometer Elite R m.
GlucoWatch Biographer m.
LifeGuide glucose m.
One Touch blood glucose m.

Supreme II blood glucose m.
TD Glucose m.
metformin
m. hydrochloride
methacholine
methadone
methamphetamine
methandrostenolone
methanol
methantheline
methasone-suppressed corticotropin-releasing hormone test
methemoglobinemia
methimazole (MMI)
methionine
m. adenosyltransferase
m. enkephalin (ME)
peptide histidine m. (PHM)
method
bleach m.
carbodiimide modified heteroduplex screening m.
colorimetric m.
Falck-Hillarp histofluorescence m.
FISH m.
fluorescent in situ hybridization m.
Gaur m.
glucose clamp m.
Gomori staining m.
interposition m.
paracetic acid-based m.
ribonuclease A cleavage m.
sandwich enzyme immunoassay m.
Sanger dideoxy sequencing m.
symptothermal rhythm m.
Uchida m.
uricase m.
Ziehl-Neelsen m.
methotrexate
methotrimeprazine
methoxychlor
methoxyflurane
methoxyhydroxyphenylglycol
5-methoxyindoleacetic acid
methoxyisobutylisonitrile (MIBI)
5-methoxytryptamine
5-methoxytryptophol
methscopolamine
methyclothiazide
methyl
m. chloride
Oreton M.
m. oxidase
2-methylacetoacetate
methylation
2-methylbutyric acid
methyl chloride
methylcrotonyl
3-m. carboxylase
3-m.-CoA carboxylase deficiency
3-methylcrotonylglycine
2-methyl-d-hydroxybutyrate
methyldopa
methylene blue
methylenetetrahydrofolate reductase
3-methylglutaconate
3-methylglutarate
3-methylhistidine
methylisobutylxanthine (MIX)
methylmalonic
m. acid
m. acidemia
m. acidemia with homocystinemia
m. aciduria
methylmalonyl-CoA mutase
methylmercaptoimidazole (MMI)
methylmethacrylate
methylprednisolone
methylprednisone
methyl-sulfated neostigmine
methyltestosterone
Premarin with m.
methylxanthine drug
methysergide
Meticorten
metoclopramide
m. hydrochloride
metolazone
metoprolol
metrapone stimulation test
metrizamide
Metrodin
metronidazole
metrorrhagia
metyrapone
m. test
m. testing
m. therapy
metyrapone-induced hypercortisolism
metyrosine
Mevacor
mexiletine

NOTES

M

Meynert
nucleus basalis of M.
Mg^{2+}
free M.
total M.
MGDI
mammary-derived growth inhibitor
MGP
matrix Gla protein
MGSA
melanoma growth stimulatory activity
MHC
major histocompatability complex
myosin heavy chain
MHC class I molecule
MI
maturation index
Miacalcin
MIB-1
M. antibody
MIBG
metaiodobenzylguanidine
^{131}I-labeled MIBG
^{131}I-labeled metaiodobenzylguanidine
MIBG scan
MIBG-negative pelvic pheochromocytoma
MIBI
methoxyisobutylisonitrile
Tc-99m MIBI
mice
Ames dwarf m.
Snell dwarf m.
micelle
Michigan
M. Diabetic Neuropathy Score
M. Neuropathy Screening Test
Miconazole
Micral
M. Chemistrip
M. urine dipstick test
microadenoma
nonfunctioning m.
pituitary m.
silent m.
microadenomectomy
transsphenoidal m.
microalbumin
microalbuminuria
microalteration in muscle tissue
microaneurysm
microangiopathy
diabetic m.
microarchitectural
microcalorimetry
microcarcinoid
bronchial m.
microcatheter
microcephaly
microchimerism
microclip
dural m.
microcornea
microcyst
subcapsular follicular m.
microcytic anemia
microcytosis
microdactyly
microdeletion
Y chromosome m.
microdialysis
m. probe
microdissector
bayoneted Jannetta m.
45-degree angled Jannetta m.
microelectrode
voltammetric m.
microencephaly
microfilament-mediated process
microfilaria
Microflo
M. glucose monitoring test strip
M. test strip
microfollicular pattern
micrognathia
microhematuria
microheterogeneity
microinfusion pump
Microlet Vaculance
microlithiasis
occult biliary m.
microlymphography
fluorescence m.
micromelia
micrometastasis
Micro-monitor
Tracer Blood Glucose M.-m.
Micronase
microNefrin
Micronesia
microneurographic
micronized
m. estradiol
m. progesterone
micronodular
m. adrenal disease
m. hyperplasia
Micronor
micronutrient
micropenis
microperfusion
microphallus
microphthalmia
microphthalmic
m. cyst
osteopetrotic m.

micropinocytosis
micropinocytotic
micropituitary rongeur
MicroPor
  Altea M.
microprolactinoma
micropsia
micropuncture
microsatellite
  m. instability
  m. marker
microscissors
  single-bladed Kurze m.
microscope
  operating m.
microscopy
  intraviral m.
  Nomarski m.
  polarized light m.
microsomal
  m. antibody
  m. antibody titer
  m. antigen
microsome
microsurgery
  pituitary m.
microsurgical resection
microtome
  sectioning m.
microvascular disease
microvilli
microwave
  m. hyperthermia
  m. hyperthermia of the prostate
Microzide
MIDA
  mass isotopomer distribution analysis
Midamor
Midas Rex drill
midbrain
  m. raphe nucleus
midcycle spotting
MIDD
  maternally inherited diabetes and deafness
midgut
midline
  m. central neuraxis
  m. jugum sphenoidale
  m. zone
midnight plasma cortisol concentration
Midol
  M. IB
  M. PM
midparental height (MPH)
midrodrine
midsagittal image
MIF
  migration inhibitory factor
Mifegyne
mifepristone
miglitol
migration inhibitory factor (MIF)
MIH
  müllerian-inhibiting hormone
  müllerian inhibitory hormone
mild
  m. overt thyrotoxicosis
  m. thyroid failure
milia
  multiple m.
miliary tuberculosis
milieu
  androgen m.
  hormonal m.
  hypoandrogenic m.
  m. interieur
  internal m.
  reproductive m.
milk
  breast m.
  m. ejection
  m. let down
  m. let-down reflex
  m. line
  uterine m.
milk-alkali syndrome
Milkman syndrome
Miller-Dicker syndrome
Miller syndrome
millimeter (mm)
Milophene
milrinone
Milroy disease
mimicry
  molecular m.
mineral
  m. apposition rate (MAR)
  bone m.
  m. deficiency
  m. flux
  m. homeostasis

NOTES

mineralization
m. defect
m. front
m. impairment
m. lag time
matrix m.
mineralized
m. bone histology
m. matrix
mineralocorticoid
adrenal corticosteroid (m.)
m. agonist
m. excess
m. hormone
m. receptor (MR)
m. replacement
m. replacement therapy
miniature-type congenital adrenal hypoplasia
minihelix
mini hormone
minimal detectable concentration (MDC)
minimally symptomatic hypothyroidism (MSH)
MiniMed
M. continuous glucose sensor
M. 508 insulin pump
M. 511 insulin pump
minipill
Minipress
minipuberty of infancy
minipump
osmotic m.
minisequencing
solid-phase m.
Minnesota Multiphasic Personality Inventory (MMPI)
minocycline-associated pigment
minor
m. mechanical debridement
m. tranquilizer
minora
minoxidil
Minoxigaine
miosis
MIP
maximum intensity projection
membrane integral protein
MIP-1-alpha
macrophage inflammatory protein-1-alpha
MIP-1-beta
macrophage inflammatory protein-1-beta
MIS
müllerian-inhibiting substance
MIS II receptor
misfolded protein
misoprostol
misplaced exocytosis
missense
MIT
monoiodinated tyrosine
monoiodotyrosine
3-monoiodotyrosine
MIT:DIT ratio
mithramycin
mitochondria
tubulovesicular m.
mitochondrial
m. defect
m. deoxyribonucleic acid (mDNA, mtDNA)
m. DNA
m. enzyme
m. matrix
m. myopathy
m. P450 monooxygenase
m. porin
mitogen
mitogen-activated
m.-a. protein (MAP)
m.-a. protein kinase (MAPK)
m.-a. protein kinase cascade
m.-a. protein kinase pathway
mitogenesis
mitomycin C
mitosis
mitotane
MIX
methylisobutylxanthine
mix
antiknock m.
mixed
m. agonist-antagonist
m. bone lesion
m. GH cell-prolactin cell adenoma
m. GH-PRL cell adenoma
m. GH- and prolactin-secreting adenoma
m. gonadal dysgenesis
m. growth hormone cell-prolactin cell adenoma
m. growth hormone-prolactin cell adenoma
m. growth hormone- and prolactin-secreting adenoma
m. pattern
m. phenotype tumor
m. pituitary adenoma-gangliocytoma
m. sclerosing bone dystrophy
m. sensorimotor polyneuropathy
m. uremic osteodystrophy
mixed-function oxygenase
Mixer
Genotropin M.

mixture
racemic m.
MLC
myosin light chain
MLC kinase (MLCK)
MLCK
MLC kinase
myosin light chain kinase
MLD
metachromatic leukodystrophy
MLT
melatonin
mm
millimeter
MMC
myelomeningocele
MMI
methimazole
methylmercaptoimidazole
MMP
matrix metalloprotease
matrix metalloproteinase
MMP-12
matrix metalloproteinase-12
MMPI
Minnesota Multiphasic Personality Inventory
mnemonic
Mobenol
mobility
limited joint m. (LJM)
mobilization
plasmin m.
Möbius syndrome
MOD
maturity-onset diabetes
modality
dialysis m.
model
four-compartment m.
fuzzy logic m.
Jost m.
predictive growth m.
three-compartment m.
transgenic mouse m.
tumor xenograft m.
m. U Gamma Knife
Modem
Acculink M.
Modicon
modification
behavior m.
M. of Diet in Renal Disease (MDRD)
posttranslational m.
modified
m. University of Wisconsin (mUW)
m. University of Wisconsin solution
modifier
selective estrogen response m. (SERM)
Moducal
modulator
cAMP-response element m. (CREM)
estrogen-receptor m.
selective androgen-receptor m. (SARM)
selective estrogen-receptor m. (SERM)
serum estrogen-receptor m.
MODY
mature-onset diabetes of the young
maturity-onset diabetes in the young
maturity-onset diabetes of youth
mofetil
mycophenolate m.
moiety
adenylate cyclase m.
asparagine-linked glycosylation m.
carbohydrate m.
diphenyl ether m.
mole
complete hydatidiform m.
hydatidiform m.
partial hydatidiform m.
molecular
m. chaperone
m. mimicry
m. probe hybridization
molecule
accessory m.
adhesion m.
amphoteric m.
cell-cell adhesion m. (CAM)
cJun m.
class I major histocompatibility complex m.
class I MHC m.
class II major histocompatibility complex m.
class II MHC m.

NOTES

molecule *(continued)*
class III major histocompatibility complex m.
class III MHC m.
collagen m.
coregulator m.
heterotetrameric m.
intercellular adhesion m. (ICAM)
lipophilic m.
membrane-bound receptor m.
MHC class I m.
nascent collagen m.
neural cell adhesion m. (N-CAM)
poorly processed POMC m.
poorly processed proopiomelanocortin m.
procollagen m.
proinsulin-like m.
proopiomelanocortin m.
proteoglycan m.
reporter m.
molecule-1
intercellular adhesion m. (ICAM-1)
molimina
premenstrual m.
Mol-Iron
Molypen
Monafed
monamine (*var. of* monoamine)
Monckeberg sclerosis
Mondini dysplasia
monitor
BodyGem metabolism m.
Diasensor 2000 glucose m.
Duet glucose control m.
Glucometer DEX blood glucose m.
GlucoWatch glucose m.
Medisense Pen 2 self-blood glucose m.
m. peptide
Rigi-Scan m.
SpectRx glucose m.
SureStep glucose m.
monitoring
blood glucose m.
capillary blood glucose m.
self-blood glucose m. (SBGM)
monoallelic
m. expression
m. transcription
monoamine, monamine
brain m.
m. oxidase (MAO)
m. oxidase inhibitor
m. pathway
m. serotonin (5-HT)
monoclonal
m. antibody (MAb, Mab)
m. anti-T-cell antibody
monoclonus
monocular temporal arcuate defect
monocyte
m. chemoattractant protein-1
m. chemotactic protein-1 (MCP-1)
marrow m.
peripheral blood m. (PBM)
monocytopenia
monodeiodinase
m. activity
5′-m. activity
5′-m. type I
monodeiodination activity
monofilament
Semmes-Weinstein 5.07 m.
monofilament pressure esthesiometer
monofluorophosphate
monofollicular feedback
monogenic disorder
Mono-Gesic
monohydrate
sibutramine hydrochloride m.
monohydrogen phosphate
monoiodinated tyrosine (MIT)
monoiodotyrosine (MIT)
3-monoiodotyrosine (MIT)
Monojector
M. fingerstick device
M. fingerstick device for blood glucose testing
monokine
monolayer culture
monomer
calcitonin m.
collagen m.
thyroid hormone receptor m.
TR m.
triiodothyronine m.
monomorphic
monomorphous
mononeuritis
m. multiplex
mononeuropathy
compressive m.
diabetic m.
hypothyroid m.
m. multiplex
mononucleosis
infectious m.
monoovarial feedback
monooxygenase
mitochondrial P450 m.
peptidylglycine alpha-amidating m. (PAM)

peptidylglycine alpha-hydroxylating m. (PHM)
monophasic
monophosphate
adenosine 5′ m. (AMP)
adenosine cyclic m.
cyclic adenosine m. (cAMP)
cyclic 3′,5′-adenosine m. (cAMP)
cyclic arginine m. (cAMP)
cyclic guanosine m. (cGMP)
cyclic 3′,5′-guanosine m. (cGMP)
5′-cyclic guanosine m. (cGMP)
dibutyryl cyclic arginine m.
guanosine m. (GMP)
nephrogenous cyclic adenosine m.
monophosphate-phosphodiesterase
cyclic guanosine m.-p.
monosaturated fatty acid
monostotic
m. disease
m. form
monosymptomatic hyperthyroidism
monosystemic hyperthyroidism
monotherapy
estrogen m.
troglitazone m.
monovalent
monozygotic
m. twins
Monro
foramen of M.
mons pubis
Month
Lupron Depot-3 M.
Lupron Depot-4 M.
moon
m. face
m. facies
morbid obesity
Morgagni syndrome
morning
m. corticotropin-releasing hormone test
m. cortisol
m. CRH test
m. glory disc
morning-after pill
morphine
endogenous m.
m. sulfate
morphogen
morphologic
m. differentiation
m. manifestation
morphology
colony m.
spindle-shaped fibroplastic m.
morphometry
Morquio syndrome
Morris syndrome
morula
mosaic
47,XXY m.
46,XY m.
mosaicism
chromosomal m.
gonadal m.
trisomy X m.
Turner m.
XO/XY m.
Y chromosome m.
MOS protooncogene
Mostofi classification of testicular tumor
motif
glycosylation consensus m.
nuclear localization signal m. (NLS)
ribonucleic acid-binding m. (RBM)
RNA-binding m. (RBM)
Y chromosome RNA recognition m. (YRRM)
zinc-finger m.
motilin
motility
aberrant m.
ocular m.
Motrin
M. IB
Junior Strength M.
movement
abnormal ocular m.
athetoid m.
choreiform m.
flagellar m.
moxestrol
MPA
medroxyprogesterone acetate
MPD
main pancreatic duct
MPF
major proglucagon fragment
MPH
midparental height

NOTES

M6P/IGF-2R
mannose-6-phosphate/IGF-2 receptor
MPLV
myeloproliferative leukemia virus
MPO
myeloperoxidase
M-Prednisol Injection
MPS I
mucopolysaccharidosis I
MR
mineralocorticoid receptor
MRC
magnetic resonance cholangiography
MRCP
magnetic resonance cholangiopancreatography
MRE
magnetic resonance elastography
MRF
melanocyte-stimulating factor
MRH
melanocyte-releasing hormone
MRI
magnetic resonance imaging
gadolinium-enhanced MRI
mRNA
messenger ribonucleic acid
messenger RNA
GnRH mRNA
receptor mRNA
TRH mRNA
MRS
magnetic resonance spectroscopy
MS-8
Pancrecarb M.
MS Contin Oral
MSH
melanocyte-stimulating hormone
minimally symptomatic hypothyroidism
MSH peptide
MSIR Oral
MT
metallothionein
Pancrease MT
Ultrase MT
MTC
medullary thyroid cancer
medullary thyroid carcinoma
mtDNA
mitochondrial deoxyribonucleic acid
M.T.E.-4
M.T.E.-5
M.T.E.-6
mTOR
mammalian target of rapamycin
MTV
mammary tumor virus
mucification
mucin
mucinosis
follicular m.
papular m.
reticular erythematous m.
mucinous
m. cystadenocarcinoma
m. cystadenoma
m. cystic tumor
mucin-producing
m.-p. adenocarcinoma
m.-p. tumor of the pancreas
mucocele
mucocutaneous
m. candidiasis
m. rash
mucoepidermoid carcinoma
Muco-Fen-DM
Muco-Fen-LA
mucoid wedge
mucolipidosis
m. II
mucolipidosis II
Mucomyst
Mucoplex
mucopolysaccharide
mucopolysaccharidosis, pl. **mucopolysaccharidoses**
m. I (MPS I)
m. types I, II, III, IIIB, IIID, IVA, IVB, VI, VII
mucoprotein
Mucor
mucormycosis
bone m.
cardiac m.
disseminated m.
gastrointestinal m.
pulmonary m.
renal m.
rhinocerebral m.
mucosa
cervical m.
mucosa-associated lymphoid tissue (MALT)
mucosal neuroma
Mucosil
mucosulfatidosis
mucous escalator
mucus thread
Muercke line
mulibrey nanism
müllerian
m. agenesis
m. derivative
m. duct
m. duct derived structure

m. duct syndrome
m. inhibitory hormone (MIH)
müllerian-inhibiting
m.-i. hormone (MIH)
m.-i. substance (MIS)
m.-i. substance receptor
Müller muscle
MulTE-PAK-4
MulTE-PAK-5
multiantennary
multicentric
m. islet cell adenoma
m. reticulohistiocytosis
multidose insulin treatment
multidrug resistance protein (MDR)
multiexon
multiexonic gene
multiforme
erythema m.
glioblastoma m.
multigenic
multihormonal system disorder
multinodular
m. euthyroid goiter
multiple
m. anterior pituitary hormone deficiency
m. endocrine abnormalities (MEA)
m. endocrine adenomatosis
m. endocrine adenopathies (MEA)
m. endocrine neoplasia (MEN)
m. endocrine neoplasia type 1 (MEN 1)
m. endocrine neoplasia type 2 (MEN 2)
m. endocrine neoplasia type 3 (MEN 3)
m. endocrine neoplasia type 2A (MEN 2A)
m. endocrine neoplasia type 2B (MEN 2B)
m. hamartoma syndrome
m. luteinized theca cyst
m. milia
m. myeloma
m. myeloma cell line
m. pituitary hormone deficiency
M. Risk Factor Intervention Trial
m. sclerosis
m. sulfatase deficiency
m. system atrophy
multiple-injection regimen
multiplex
dysostosis m.
mononeuritis m.
mononeuropathy m.
multiplier effect
multiport collimated cobalt-60 therapy
multipotential progenitor
multisynaptic pathway
Multi Vit Drops
mu-M
mumps
m. orchitis
postpubertal m.
m. virus
Münchausen syndrome
mural trophectoderm
muramidase
murine
m. gene
m. L cell
m. osteopetrosis mutation
murmur
Means-Lerman scratch m.
muscarinic
m. agonist carbamylcholine
m. cholinergic receptor
muscimol
muscle
anterior scalene m.
bulbospongiosus m.
m. catabolism
cremaster m.
cricothyroid m.
m. effect
m. enzyme
infrahyoid m.
ischiocavernosus m.
levator palpebrae superioris m.
Müller m.
myometrial smooth m.
omohyoid m.
platysma m.
posterior cricoarytenoid m.
skeletal m.
sternocleidomastoid m.
sternohyoid m.
sternothyroid m.
strap m.
stylohyoid m.
superficial perineal m.
transverse rectus abdominis m. (TRAM)

NOTES

muscle *(continued)*
 transversus perinei superficialis m.
 white m.
muscle:fat ratio
muscular
 m. dystrophy
 m. weakness
musculoskeletal mass
mutagenesis
 site-directed m.
mutans
 Streptococcus m.
mutant allele
mutase
 methylmalonyl-CoA m.
mutated
 ataxia telangiectasia m. (ATM)
mutation
 androgen receptor gene m.
 Arg m.
 BRCA 1 m.
 BRCA 2 m.
 breast cancer antigen 1 m.
 breast cancer antigen 2 m.
 factor II m.
 factor V deficiency Leiden m.
 gain-of-function m.
 germline PTEN m.
 germline putative protein-tyrosine phosphatase m.
 germline TP53 m.
 GPCR m.
 homozygous missense m.
 inactivating m.
 Leiden m.
 loss-of-function m.
 murine osteopetrosis m.
 osteopetrotic m.
 point m.
 R257X m.
 somatic m.
 somatic PTEN m.
 thyroid-stimulating hormone receptor m.
 TSH receptor m.
mutation-enriched restriction fragment length polymorphism assay
mutism
 deaf m.
mUW
 modified University of Wisconsin mUW solution
M.V.C. 9 + 3
M.V.I.-12
M.V.I. Pediatric
myalgia
Myapap
mycobacteria
 nontuberculous m.
Mycobacterium
 M. avian-intracellulare
 M. avium-intracellulare
 M. cheloni
 M. fortuitum
 M. intracellulare
 M. kansasii
 M. leprae
 M. tuberculosis
mycobacterium
 atypical m.
mycophenolate mofetil
Mycoplasma
 M. hominis
mycotic infection
mydriasis
 anisocoria with ipsilateral m.
myelinated fiber bundle
myelin basic protein (MBP)
myelinolysis
 central pontine m.
myelodysplasia
 occult m.
myelofibrosis
myeloid
 m. leukemia inhibitory factor
 m. metaplasia
 m. precursor
myelolipoma
myeloma
 multiple m.
myelomeningocele (MMC)
myelomonocytic cell
myeloperoxidase (MPO)
myelophthisic anemia
myeloproliferative leukemia virus (MPLV)
Mykrox
Mylanta
Mylanta-II
Mylicon
myocardium
myocyte
myoedema
myoepithelial cell
myofiber diameter
myogenic regeneration
myogenin
myoglobin
myoglobinuria
 idiopathic paroxysmal m.
myoid cell
myoinositol
myokymia
myometrial
 m. oxytocin receptor

m. relaxation
m. smooth muscle
myometrium
myopathy
hypothyroid m.
lipid m.
mitochondrial m.
thyrotoxic m.
tRNA mitochondrial m.
X-linked myotubular m.
myopathy, encephalopathy, lactic acidosis, stroke-like episodes (MELAS)
myosalpinx
myosin
m. heavy chain (MHC)
m. light chain (MLC)
m. light chain kinase (MLCK)
Myotonachol
myotonia dystrophica
myotonic dystrophy
myotropic hormone
myxedema
m. ataxia
m. coma
idiopathic m.
m. ileus
localized m.
preclinical m.
preradial m.
pretibial m.
primary m.
myxedematosus
lichen m.
myxedematous
m. cretinism
m. endemic cretinism
m. face
myxoma
atrial m.
cutaneous m.
ventricular m.

NOTES

N
norepinephrine
Humulin N
Nabadial
nabilone
Nabolin
nabothian cyst
nabumetone
***N*-acetylated**
***N*-acetyl-beta-glucosaminidase**
***N*-acetylglucosamine (GlcNAc)**
N.-a. receptor
***N*-acetyl-5-methoxykynurenamine**
***N*-acetyl-5-methoxytryptamine**
***N*-acetylserotonin**
***N*-acetyltransferase**
serotonin -a.
NAD
nicotinamide-adenine dinucleotide
NAD kinase
nadir
cortisol n.
n. hypoglycemia
nadolol
NADPH
nicotinamide adenine dinucleotide phosphate
NADPH-cytochrome P450 reductase
naeslundii
Actinomyces n.
nafarelin
nafenopin
nafomostat mesylate
nafoxidine
Nägele rule
Nager syndrome
Na^+/H^+-ion exchanger
nail
hypoplastic n.
pitting of n.
Plummer n.
Terry n.
nail-patella syndrome
naïve
cold n.
Najjar syndrome
nalbuphine
Naldecon
N. Senior DX
N. Senior EX
Nalfon
nalidixic acid
naloxone
naltrexone
nandrolone
n. decanoate
n. phenylpropionate
nanism
mulibrey n.
Na^+-phosphate cotransporter
Naprosyn
naproxen
NAPRTCS
North American Pediatric Renal Transplant Cooperative Study
Naqua
narcolepsy
narcotine analog
nasal
n. cavity
n. insulin
n. limbus
n. speculum
nascent
n. collagen molecule
n. protein
n. protein chain
nasogastric (NG)
nasogastric tube
nasogastrojejunal tube (NGJT)
nasotuberculum line
Natabec
N. FA
N. Rx
Natalins
N. Rx
nateglinide
National
N. Center for Health Statistics (NCHS)
N. Cholesterol Education guidelines
N. Cholesterol Education Program criteria
N. Cholesterol Evaluation Program (NCEP)
N. Cooperative Growth Study (NCGS)
N. Diabetes Data Group (NDDG)
N. Health and Nutrition Examination Survey (NHANES)
N. Institutes of Health (NIH)
N. Osteoporosis Foundation (NOF)
native pancreas
natriuresis
natriuretic
n. hormone
n. peptide
n. peptide receptor (NPR)
natruresis

natural
n. killer (NK)
n. killer cell
nature
pleiotropic n.
Naturetin
nausea
N-CAM
neural cell adhesion molecule
NCEP
National Cholesterol Evaluation Program
NCEP criteria
NCGS
National Cooperative Growth Study
NCHS
National Center for Health Statistics
Nck protein
NCoA-1 coactivator
NCoA-2 coactivator
N-CoR
NCV
nerve conduction velocity
NDDG
National Diabetes Data Group
NDI
nephrogenic diabetes insipidus
NE
norepinephrine
near-total thyroidectomy
nebenkern
neck
n. of pancreas
webbed n.
neck-to-thigh ratio (N/T)
necrobiosis lipoidica diabeticorum (NLD)
necrolysis
epidermal n.
toxic epidermal n.
necrolytic migratory erythema (NME)
necropsy
necrosis
adrenal n.
aseptic n.
brain n.
central n.
disseminated fat n.
fat n.
focal tumor n.
frank n.
hepatic n.
idiopathic ischemic n.
infected pancreatic n.
ischemic n.
papillary n.
pituitary n.
pituitary growth hormone-secreting adenoma n.
postpartum pituitary n.
pressure n.
renal pupillary n.
spontaneous pituitary n.
subcutaneous fat n.
thyroid n.
necrospermia
necrotic palatal ulcer
necrotizing
n. cellulitis
n. fasciitis
N.E.E. 1/35
needle
n. catheter jejunostomy
fine n.
Howell aspiration n.
osteodysplasia of Melnick and N.'s
Tru-Cut n.
Vim-Silverman n.
needlescopic procedure
NEFA
nonesterified fatty acid
negative
n. arterial-portal glucose gradient
n. feedback
n. feedback loop
n. feedback regulation
hormone-binding n.
n. T_3 response element (TRE)
n. triiodothyronine response element
Neisseria
N. gonorrhoeae
Nelova
N. 10/11
N. 0.5/35E
N. 1/50M
Nelson syndrome
NEM
N-ethylmaleimide
Neo-Calglucon
neocortex
frontal n.
Neo-Durabolic
Neo-Estrone
neoformans
Cryptococcus n.
neointimal hyperplasia
neologism
neonatal
n. adrenoleukodystrophy
n. exchange transfusion
n. goiter
n. Graves hyperthyroidism
n. hypocalcemia
n. hypothyroidism
n. severe hyperparathyroidism (NSHPT)
n. thyroid dysfunction

neoplasia
familial multiple endocrine n.
multiple endocrine n. (MEN)
multiple endocrine n. type 1 (MEN 1)
multiple endocrine n. type 2 (MEN 2)
multiple endocrine n. type 3 (MEN 3)
multiple endocrine n. type 2A (MEN 2A)
multiple endocrine n. type 2B (MEN 2B)
neoplasm
androgen-secreting n.
clonal n.
follicular n.
germ-cell n.
gestational trophoblastic n. (GTN)
hepatic n.
histiocytic n.
Hürthle cell n.
hyalinizing trabecular n.
intraductal oncocytic papillary n. (IOPN)
intraductal papillary mucinous n. (IPNM)
lymphoreticular n.
pancreatic endocrine n. (PEN)
peripancreatic n.
plurihormonal neuroendocrine n.
trophoblastic n.
neoplastic
n. adenohypophysial cell
n. pathologic lesion
Neoral
Neosar
Neosten
neostigmine
methyl-sulfated n.
neotenin
Neotrace-4
NeoVadrin
N. B Complex
neovascularization
n. of disc (NVD)
n. elsewhere in retina (NVE)
nephrectomy
nephritis
chronic interstitial n.
thyroid antigen-antibody n.
Nephro-Calci
nephrocalcin
nephrocalcinosis
papillary n.
Nephrocaps
Nephro-Fer
nephrogenic
n. diabetes
n. diabetes insipidus (NDI)
nephrogenous
n. cAMP
n. cyclic adenosine monophosphate
nephrolithiasis
nephrolithotomy
percutaneous n.
nephron
cortical n.
renal n.
nephropathic cystinosis
nephropathy
acute uric acid n.
diabetic n.
tubulointerstitial n.
urate n.
nephrotic syndrome
Nephrox Suspension
neprilysin
Nernst equation
nerve
abducent n.
ansa cervicalis n.
ansa hypoglossal n.
buffer n.
cervical sensory n.
n. conduction velocity (NCV)
N. Disability Score
n. growth factor (NGF)
hypertrophied corneal n.
hypoglossal n.
intercostal n.
laryngeal n.
ocular motor cranial n.
oculomotor n.
optic n.
parasympathetic n.
phrenic n.
preganglionic sympathetic n.
pudendal n.
recurrent laryngeal n.
spinal accessory n.
splanchnic n.
sympathetic n.
N. Symptom Score

NOTES

nerve *(continued)*
trigeminal n.
trochlear n.
vagus n.
nervorum
vasa n.
nervosa
anorexia n.
bulimia n.
pars n.
nesidioblastoma
nesidioblastosis
nesidiodysplasia
NESP55
neuroendocrine secretory protein 55
NESP55 protein
nest
solid cell n.
squamous cell n.
Nestrex
NET
norepinephrine transporter
norethisterone
net
n. calcium absorption
n. calcium influx
n. efflux
n. hepatic glucose uptake (NHGU)
N-ethylmaleimide (NEM)
network
cis Golgi n.
endoplasmic reticulum-Golgi n.
Golgi n.
intraglandular lymphatic n.
trans-Golgi n.
Neucalm-50 Injection
***neu* oncogene**
neural
n. cell adhesion molecule (N-CAM)
n. crest
n. lobe
n. relationship
n. stalk
n. tube
n. tumor
neuraminidase treatment
neuraxis
midline central n.
neurilemoma
cystic n.
neurinoma
neurite outgrowth
neuritis
chiasmal n.
lactation optic n.
neuroanatomic technique
neuroarthropathy
neuroblast
neuroblastoma
neurocircuit
neurocrest
neurodegenerative disease
neurodevelopmental delay
neurodiagnostic study
neuroectoderm
neuroendocrine
n. cell
n. control
n. control loop
n. programming
n. reflex
n. secretory protein 55 (NESP55)
n. tumor
neuroendocrine system
neuroendocrinology
neurofibroma
neurofibromatosis
n., type I
n., type II
neurofilament
neurogenic
n. atrophy
n. diabetes insipidus
n. hypogonadism
n. precocious puberty
n. pulmonary edema
neuroglia
n. cell
peripheral n.
neuroglucopenia
neuroglycopenia
neuroglycopenic symptom
neurogranin
neurohormonal
n. cell
neurohormone
neurohumoral
neurohypophysial, neurohypophyseal
n. diabetes insipidus
n. hormone
n. nerve terminal
n. peptide
n. stalk
neurohypophysis
neuroimaging study
neuroimmunology
neuroimmunomodulation
neurokinin
n. A
n. B
neuroleptic
n. malignant syndrome
neurologic endemic cretinism
neuroma
mucosal n.

neuromedin K
neuromodulator
neuromuscular junction disorder
neuromyotonia
ocular n.
neuron
cholinergic n.
dopaminergic n.
hippocampal n.
hypophysiotropic n.
hypothalmo-neurohypophyseal n.
intrinsic gut n.
magnocellular cholinergic n.
magnocellular hypothalamohypophyseal n.
magnocellular neurosecretory n.
oxytocinergic n.
paraventricular n.
parvocellular n.
peptidergic n.
postganglionic sympathetic n.
preganglionic sympathetic n.
primary afferent nociceptor n. (PAN)
thermosensitive n.
tuberohypophyseal n.
tuberohypophyseal dopaminergic n. (THDA)
tuberoinfundibular n.
tuberoinfundibular dopaminergic n. (TIDA)
neuronal
n. cytosol
n. hamartoma
n. shock
neuron-specific enolase
Neurontin
neuroophthalmologic manifestation
neuroophthalmology
neuropathic
n. arthropathy
n. cachexia
n. ulcer
neuropathy
autonomic n.
compression n.
compressive n.
cranial n.
demyelinative n.
diabetic autonomic n.
distal symmetric diabetic n.
gastrointestinal autonomic n.
genitourinary autonomic n.
large fiber n.
Leber hereditary optic n.
nondiabetic immune-mediated n.
optic n.
optic and chiasmal n.
peripheral n.
progressive multifocal axonal n.
proximal diabetic n.
proximal motor n.
radiation optic n.
neuropeptide
n. B
n. gamma
n. immunocytochemistry
n. K
n. Y (NPY)
neuropharmacology
neurophysin
hormone-specific n.
n. II
n. protein
vasopressin n. II
neurophysin I
neurophysin-positive varicosity
neurophysiology
neuropsychiatric
n. disorder
n. effect
neuroradiologic imaging procedure
neuroradiology
neurosarcoidosis
neurosecretion
neurosecretory
n. cell
n. gland
n. granule (NSG)
n. vessel
neurosteroid
neurosurgeon
pituitary n.
neurotensin
neurotransmitter
bioamine n.
primary sympathetic n.
neurotrophic
n. factor
n. hormone
n. therapy

NOTES

neurotrophin
neurotrophin-3 (NT-3)
neurotrophin-4 (NT-4)
neurotrophin-5 (NT-5)
neurturin (NTN)
Neut
neutral
n. endopeptidase
n. protamine Hagedorn (NPH)
n. protamine Hagedorn insulin
neutrophil
n. activation
n. chemotaxis
n. respiratory burst activity (NRBA)
nevoid basal cell carcinoma
Newcastle bone disease
NF-1 transcription factor
NF-kappa-B
nuclear factor-κB
NF-kappa-B element
receptor activator of NF-κB (RANK)
NFPA
nonfunctioning pituitary adenoma
NG
nasogastric
NGF
nerve growth factor
NGJT
nasogastrojejunal tube
N-glycosylation
NGM
norgestimate
NG tube
NHANES
National Health and Nutrition Examination Survey
NHANES I
NHANES II
NHGU
net hepatic glucose uptake
niacin
niacinamide
Niaspan
Nicobid
Nicoderm Patch
Nicolar
Nicorette
N. DS Gum
N. Gum
nicotinamide
n. adenine dinucleotide phosphate (NADPH)
nicotinamide-adenine dinucleotide (NAD)
nicotine-stimulated pathway
Nicotinex
nicotinic
n. acid
n. cholinergic receptor
n. receptor
nicotinic-type receptor
Nicotrol
N. Patch
NIDDM
noninsulin-dependent diabetes mellitus
nonobese type 2 NIDDM
obese type 2 NIDDM
nidus
Niemann-Pick disease
nifedipine
Niferex
Niferex-PN
night-day rhythm
nigra
substantia n.
nigricans
acanthosis n. (AN)
hyperandrogenism, insulin resistance, acanthosis n. (HAIRAN)
nigrostriatal bundle
NIH
National Institutes of Health
Nilandron
Nilevar
nilutamide
nimesulide
nipples
hypoplasia of n.
supranumerous mammary glands and n.
NIS
sodium-iodide symporter
Nissl substance
Nitabuch layer
nitrate
gallium n.
nitric
n. oxide (NO)
n. oxide synthase (NOS)
nitrite
sodium n.
nitroblue tetrazolium test
nitrocellulose membrane
nitrofurantoin
nitrogen
n. balance
blood urea n. (BUN)
n. retention
total body n.
n. wasting
nitroglycerin
nitroprusside
nitrosonaphthol
nitrosourea

nitrous oxide-donor drug
nizatidine
NK
natural killer
NK cell
NK1 receptor
NK2 receptor
NK3 receptor
NKCC2
sodium-potassium-2 chloride cotransporter
NKH
nonketotic hyperglycemia
NLD
necrobiosis lipoidica diabeticorum
N-linked glycosylation
NLS
nuclear localization signal motif
NMDA
N-methyl-D-aspartate
NME
necrolytic migratory erythema
N-methyl-D-aspartate (NMDA)
N-methyl D-aspartic acid
N-methyltransferase
phenylethanolamine N.-m. (PNMT)
NMR
nuclear magnetic resonance
***n-myc* gene**
NO
nitric oxide
NO synthase (NOS)
No
N. Pain-HP
No. 1
Valertest N.
Nocardia
N. asteroides
nociceptin/orphanin
n. FQ (N/OFQ)
n. FQ peptide
nocturnal
n. arrhythmogenesis
n. emission
n. hypoglycemia
n. penile tumescence (NPT)
n. penile tumescence testing
n. rhythm
n. thyroid-stimulating hormone surge
n. TSH surge
n. vasopressin release
node
Delphian lymph n.
juxtathyroid n.
lymph n.
paraaortic lymph n.
parasternal n.
sentinel lymph n.
Sister Mary Joseph n.
upper pretracheal n.
node-based malignant lymphoproliferative disease
NO-donor drug
nodosa
periarteritis n.
polyarteritis n.
trichorrhexis n.
nodosum
erythema n.
nodular
n. autonomy
n. fasciitis
n. goiter
nodule
autonomous n.
autonomously functioning thyroid n. (AFTN)
autonomous toxic n.
cold n.
cool n.
cystic n.
distinct n.
dominant thyroid n.
functioning n.
hamartomatous n.
hemorrhagic n.
hot n.
ill-defined n.
Kimmelstiel-Wilson n.
single thyroid n.
soft tissue n.
solitary nontoxic n.
thyroid n.
toxic solitary n.
toxic thyroid n. (TTN)
warm n.
NOF
National Osteoporosis Foundation
N/OFQ
nociceptin/orphanin FQ
N/OFQ peptide
Nomarski microscopy
nomegestrole acetate

NOTES

nomogram
non
  sine qua n.
nonaggressive tumor
nonandrogen
nonandrogenic progestin
nonapeptide
non-aureus
  Staphylococcus n.-a.
nonautoimmune
  n. familial hyperthyroidism
  n. nontoxic diffuse goiter
nonbeta cell tumor
noncalcareous stone
noncalcemic
  n. analog
noncaseating granuloma
noncholecystokinin substance
nonclassical
  n. hydroxylase deficiency
  n. 21-hydroxylase deficiency
nonclostridial anaerobic cellulitis
noncollagen bone matrix
noncollagenous protein
noncontraceptive estrogen
noncontractile cell
noncornified cell
noncovalent bond
nondiabetic immune-mediated neuropathy
nondissociated acid
nondysjunction
  meiotic n.
nonencapsulated
nonendocrine disease
nonenzymatic
  n. photolysis
  n. protein glycation
nonergot
  n. long-acting prolactin inhibitor
nonesterified fatty acid (NEFA)
nonestrogenic stereoisomer 17-alpha estradiol
nonfamilial parathyroid adenoma
nonfunctional pituitary adenoma
nonfunctioning
  n. adrenal carcinoma
  n. microadenoma
  n. pheochromocytoma
  n. pituitary adenoma (NFPA)
  n. pituitary tumor
nongenomic
  n. action
  n. effect
  n. factor
nongoitrous
nongranular clear chromophobe cell
non-Graves disease hyperthyroidism
nongrowth hormone deficient short stature
non-histocompatibility locus antigen-associated form
nonhistone protein
non-HLA-associated form
nonhomologous recombination
nonhormonal regulator
nonhuman leukocyte antigen associated form
noninsulin-dependent diabetes mellitus (NIDDM)
noninsulinoma pancreatogenous hypoglycemia
nonionic
  n. contrast radiography
  n. iodinated contrast
nonislet cell tumor
nonislet-cell tumor-induced hypoglycemia
nonketotic
  n. hyperglycemia (NKH)
  n. hyperglycinemia
  n. hyperosmolar coma
  n. hyperosmolar state
  n. hypoglycemic acidosis
nonneoplastic pathologic lesion
nonobese
  n. diabetic
  n. type 2 NIDDM
nonoral estradiol delivery system
nonosmotic stimulus
nonpapillary thyrogenic carcinoma
nonpeptide antagonist
nonphotic
  n. cue
  n. entrainment
nonpituitary thyrotropin
nonprolactinoma
nonproliferative diabetic retinopathy
nonpurulent fluid
nonpyknotic nucleus
nonresorbable resin
nonsalt-wasting congenital adrenal hyperplasia
nonsecreting
  n. pituitary adenoma
  n. pituitary tumor
nonsecretory
  n. adenoma
  n. adrenal adenoma
nonselective arterial digital angiography
nonshivering thermogenesis
nonsmall cell carcinoma
nonspecific binding (NSB)
nonsteroidal
  n. antiinflammatory agent
  n. antiinflammatory drug (NSAID)
  n. estrogen

nonsuppressible
n. insulinlike activity (NSILA)
n. insulinlike activity factor
nonsustained erection
nonsyndromic
n. autosomal recessive disorder
n. coronal craniosynostosis
n. familial enlarged vestibular aqueduct
nonsyndromic deafness
nonthyroid
n. disease
nonthyroidal
n. illness (NTI)
n. illness syndrome
nonthyroid illness
nonthyromimetic
nontoxic
n. multinodular goiter
n. nodular goiter
n. sporadic goiter
n. thyroid adenoma
nontropical sprue
nontropic sprue
nontuberculous mycobacteria
Noonan syndrome
noradrenaline
noradrenergic
n. afferent
n. blocker
n. receptor
norandrostenolone
Norcet
nor-derivative progestin
Nordette
NordiPen
Norditropin
N. SimpleXx
norepinephrine (N, NE)
n. perikaryon
n. transporter (NET)
norethandrolone
Norethin
N. 1/35E
N. 1/50M
norethindrone
n. acetate
estradiol and n.
ethinyl estradiol and n.
mestranol and n.
norethisterone (NET)
norethynodrel
noretisterone
norfloxacin
Norgesic
N. Forte
norgestimate (NGM)
ethinyl estradiol and n.
norgestrel
conjugated equine estrogen plus n. (CEEP)
ethinyl estradiol and n.
Norinyl
N. 1+35
N. 1+50
Norlutin
normal gonadal steroid level
normetanephrine
normocalcemia
normocalcemic
n. hypercalciuria
n. primary hyperparathyroidism
normocholesterolemia
normocortisolemia
normocytic normochromic anemia
Normodyne
normofunctioning
normoglycemia
normoglycemic
normokalemia
normolipidemic
normomagnesemic
normoprolactinemia
normoprolactinemic woman
normothermic
Norplant II
Norprolac
norpseudoephedrine
NOR-QD
Norrie disease
nortestosterone
Nor-tet Oral
North
N. America blastomycosis
N. American Pediatric Renal Transplant Cooperative Study (NAPRTCS)
Northern
N. blot
N. blot analysis
NOS
nitric oxide synthase
NO synthase

NOTES

N

nose
beaked n.
notochord
Nottingham Health Profile
Novartis
Novo-Butamide
NovoFine
Novogen
Novo-Glyburide
Novolin
N. 70/30
N. ge
N. L
N. N
N. 85/15 PenFill cartridge
N.-Pen II
N. R
NovoLog
Novo-Metformin
Novo-Methacin
NovoNorm
NovoPen 3
Novo-Prednisolone
Novo-Prednisone
Novo-Profen
Novo-Propamide
NovoRapid
Novo-Spiroton
NP-59
N. iodonocholesterol scan
N. scintigraphy
NPH
neutral protamine Hagedorn
NPH Iletin I
NPH insulin
Pork NPH
NPH-N
NP-59 isotope
NPR
natriuretic peptide receptor
NPT
nocturnal penile tumescence
NPT testing
NPY
neuropeptide Y
N-3-pyridyl-methyl-N-*p*-nitrophenylurea
NR
nuclear receptor
NRBA
neutrophil respiratory burst activity
NS
Stadol NS
NSAID
nonsteroidal antiinflammatory drug
NSB
nonspecific binding
NSG
neurosecretory granule
NSHPT
neonatal severe hyperparathyroidism
NSILA
nonsuppressible insulinlike activity
NT-3
neurotrophin-3
NT-4
neurotrophin-4
NT-5
neurotrophin-5
N/T
neck-to-thigh ratio
N/T ratio
N-telopeptide collagen
N-telopeptide/creatine
***N*-terminal**
N-t. peptide
N-t. telopeptide of type I collagen
N-termini
N-terminus
NTI
nonthyroidal illness
NTN
neurturin
NTS
nucleus of the tractus solitarius
nucleus tractus solitarius
Nubain
nuclear
n. accessory hormone
n. angiography
n. atypia
n. factor-κB (NF-kappa-B)
n. factor-kappa B element
n. factor-kB
n. hormone receptor
n. localization signal motif (NLS)
n. magnetic resonance (NMR)
n. pore complex
n. receptor (NR)
n. receptor corepressor
n. runoff assay
n. scintigraphy
n. transcription factor
n. translocation
nucleation
nucleotide
antisense n.
guanyl n.
n. triphosphate
nucleus, pl. **nuclei**
arcuate n.
n. basalis of Meynert
cortical amygdaloid n.
dorsal motor n.
dorsomedial n. (DMN)
Edinger-Westphal n.
ghost n.

heterochromatic n.
hypothalamic paraventricular n.
intermediate n.
lacrimal n.
midbrain raphe n.
nonpyknotic n.
osteoclastic n.
paramagnetic n.
paramedian reticular n.
paraventricular n. (PVN)
paraventricular thalamic n. (PVT)
premammillary n.
pyknotic n.
Raphe n.
salivatory n.
sexually dimorphic n.
stress-relevant amygdalar n.
suprachiasmatic n. (SCN)
suprachiasmic n.
supraoptic n.
thalamic n.
n. of the tractus solitarius (NTS)
n. tractus solitarius (NTS)
vagal n.
n. ventralis anterior of thalamus
ventromedial n. (VMN)

Nucofed
Nucotuss
Nu Gauze
Nu-Glyburide
Nu-Ibuprofen
Nu-Indo
Nu-Iron
null
n. cell
n. hypothesis
null-cell adenoma
nulliparous
numbness
circumoral n.
Numorphan
Nuprin
Nu-Propranolol
nutans
spasmus n.
Nutraplus Topical
nutrition
parenteral n.
total parenteral n. (TPN)
nutritional rickets
Nutropin
N. AQ
N. Depot
NVD
neovascularization of disc
NVE
neovascularization elsewhere in retina
NX
Talwin NX
nyctohemeral rhythm
nystagmus
roving n.
see-saw n.

NOTES

N

O
cathepsin O
streptolysin O
O_2
oxygen
OA
open adrenalectomy
osteoid area
OB
Chromagen OB
obese
o. type 2 NIDDM
o. type 2 noninsulin-dependent diabetes mellitus
obesity
abdominal o.
android o.
central o.
centripetal o.
clinical o.
diet-induced o.
genetic o.
gynecoid o.
hypothalamic o.
morbid o.
truncal o.
obesity-related hyposomatotropism
obesity/type 2 diabetes syndrome
ob gene
obligatory thermogenesis
oblique arytenoid
obliterans
arteriosclerosis o.
oblongata
medulla o.
obstruction
superior ophthalmic vein o.
obstructive intestinal disease
obtundation
Oby-trim
OC
Osteocalcin
OCA
oculocutaneous albinism
occludens
zone o.
zonula o.
occlusion
acute arterial o.
branch retinal vein o.
occult
o. biliary microlithiasis
o. carcinoma
o. diabetes
o. myelodysplasia
occupancy
receptor o.
ochronosis
Ochsner clamp
OCIF
osteoclastogenesis inhibitory factor
Oct-1
octamer-binding
Oct-1 transcription factor
octacalcium phosphate
octamer-binding (Oct-1)
o.-b. transcription factor
Octamide
[13C]-octanoic acid test
octapeptide
Octostim
OctreoScan
octreotide
In-111 o.
o. LAR
o. long-acting release
o. scan
somatostatin analogue o.
o. therapy
Ocufen Ophthalmic
ocular
abnormal o. movement
o. albinism
o. calcification
o. complications of diabetes
o. dysmotility
o. histidinemia
o. motility
o. motor cranial nerve
o. neuromyotonia
o. pain
o. paresis
oculocutaneous
o. albinism (OCA)
o. albinism type I
oculodentoosseous dysplasia
oculomotor
o. nerve
o. nerve palsy
oculopharyngeal muscular dystrophy
ODC
ornithine decarboxylase
odds
logarithm of o.
ODF
osteoclast differentiation factor
O_2 disposable boot device
odontoblast
odontohypophosphatasia

odor
apocrine body o.
excessive body o.
oestradiol
Oestrillin
ofloxacin
Ogen
O. Oral
O. Vaginal
OGF
opioid growth factor
ovarian growth factor
OGTT
oral glucose tolerance test
24-OHase
vitamin D 24-hydroxylase
Ohase
hydroxylase
17-OHCS
17-hydroxycorticosteroid
OHL
hydroxylysine
17-OHP
17-hydroxyprogesterone
OHSS
ovarian hyperstimulation syndrome
1,25$(OH)_2$-VitD
1,25-dihydroxyvitamin D
25OH-VitD
25-hydroxyvitamin D
OI
osteogenesis imperfecta
oil
evening primrose o.
iodized o.
progesterone o.
okadaic acid
OKT3
ornithine-ketoacid transaminase
oleic acid
olfaction
olfactory
accessory o. bulb (AOB)
o. bulb
o. placode
oligoanovulation
oligoanuric
oligoasthenozoospermia
oligoclonal
oligoclonality
oligodeoxynucleotide
o. antisense probe
21-mer phosphorothioate antisense o.
oligodontia
oligomenorrhea
o. with anovulatory menses
oligonucleotide
allele-specific o. (ASO)
o. inhibition
o. probe
oligosaccharide
o. chain
high-mannose o.
o. transferase enzyme
oligospermia
oligozoospermia
olivopontocerebellar atrophy
OM
oncostatin M
omega-3 polyunsaturated fatty acid
omega-conotoxin-sensitive pathway
omentum
Cushing disease of the o.
omeprazole
O-methylation
Omnican Piston syringe for insulin
Omnicef
Omnipen
Omnipen-N
omohyoid muscle
OMS Oral
onapristone
Oncet
oncocyte
oncocytic
o. adenoma
o. variant
oncocytoma
oncocytosis
oncogene
B o.
c-*fms* o.
c-myc o.
erb o.
Harvey-Ras o.
kit o.
mas o.
neu o.
RAS o.
rearranged during transformation o.
RET o.
ros o.
v-*erb* A o.
viral o.
oncogenesis
oncogenic
o. osteomalacia
o. rickets
oncogenous
o. osteomalacia
oncosis
oncostatin M (OM)
oncotic pressure
ondansetron

ONDST
overnight high-dose dexamethasone suppression test
One
O. Touch Basic
O. Touch blood glucose meter
O. Touch Fast Take meter kit
O. Touch II hospital blood glucose monitoring system
O. Touch Profile
One-Alpha
ontogenesis
ontogeny
B-cell o.
osteoblast o.
onycholysis
oocyesis
oocyte
o. maturation-inhibiting factor
o. meiotic inhibitor
primary o.
secondary o.
oogonia
oolemma
oophorectomize
oophorectomy
oophoritis
autoimmune o.
oophorus
cumulus o.
open
o. adrenalectomy (OA)
o. posterior fontanelle
o. reading frame (ORF)
opening
diaphragmal o.
operating microscope
operation
Billroth II o.
Frey o.
Karydakis o.
Partington o.
Sistrunk o.
OPG
osteoprotegerin
OPGF
osteoprotegerin factor
OPGL
osteoprotegerin ligand
17-OPH
17-hydroxyprogesterone
ophthalmic
Acular O.
o. administration of insulin
o. artery
o. Graves disease
Ocufen O.
ophthalmopathy
endocrine o.
euthyroid o.
Graves o. (GO)
infiltrative o.
radioiodine-induced exacerbation of o.
thyroid o.
thyroid-associated o. (TAO)
ophthalmoplegia
external o.
internal o.
ophthalmyopathy
opioid
endogenous o.
o. growth factor (OGF)
o. peptide
opioidergic
opioid-stimulated pathway
opisthotonus
opium
o. alkaloid
belladonna and o.
o. tincture
opsonization
optic
o. apparatus glioma
o. canal
o. chiasm
o. and chiasmal neuropathy
o. disk pallor
o. glioma
o. hypocalcemia
o. nerve
o. neuropathy
o. radiation
o. recess
o. tract
o. tract pituitary tumor
opticochiasmatic glioma
Optiquant assay
OR
ovary reserve
Oragrafin
oral
o. administration of insulin

O

NOTES

oral *(continued)*
AllerMax O.
Amen O.
o. antidiabetic agent
Anxanil O.
Aristocort O.
Atarax O.
Atolone O.
Atozine O.
Banophen O.
Belix O.
Benadryl O.
Calm-X O.
Cataflam O.
Celestone O.
o. cholecystographic dye
Cleocin HCl O.
Cleocin Pediatric O.
Cortef O.
Curretab O.
Cycrin O.
Cytomel O.
Decadron O.
Delta-Cortef O.
Dilaudid O.
Dimetabs O.
Dormarex 2 O.
Dormin O.
Dramamine O.
Durrax O.
Estrace O.
Flagyl O.
Genahist O.
o. glucose tolerance test (OGTT)
o. hamartoma
Hydrocortone O.
Hy-Pam O.
o. hypoglycemic agent
Indocin SR O.
Kenacort O.
Marmine O.
Medrol O.
Mephyton O.
MS Contin O.
MSIR O.
o. multiple vitamin
Nor-tet O.
Ogen O.
OMS O.
Oramorph SR O.
Orinase O.
Ortho-Est O.
Panmycin O.
Pediapred O.
Phenergan O.
Prelone O.
Proglycem O.
Protostat O.
Provera O.
Robitet O.
Roxanol SR O.
Sumycin O.
Tega-Vert O.
Tetracap O.
Vamate O.
Vancocin O.
Vistaril O.
Voltaren O.
Voltaren-XR O.

Oralet
Fentanyl O.

Oralgen

Oralin

Oramorph SR Oral

Oramyd

Orasone

orbital
o. apex syndrome
o. cellulitis
o. fat
o. fibroblast
o. tissue

orbitopathy
dysthyroid o.
infiltrative o.
thyroid o.

orchidometer
Prader o.

orchiectomy

orchis

orchitis
mumps o.
tuberculous o.
viral o.

orciprenaline

Oretic

Oreton Methyl

orexigenic
o. agent
o. peptide

Orexin
O. A
O. B

ORF
open reading frame

Org 31806

Org 32376

organ
circumventricular o. (CVO)
effector o.
peripheral o.
subcommissural o. (SCO)
subfornical o. (SFO)
ultimobranchial o.
vomeronasal o.
o. of Zuckerkandl

organic
o. impotence
o. matrix
o. osmolyte
Organidin
O. NR
organification
o. defect
Organization
Pan American Health O. (PAHO)
World Health O. (WHO)
World Health O. (type I, II, III)
organochlorine insecticide
organogenesis
organomegaly
organum
o. vasculosum
o. vasculosum laminae terminalis (OVLT)
o. vasculosum of the lamina terminalis (OVLT)
orgasm
female o.
male o.
origin
gonadotroph cell o.
Schwann cell o.
somatropin of rDNA o.
original University of Wisconsin (oUW)
original University of Wisconsin solution (UW solution)
Orinase
O. Diagnostic Injection
O. Oral
ORL-1 receptor
orlista
orlistat
Ormazine
ornithine
o. carbamoyltransferase
o. cycle
o. decarboxylase (ODC)
o.-ketoacid transaminase (OKT3)
o. transaminase
o. transcarbamylase (OTC)
o. transcarbamylase deficiency
orosomucoid
orotic acid
orphan
O. Annie eye
o. receptor
orphenadrine, aspirin, and caffeine
Ortho-Cept
Ortho-Cyclen
Ortho-Est Oral
orthoiodine atom
Ortho-Novum
O.-N. 1/35
O.-N. 1/50
O.-N. 7/7/7
O.-N. 10/11
orthophosphate
inorganic o. (P_i)
Ortho-Prefest
orthorhombic
orthostasis
orthostatic hypotension
orthotic
custom-healing o.
orthotopic liver transplantation
Ortho Tri-Cyclen
orthotyrosyl iodine atom
Orudis
O. KT
Oruvail
OS
Ensure Glucerna OS
Os-Cal 500
oscillation
ultradian o.
oscillator
circadian o.
oscillatory behavior
Oshaburi-Kombu
Osler-Rendu-Weber disease
Osmitrol Injection
Osm/kg
osmoles per kilogram
Osm/L
osmoles per liter
osmolality
body fluid o.
body water o.
cytosolic o.
o. dehydration test
effective o.
interstitial o.
plasma o. (POSM)
serum o.
urine o.
osmolar
o. clearance
o. gap

NOTES

osmolarity
extracellular fluid o.
osmole
idiogenic o.
osmoles
o. per kilogram (Osm/kg)
o. per liter (Osm/L)
osmolyte
organic o.
osmoreceptor
osmoregulation
osmoregulatory defect
osmostat
osmotic
o. cell injury
o. demyelination
o. diarrhea
o. diuresis
o. diuretic
o. equilibrium
o. hemostasis
o. homeostasis
o. minipump
o. regulation
o. stimulus
o. threshold
osseous
o. fragmentation
o. matrix
ossification
endochondral o.
intramembranous o.
periosteal o.
ossium
fibrogenesis imperfecta o.
Ostaderm
osteitis
o. deformans
o. fibrosa
o. fibrosa cystica
o. fibrosa cystica generalisata of von Recklinghausen
osteoarthritis
osteoarthropathy
hypertrophic o.
primary hypertrophic o.
pulmonary o.
secondary hypertrophic o.
osteoarticular destruction
osteoblast
o. heterogenicity
o. ontogeny
o. phenotype
o. progenitor proliferation
o. proliferation
osteoblastic
o. phenotype
o. resorption
o. tumor
osteoblast-like osteosarcoma cell
osteoblast-mediated bone formation
Osteocalcin (OC)
O. level
O. secretion
serum O.
osteochondrodysplasia
osteoclast
o. activity
o. apoptosis
bone-resorbing o.
o. differentiation factor (ODF)
o. precursor
o. ultrastructure
osteoclast-activated bone resorption
osteoclast-driven bone resorption
osteoclastic
o. activity
o. bone
o. bone resorption
o. function
o. nucleus
o. osteolysis
o. resorption lacuna
o. stimulation
osteoclast-mediated bone resorption
osteoclastogenesis
o. inhibitory factor (OCIF)
osteocyte
osteocytic
o. membrane system
o. osteolysis
osteodysplasia of Melnick and Needles
osteodysplastic primordial dwarfism
osteodystrophy
Albright hereditary o. (AHO)
aplastic uremic o.
mixed uremic o.
pediatric renal o.
renal o.
thyrotoxic o.
uremic o.
osteoectasia with hyperphosphatasia
osteofibrosis
osteogenesis
o. imperfecta (OI)
O. Imperfecta Foundation
o. imperfecta types I, II, III, IV
osteogenic protein-2
osteoid
o. accumulation
o. area (OA)
o. seam
o. seam thickness
o. surface

unmineralized lamellar o.
woven o.
osteoinduction
osteolysis
carpotarsal o.
familial expansile o. (FEO)
Gorham massive o.
idiopathic o.
osteoclastic o.
osteocytic o.
osteolytic
o. flame
o. lesion
osteoma
osteomalacia
aluminum-associated o.
aluminum-induced o.
aluminum-related o.
axial o.
calvarial o.
hypophosphatemic o.
oncogenic o.
oncogenous o.
o. syndrome
vitamin D-deficiency o.
Osteomark
osteomesopyknosis
osteomyelitis
temporal bone o.
osteon
osteonecrosis
osteonectin
osteopathia striata
osteopenia
corticoid-induced o.
cyclosporine A-induced o.
posttransplantation o.
progressive o.
trabecular o.
osteopetrosis
human malignant o.
infantile o.
osteopetrotic
o. microphthalmic
o. mutation
o. phenotype
osteophyte
osteopoikilosis
osteopontin
osteoporosis
age-related o.
o. circumscripta
glucocorticoid-induced o.
idiopathic juvenile o.
involutional o.
low-turnover o.
postmenopausal o.
posttraumatic o.
steroid-induced o.
osteoporotic cytokine
osteoprogenitor
o. cell
osteoprotegerin (OPG)
o. factor (OPGF)
o. ligand (OPGL)
osteosarcoma
osteosclerosis
autosomal dominant o.
hepatitis C-associated o.
osteostatin
osteotomy
cranioorbitozygomatic o. (COZ)
Ostoforte
OT
oxytocin
OTC
ornithine transcarbamylase
OTC deficiency
otitis
malignant external o.
ouabain
ouabain-like hormone
ouabain-sensitive Na^+-K^+ ATPase
outcome
visual o.
outgrowth
neurite o.
output
cardiac o. (CO)
hepatic glucose o. (HGO)
urine o.
oUW
original University of Wisconsin
oUW solution
ova
primordial o.
ovale
foramen o.
ovarian
o. ablation
o. cortex
o. cycle
o. dysgenesis
o. endometriosis cyst

NOTES

ovarian *(continued)*
o. failure
o. fimbria
o. follicle
o. goiter
o. granulosa cell
o. growth factor (OGF)
o. hyperandrogenesis
o. hyperandrogenism
o. hyperstimulation syndrome (OHSS)
o. hyperthecosis
o. hypoandrogenism
o. ligament
o. steroidogenesis
o. steroidogenic dysfunction
o. teratoma
o. tumor
o. venous plasma oxytocin
ovariectomy
ovarii
struma o.
ovary
Chinese hamster o. (CHO)
cystic o.
granulosa cell tumor of the o.
polycystic o. (PCO)
o. reserve (OR)
resistant o.
streak o.
syndrome of polycystic o.
Ovcon
O. 35
O. 50
overactivity
thyroid o.
overexpressed
overexpression
gene o.
overgrowth
acral o.
articular o.
bacterial o. (BO)
overinvolution
overlap syndrome
overload
aluminum o.
iron o.
overnight
o. high-dose dexamethasone suppression test (ONDST)
o. metyrapone test
o. 1-mg dexamethasone suppression test
oversuppression
overt glycosuria
overtreatment
overworked B-cell hypothesis
Ovidrel
oviduct
ovine corticotropin-releasing hormone
OVLT
organum vasculosum laminae terminalis
organum vasculosum of the lamina terminalis
Ovol
ovotestis
Ovral
Ovrette
ovulation
o. induction
paracyclic o.
ovulatory
o. cycle
o. follicle
OX40 ligand (OX40L)
oxalate
calcium o.
Oxandrin
oxandrolone
oxaprozin
oxidase
corticosterone methyl o. (CMO)
corticosterone methyl o. II
cytochrome o.
diamine o. (DAO)
enzyme lysyl o.
hydroxyproline o.
immunogenic glucose o.
lysyl o.
methyl o.
monoamine o. (MAO)
proline o.
terminal o.
18-oxidase
oxidase-platin
glucose o.-p.
oxidation
fatty acid o.
glucose o.
oxidative
o. damage
o. phosphorylation
oxide
intrapenile nitric o.
magnesium o.
nitric o. (NO)
phenylarsine o.
zirconium o.
oxilorphan
OX40L
OX40 ligand
oxoacid
2-o.
3-o.-CoA transferase
18-oxocortisol

5-oxoproline
oxtriphylline
oxycodone
o. and acetaminophen
o. and aspirin
OxyContin
oxygen (O_2)
o. disposable boot device
o. free radical
hyperbaric o.
singlet o.
oxygenase
mixed-function o.
OxyIR
oxymetazoline hydrochloride
oxymetholone
oxymorphone
oxyphenbutazone
oxyphil cell
oxyphilic
o. adenoma
o. change
o. metaplasia
oxytocic
o. fraction
oxytocin (OT)
ovarian venous plasma o.
o. secretion
oxytocinergic
o. cell body
o. neuron
oxytocin-neurophysin
Oyst-Cal 500
Oystercal 500

NOTES

P
progesterone
substance P
P450
P450 arom
aromatase P450
P450 aromatase (placental) deficiency
cytochrome P450
P450 side chain cleavage (P450SCC)
P450 side chain cleavage enzyme
P_i
inorganic orthophosphate
17p12-13
chromosome 17p12-13
p53
p. gene
p. tumor-suppressor gene
p160 family of coactivators
P21 gene
$p21^{WAF1}$ tumor-suppressor gene
P450arom gene
P450c21 deficiency
P450SCC enzyme
p57KIP2 gene
p75 protein
PAAF
pancreatitis-associated ascites fluid
PAAP
percutaneous alcohol ablation of the parathyroid gland
PABM
peak adult bone mass
PAC
pancreatic adenocarcinoma
plasma aldosterone concentration
PAC lateralization ratio
PACE
pulmonary angiotensin I converting enzyme
pacemaker
accurate p.
endogenous circadian p.
idioventricular p.
sloppy p.
universal p.
X p.
Y p.
pachydermoperiostosis
packing
cotton pledget p.
paclitaxel
PAC/PRA
plasma aldosterone concentration/plasma renin activity
PAC/PRA ratio
PAD
peripheral arterial disease
pad
cervicodorsal fat p.
clavicular fat p.
dorsocervical fat p.
infraclavicular fat p.
supraclavicular fat p.
thinning fat p.
PAF
platelet-activating factor
PAG
pineal antigonadotropin
Paget
P. disease
P. disease of bone
pagetic
p. bone
p. bone lesion
PAH
prealbumin-associated hyperthyroxinemia
PAHO
Pan American Health Organization
PAHO grade 0, 1, 2
PAHO stage 0, Ia, Ib, II, III
PAI
plasminogen activator inhibitor
PAI-1
plasminogen activator inhibitor-1
pain
bone p.
C-fiber p.
ocular p.
painful
p. subacute thyroiditis
p. thyroiditis
Pain-HP
No P.-H.
painless
p. cold-sensitive digital vasospasm
p. hyperthyroidism
p. postpartum thyroiditis
paint
luminescent p.
paired
p. box homeotic 3 (PAX3)
p. box homeotic 8 (PAX8)
PAK
pancreas after kidney
PAK transplantation

PAL
peptidyl-alpha-hydroxyglycine alpha-amidating lyase
palate
high-arched p.
pallidus
globus p.
Pallister-Hall syndrome
pallor
disk p.
optic disk p.
palmar keratosis
Palmitate-A 5000
palmitic acid
palmitoleic acid
palmitoyltransferase
carnitine p. I (CPTI)
carnitine p. II (CPTII)
palmoplantar keratosis
palpation thyroiditis
palsy
cerebral p.
cranial nerve p.
hereditary neuropathy with liability to pressure p. (HNPP)
lateral rectus p.
oculomotor nerve p.
superior oblique p.
PAM
peptidylglycine alpha-amidating monooxygenase
pamidronate
intravenous p.
Pamine
PAMP
proadrenomedullin N-20 terminal peptide
pampiniform plexus
Pamprin IB
PAN
primary afferent nociceptor neuron
Pan
P. American Health Organization (PAHO)
P. American Health Organization grade (0–2)
Panadol
panadrenal insufficiency
Panasal 5/500
PANCH
pituitary adenoma-adenohypophyseal neuronal choristoma
pancreas
p. after kidney (PAK)
p. after kidney transplantation
annular p.
bioartificial p.
cadaver p.
p. cancer
cortex p.
p. divisum
endocrine p.
exocrine p.
head of p.
mucin-producing tumor of the p.
neck of p.
remnant p.
retention cyst of the p.
serous cystadenoma of the p.
Starling curve of the p.
p. transplantation alone (PTA)
Pancrease
P. MT
pancreastatin
pancreatectomy
distal subtotal p.
total p.
pancreatic
p. acinar cell
p. adenocarcinoma (PAC)
p. alpha-cell tumor
p. cholera
p. denervation
p. diabetes
p. digestive zymogen
p. disorder
p. duct cell carcinoma (PDC)
p. endocrine neoplasm (PEN)
p. endocrine tumor
p. enzyme
p. exocrine deficit
p. functioning diagnostant (PFD)
p. functioning diagnostant test
p. islet beta cell
p. islet cell-specific enhancer sequence (PICSES)
p. islet cell tumor
p. juice
p. parenchyma
p. parenchymal perfusion
p. polypeptide (PP)
p. polypeptide-secreting tumor (PPoma)
p. steatorrhea
p. stone
p. tuberculosis
pancreaticoblastoma
pancreaticojejunostomy
side-to-side p.
pancreatin
pancreatis insufficiency
pancreatitis
acute hemorrhagic p. (AHP)
acute necrotizing p.
acute recurrent p. (ARP)
alcohol-related chronic p. (ARCP)
chronic alcoholic p. (CAP)
early-onset idiopathic chronic p.
eosinophilic p.
groove p.

hereditary p. (HP)
idiopathic p.
late-onset idiopathic chronic p.
mass-forming p.
severe acute p. (SAP)
tropical calcific p. (TCP)
tumor-forming p.

pancreatitis-associated
p.-a. ascites fluid (PAAF)
p.-a. protein (PAP)

pancreatoduodenectomy (PD)
pylorus-preserving p. (PPPD)

pancreatogram

pancreatography
computed tomography under endoscopic retrograde p. (ERP-CT)

pancreatopathy
fibrocalculous p.

pancreatoscope
ultrathin p.

pancreatoscopy
peroral p.

Pancrecarb
P. MS-8

pancrelipase

pancreolauryl test

pancreozymin
p. secretin (PS)
p. secretin test

pancytopenia

pandemic
encephalitis p.

panhypopituitarism
hereditary p.

Panmycin Oral

Panomat microinfusion pump

panophthalmitis

panoramic visualization

Pantopon

pantothenic acid

PAP
pancreatitis-associated protein

Pap
Papanicolaou
Pap smear

Papanicolaou (Pap)
P. smear
P. Society of Cytopathology
P. stain

PAPase
phosphatidate phosphohydrolase

papaverine

papilla
dental p.
dermal p.
fungiform p.
renal p.

papillary
p. adenoma
p. craniopharyngioma
p. necrosis
p. nephrocalcinosis
p. renal carcinoma
p. stenosis
p. thyroid cancer
p. thyroid carcinoma (PTC)
p. tumor projection

papilledema

papilloma
intraductal p.

papillomatosis
juvenile p.

papillomatous papule

papular mucinosis

papule
papillomatous p.

PAR
plasma appearance rate

paraadenomatous corticotroph hyperplasia

paraaminobenzoic acid

paraaminosalicylic acid

paraaortic lymph nodes

parabasal cell

parabolic reflector

paracellular calcium resorption

paracentesis
abdominal p.
large-volume p. (LVP)

paracetamol

paracetic acid-based method

paracoccidioidomycosis

paracrine
p. action
p. agent
p. cell
p. effect
p. factor
p. regulation
p. secretion
p. suppressor
p. system

paracyclic ovulation

NOTES

paraendocrine
paraffin-embedded semithin section
parafollicular
p. calcitonin-producing cell
p. duct
paraganglia
paraganglioma
adrenal medullary p.
extraadrenal p.
paragonimiasis
parahormone
paralactin
parallel
p. development of axillary hair
p. development of pubic hair
p. hole collimation
paralysis
familial periodic p.
hyperthyroid periodic p.
hypokalemic periodic p.
thyrotoxic periodic p.
vocal cord p.
paralytic ileus
paramagnetic
p. metal
p. nucleus
paramedian reticular nucleus
paramesonephric duct
paramethasone acetate
paraneoplastic
p. growth hormone
p. syndrome
p. tumor
paraneurone
parapineal
parapituitary
p. area
paraplegia
Basedow p.
spastic p.
paraquat
parasellar
p. meningioma
p. region
p. syndrome
p. tissue
p. tumor
parastatin
parasternal node
parasympathetic
p. nerve
p. nervi erigentes
p. nervous system
paraterminal gyrus
Parathar
parathion
parathormone (PTH)
parathyrin
parathyroid
abnormal p. gland
p. adenoma
p. autotransplantation
p. carcinoma
p. cell
p. cell membrane
p. computed tomography
congenital aplasia of the p.
p. crisis
p. cyst
p. extracellular calcium-sensing receptor
p. gland
p. gland dysfunction
p. gland hyperplasia
p. hormone (PTH)
p. hormone assay
p. hormone excess
p. hormone gene transcription
p. hormonelike polypeptide (PTH-LP)
p. hormonelike protein
p. hormone-mediated calcium efflux
p. hormone-related peptide (PTHrP, PTH-RP)
p. hormone-related protein
p. hormone-related protein-transfected RIN-141 cell
p. hormone resistance syndrome
p. hormone secretion
p. insufficiency
p. scintigraphy
p. ultrasound
parathyroidal abscess
parathyroidectomy (PTX)
subtotal p.
total p.
parathyroiditis
paraventricular
p. neuron
p. nucleus (PVN)
p. nucleus of the hypothalamus
p. thalamic nucleus (PVT)
paregoric
parenchyma
breast p.
pancreatic p.
thyroid p.
parenchymal brain injury
parenchymography
cephalic p.
parenteral
p. iron dextran
p. nutrition
parents
consanguineous p.

paresis
ocular p.
paresthesia
paricalcitol
p. injection
parietalis
decidua p.
Parinaud syndrome
Parkinson disease
parkinsonism
idiopathic p.
Parlodel
P. LAR
parolfactory gyrus
parotid
p. gland
p. hormone
p. sialography
parotitis
paroxetine
paroxysm
lethal p.
paroxysmal
p. hypersexuality
p. hypertension
p. hyperthermia
p. hypothermia
p. nocturnal hemoglobinuria
p. pain disorder
Parry disease
pars
p. arcuata
p. distalis
p. infundibularis
p. infundibulum
p. intermedia
p. intermedia cyst
p. nervosa
p. posterior
p. recta
p. tuberalis
part
intramural uterine p.
thickened acral p.
partial
p. agonist
p. agonist-partial antagonist
p. androgen insensitivity
p. androgen sensitivity
p. hydatidiform mole
p. 21-hydroxylase deficiency
p. hypopituitarism
p. insulin resistance
p. resection
p. thyroid-stimulating hormone hyporesponsiveness
p. TSH hyporesponsiveness
partial labioscrotal fusion
particle
hydroxyapatite/tricalcium phosphate p.
Partington operation
parturition
parvocellular
p. division
p. neuron
parvovirus B19
PAS
periodic acid-Schiff
PAS resistant
passive immunity
patch
Androderm testosterone transdermal p.
blue p.
gray p.
Habitrol P.
Nicoderm P.
Nicotrol P.
Peyer p.
ProStep P.
scrotal matrix p.
signal p.
testosterone skin p.
transdermal scrotum testosterone p.
transdermal torso testosterone p.
patent ductus arteriosus
path
embryonal p.
Pathilon
pathogen
blood-borne p.
pathognomic
pathognomonic
p. Askanazy cell
p. black eschar
pathologic
p. calcification
p. hypercortisolemia
p. parathyroid disease
pathological endocrine tissue
pathophysiological condition
pathway
adenylyl cyclase p.

NOTES

pathway *(continued)*
afferent p.
apoptosis p.
L-arginine:nitric oxide p.
cholinergic p.
cyclooxygenase p.
17-deoxy p.
energy p.
G-protein signaling p.
Gs-cAMP p.
inositol phosphate p.
insulin signaling p.
lipoxygenase p.
MAPK p.
MAP kinase p.
mitogen-activated protein kinase p.
monoamine p.
multisynaptic p.
nicotine-stimulated p.
omega-conotoxin-sensitive p.
opioid-stimulated p.
pentose phosphate p.
phosphoinositide-protein kinase A p.
phospholipase C p.
polyol p.
proteolytic p.
serine phosphorylation p.
signal-transduction p.
steroidogenic p.
type 2 energy p.
ubiquitin-proteasome p.
patient
acromegalic p.
Bercu p.
Bercu p. of Kindred S
chronic dialysis p.
euvolemic p.
Refetoff p.
testosterone-deficient p.
pattern
bimodal p.
birefringent p.
chromophobic p.
circadian p.
glandular p.
insular p.
macrofollicular p.
marble bone p.
microfollicular p.
mixed p.
sinusoidal p.
trabecular p.
undifferentiated p.
pauciclonal
pause and squeeze technique
PAX3
paired box homeotic 3
PAX3 gene
PAX8
paired box homeotic 8
PAX8 factor
PBB
polybrominated biphenyl
PBL
peripheral blood lymphocyte
PBM
peripheral blood monocyte
P-box
PBR
peripheral-type benzodiazepine receptor
PC
proprotein convertase
PC1
prohormone convertase 1
PC2
prohormone convertase 2
PC3
prohormone convertase 3
PCB
polychlorinated biphenyl
P450c17 deficiency
p/CIP coactivator
PCNA
proliferating cell nuclear antigen
PCNS
primary central nervous system
PCNS lymphoma
PCO
polycystic ovary
PCO syndrome (PCOS)
PCOD
polycystic ovary disease
PCOS
PCO syndrome
polycystic ovarian syndrome
polycystic ovary syndrome
PCPB
procarboxypeptidase B
PCR
plasma clearance rate
polymerase chain reaction
PCT
proximal convoluted tubule
PD
pancreatoduodenectomy
peritoneal dialysis
PDC
pancreatic duct cell carcinoma
PDE5
phosphodiesterase 5
PDGF
platelet-derived growth factor
PDGF gene
PDGF protein
PDGF-A
platelet-derived growth factor A

PDH
pyruvate dehydrogenase
PDI
protein disulfide isomerase
PDI-mediated disulfide bond reduction
PDK
3-phosphoinositide-dependent protein kinase
PDM
Bontril P.
PDR
proliferative diabetic retinopathy
PDS
Pendred syndrome
PDS gene
PDX-1
PE-3
phosphatidylinositol
peak
p. adult bone mass (PABM)
estradiol p.
p. thyroid-stimulating hormone response
p. TSH response
pearl
P. Hypoglycemic capsule
pheochromocytoma p.
Pearson syndrome
pebble
fiber p.
pectoralis fascia
Pedersen hypothesis
Pediacof
Pediapred Oral
Pedia-Profen
Pediatric
M.V.I. P.
P. Triban
pediatric
p. multiple vitamin
p. renal osteodystrophy
pedicle
superior vascular p.
pedigree
p. analysis
X-linked dominant p.
Pedituss
PedTE-PAK-4
Pedtrace-4
peduncle
cerebral p.
mammillary p.
Zuckerkandl p.
pedunculi
basis p.
PEG-ADA
polyethylene glycol-adenosine deaminase
pegademase
p. bovine
pegvisomant
p. for injection
Trovett p.
peliosis
p. hepatis
Pelizaeus-Merzbacher disease
pellagra
Pellet
Testopel P.
pellucida
zona p.
zona p. 1 (ZP1)
zona p. 2 (ZP2)
zona p. 3 (ZP3)
pellucidum
septum p.
pelvic
p. infertility factor
p. inflammatory disease
p. rhabdomyosarcoma
pelvis
renal p.
PEM
protein-energy malnutrition
Pemberton
P. sign
pemphigoid
bullous p.
pemphigus vulgaris
PEN
pancreatic endocrine neoplasm
pen
Disetronic P.
Genotropin P. 5
Humalog P.
Humulin Mix 75/25 P.
Humulin R p.
insulin p.
Pendred
P. syndrome (PDS)
P. syndrome gene
pendrin
p. protein
PenFill

NOTES

P

penicillamine
penicillin v potassium
penile
p. brachial index
p. length
p. prosthesis
p. self-injection
p. urethra
penis
p. at twelve syndrome
bulbus p.
crus p.
glans p.
penoscrotal hypospadias
pentachlorophenol
pentagastrin
p. provocation test
pentalaminar tubular structure
pentameric
p. GH
p. growth hormone
pentamidine
pentapeptide
pentavalent dimercaptosuccinate (DMSA)
pentazocine
p. compound
pentetreotide
indium-111 p.
pentolinium tartrate
pentose phosphate pathway
pentosuria
Pentothal
pentoxifylline
Pen-Vee K
Pepcid
P. AC
P. RPD
PEPCK
phosphoenolpyruvate-carboxykinase
PEPI
Postmenopausal Estrogen/Progestin Interventions Trial
Peptavlon
peptic ulcer disease
peptid
signal p.
peptidase
dipeptidyl p.
exopeptidase dipeptidyl p. I, II
pyroglutamyl p. II
signal p.
peptide
agouti-related p.
amyloid p.
atrial natriuretic p. (ANP)
bombesin-like p.
brain-gut p.
brain natriuretic p. (BNP)
C p.
calcitonin gene-related p. (CGRP)
connecting p.
corticotropin-like intermediate lobe p. (CLIP)
C-type natriuretic p. (CNP)
endogenous opioid p. (EOP)
gastric inhibitory p. (GIP)
gastrin-releasing p. (GRP)
GH-releasing p. (GHRP)
glucagon-like p. (GLP)
glucagon-like p.-1 (GLP-1)
GnRH-associated p. (GAP)
gonadal p.
gonadotropin-associated p.
p. growth factor
growth hormone-releasing p. (GHRP)
growth hormone-releasing p. (GHRP)
gut p.
gut-brain p.
helix-bundle p. (HBP)
p. histidine isoleucine (PHI)
p. histidine methionine (PHM)
p. hystidyl-methionine-27 (PHM-27)
intervening p. (IP)
latency-associated p. (LAP)
MB-35 p.
monitor p.
MSH p.
natriuretic p.
neurohypophysial p.
nociceptin/orphanin FQ p.
N/OFQ p.
N-terminal p.
opioid p.
orexigenic p.
parathyroid hormone-related p. (PTHrP, PTH-RP)
pituitary adenylyl cyclase-activating p.
proadrenomedullin N-20 terminal p. (PAMP)
procollagen-III p. (pIIIp)
proopiomelanocortin-derived p.
regulatory p.
signal p.
thrombin receptor-activating p. 6 (TRAP-6)
thymosin p.
trypsinogen-activating p. (TAP)
type 1 procollagen p.
urinary gonadotropin p. (UGP)
vasoactive intestinal p. (VIP)
vasodilator p.
p. YY
peptide-1
peptide-4
human neutrophil p. (HNP-4)

peptide-6
peptide-amino acid hormone
peptidergic neuron
peptidoglycan
peptidyl-alpha-hydroxyglycine alpha-amidating lyase (PAL)
peptidylglycine alpha-amidating monooxygenase (PAM)
peptidylglycine alpha-hydroxylating monooxygenase (PHM)
PER
period
PER gene
PER protein
peracetic acid
perception
depth p.
thermal p.
perchlorate
p. discharge test
Percocet
Percodan
Percodan-Demi
Percogesic
Percoll gradient
Percolone
percutaneous
p. alcohol ablation of the parathyroid gland (PAAP)
p. alcohol serotherapy
p. biopsy
p. bone marrow injection
p. choledochoscopy
p. femoral vein
p. fine-needle ethanol injection (PFNEI)
p. nephrolithotomy
perforin
perfusion
pancreatic parenchymal p.
peripheral p.
pergolide
p. mesylate
Pergonal
Perheentupa syndrome
Peri
Genotropin P. 12
Periactin
periampullary malignancy
periaqueductal gray area
periarteritis nodosa
pericardial bioprosthetic tissue
perichondrium
perifornical region
perikarya
perikaryal
p. cytoplasm
p. group
perikaryon
magnocellular p.
norepinephrine p.
periluminal
perilymph
p. fluid
perimenarchal period
perimenopausal period
perimenopause
perimetric technique
perimetrium
perimetry
automated p.
Goldmann p.
perimysial fibroblast
perineoplastic thyroiditis
perineoscrotal hypospadias
perinephric fat
period (PER)
p. gene
last menstrual p. (LMP)
perimenarchal p.
perimenopausal p.
p. protein
somatosensory-evoked potential recovery p.
periodic
p. acid-Schiff (PAS)
p. acid-Schiff-positive
p. acid-Schiff resistant
periodically fluctuating protein kinase (PFK)
periodontal membrane
perioral dermatitis
periorbital
p. edema
p. puffiness
periosteal
p. envelope
p. hypertrophy
p. ossification
periosteocytic space
periosteum
periovarian adhesion
periovulatory phase

NOTES

P

peripancreatic
p. neoplasm
p. pseudoaneurysm
peripapillary staphylomata
peripheral
p. arterial disease (PAD)
p. blood lymphocyte (PBL)
p. blood monocyte (PBM)
p. cytotrophoblast cell
p. diabetes insipidus
p. glucocorticoid deficiency
p. insulin sensitivity
p. nervous system (PNS)
p. neuroglia
p. neuropathy
p. organ
p. perfusion
p. scalloping
p. T_4
p. thyroid hormone metabolism
p. thyroxine
p. tissue resistance to thyroid hormone (PTRTH)
peripheral-type benzodiazepine receptor (PBR)
peristalsis
perithymic fat
perithyroidal adventitia
peritoneal
p. dialysis (PD)
p. fluid (PF)
p. oocyte and sperm transfer (POST)
peritoneovenous shunt
peritonitis
p. carcinomatosa
spontaneous bacterial p.
peritonsillar abscess
peritubular endothelial cell
peritumor glial reaction
periumbilical staining
perivasculitis
superficial dermal p.
periventricular
p. stratum
p. zone
perivitelline
p. barrier
p. space
perleche
Perles
Tessalon P.
permanent
p. diabetes insipidus
p. hypoparathyroidism
Permax
permissive factor
pernicious anemia
peroral pancreatoscopy
peroxidase
antithyroid p.
glutathione p.
thyroid p. (TPO)
peroxidation
lipid p.
peroxide
benzoyl p.
hydrogen p.
lipid p.
p. tone
peroxisomal disorder
peroxisome
p. proliferator-activated receptor (PPAR)
p. proliferator-activated receptor gene
peroxynitrite anion
perphenazine
Perrault syndrome
persephin (PSP)
persistent
p. hyperinsulinemic hypoglycemia of infancy (PHHI)
p. hyperparathyroidism
p. müllerian duct syndrome
p. polyuria
Personal Lasette
perstans
Mansonella p.
telangiectasia macularis eruptiva p.
pertechnetate (Tc-99m-TcO4)
p. scintigraphy
technetium p.
p. thyroid scan
perturbation
Pertussin
P. ES
pertussis
p. toxin
p. toxin-sensitive
PET
positron emission tomography
petrosal
p. sinus
p. sinus blood
p. sinus sampling
Peutz-Jeghers syndrome
PEX
phosphate-regulating gene with homologies to endopeptidases found at the HYP locus on the X chromosome
pexiganan acetate
Peyer patch
Peyronie disease
PF
peritoneal fluid

PFD
- pancreatic functioning diagnostant
- polyostotic fibrous dysplasia
  - PFD test

Pfeiffer syndrome

PFK
- periodically fluctuating protein kinase
- phosphofructokinase

PFNEI
- percutaneous fine-needle ethanol injection

PG
- postprandial glucose

PGA-I
- polyglandular autoimmune syndrome type I

PGA-II
- polyglandular autoimmune syndrome type II

PGC
- primordial germ cell

PGD_2
- prostaglandin D_2

PGE

PGE_2
- prostaglandin E_2

PGE_1
- prostaglandin E_1

PGF_{2a}
- prostaglandin F_{2a}

$PGF_{2\alpha}$
- prostaglandin $F_{2\alpha}$

PGG_2
- prostaglandin G_2

PGH_2
- prostaglandin H_2

PGHS
- prostaglandin H synthase

PGI

PGI2
- prostacyclin

PGI_2
- prostacyclin
- prostaglandin I_2

PGJ
- prostaglandin J

PGK
- phosphoglycerate kinase
  - PGK deficiency

P-glycoprotein (Pgp)

Pgp
- P-glycoprotein

pH
- extracellular pH
- physiologic pH
- urine pH

PHA
- phytohemagglutinin
- posterior hypothalamic area
- pseudohypoaldosteronism

PHA I
- pseudohypoaldosteronism type I

PHA II
- pseudohypoaldosteronism type II

phagedena

phagocytic
- p. activity

phagocytosis

phagolysosome

phagosome

phallic size

pharmacoepidemiologic survey

pharmacologic
- p. estrogen administration
- p. therapy
- p. treatment

pharmakinetic

pharyngeal
- p. hypophysis
- p. pituitary
- p. pouch

phase
- acrosome p.
- cap p.
- cephalic p.
- coupling p.
- estradiol-norethisterone p.
- follicular p.
- Golgi p.
- late luteal p.
- luteal p.
- periovulatory p.
- reversal p.
- shortened luteal p.
- short luteal p.
- thyrotoxic p.

Phazyme

Phenadex Senior

Phenazine Injection

phendimetrazine

phenelzine

Phenerbel-S

Phenergan
- P. Injection

NOTES

P

Phenergan *(continued)*
P. Oral
P. Rectal
P. VC with codeine
P. With codeine
phenformin
phenobarbital
phenobarbitone
phenolic
p. orthohydrogen atom
phenol sulfotransferase
phenomenon
aldosterone escape p.
Arthus p.
dawn p.
escape p.
first-passage p.
hemifield slide p.
Houssay p.
Jod-Basedow p.
Lyon p.
Somogyi p.
thyroid cork p.
Titanic p.
phenothiazine
phenotype
CD8+ p.
female p.
fibroblastic p.
male p.
osteoblast p.
osteoblastic p.
osteopetrotic p.
pituicyte hormonal p.
Reifenstein p.
somatic p.
phenotype-genotype analysis
Phenoxine
phenoxybenzamine
phentermine
phentolamine
phenylacetate
phenylalanine
phenylalanine-restricted diet
phenylarsine oxide
phenylbutazone
Phenyldrine
phenylethanolamine
p. N-methyltransferase (PNMT)
phenylhydrazine
phenylisopropyladenosine
phenylketonuria (PKU)
phenylpropionate
nandrolone p.
phenyltoloxamine
acetaminophen and p.
phenytoin
p. load
p. sodium
pheochromoblast
pheochromocyte
pheochromocytoma
adrenal p.
asymptomatic p.
benign sporadic adrenal p.
extraadrenal p.
familial p.
MIBG-negative pelvic p.
nonfunctioning p.
p. pearl
subclinical p.
pheomelanin
pheromone
signaling p.
PHHI
persistent hyperinsulinemic hypoglycemia of infancy
PHI
peptide histidine isoleucine
philtrum
phlebotomy
phlorhizin
phloroglucinol
PHM
peptide histidine methionine
peptidylglycine alpha-hydroxylating monooxygenase
PHM-27
peptide hystidyl-methionine-27
phonocardiogram
phosphatase
p. activity
alkaline p.
alkaline phosphatase antialkaline p. (APAAP)
bone alkaline p.
bone-specific alkaline p.
p. enzyme
glucose p.
phosphoprotein p.
plasma bone alkaline p.
serum alkaline p.
tartrate-resistant acid p. (TRAP)
p. and tensin homologue deleted on chromosome (PTEN)
phosphate
alpha-glycerol p.
amorphous calcium p.
p. balance
p. binder
p. binding
calcium hydrogen p.
cellulose sodium p.
p. deficiency

p. depletion
dibasic calcium p.
dihydrogen p.
dolichyl p.
glucose p.
inorganic p.
p. ion
p. load
magnesium ammonium p.
monohydrogen p.
nicotinamide adenine dinucleotide p. (NADPH)
octacalcium p.
phosphatidylinositol p.
plasma p.
potassium p.
pyridoxal p.
p. reabsorption
p. retention
sodium p.

phosphate-binding agent
phosphate-protein restriction
phosphate-regulating gene with homologies to endopeptidases found at the HYP locus on the X chromosome (PEX)
phosphatidate phosphohydrolase (PAPase)
phosphatidic acid
phosphatidylcholine
phosphatidylglycerol
phosphatidylinositide
p. metabolite
phosphatidylinositol (PE-3)
p. 4,5-bisphosphate (PIP_2)
p. 3′-kinase (PI3-K)
p. phosphate
p. signal
phosphatonin
phosphaturia
calcitonin-induced p.
phosphaturic
p. action
p. response
phosphodiester
p. linkage
phosphodiesterase
p. 5 (PDE5)
cGMP p.
cyclic nucleotide p.
p. inhibitor
phosphoenolpyruvate
p. carboxykinase gene
phosphoenolpyruvate-carboxykinase (PEPCK)
phosphoethanolamine
urinary p.
phosphofructokinase (PFK)
6-phosphofructo-2-kinase
phosphoglycerate
p. kinase (PGK)
p. kinase deficiency
p. mutase deficiency
phosphohydrolase
phosphatidate p. (PAPase)
phosphoinositide
3-p.-dependent protein kinase (PDK)
p. hydrolysis
phosphoinositide 3′kinase (PI3′K)
phosphoinositide-protein kinase A pathway
phosphokinase
serum creatine p.
Phospholine
phospholipase
p. A_2 (PLA_2)
p. C (PLC)
p. C enzyme
p. C pathway
p. D (PLD)
phospholipid
p. vesicle
phosphopenia
phosphopenic rickets
phosphoprotein
p. phosphatase
phosphoribosylpyrophosphate (PRPP)
phosphoribosylpyrophosphate synthase
phosphoribosyltransferase
adenine p.
hypoxanthine p.
hypoxanthine-guanine p. (HPRT)
21-mer phosphorothioate antisense oligodeoxynucleotide
phosphorus
p. balance
p. binding
p. content
dietary p.
p. dietary restriction
p. distribution

NOTES

P

phosphorus *(continued)*
p. homeostasis
lipid p.
p. metabolism
serum inorganic p.
phosphorus-induced
p.-i. hyperparathyroidism
p.-i. hypocalcemia
phosphorylase
p. *a*
p. *b*
p. b kinase
p. enzyme
glycogen p.
liver p.
purine nucleoside p. (PNP)
phosphorylated
p. glycolytic intermediate
p. rhodopsin function
p. serine 137
phosphorylate membrane protein
phosphorylation
estrogen receptor p.
oxidative p.
protein tyrosine p.
tyrosine p.
phosphoserine
Phospho-Soda
Fleet P.-S.
phosphotransferase
phosphotyrosine
phosphotyrosine-binding domain (PTB)
photic entrainment
photoactivation
photoactive yellow protein
photoaging
cutaneous p.
photocoagulation
photolysis
nonenzymatic p.
photometry
flame p.
photomotogram
photooncogene
photoperiodic
p. environment
p. mechanism
photoperiodism
photosensitivity
photosensitization reaction
phototherapy
PHP
pseudohypoparathyroidism
PHP-1a
PHP-1b
PHPT
primary hyperparathyroidism
phrenic nerve
phycomycosis
Phyllocontin
phylloides
cystosarcoma p.
phylogeny
physalaemin
physical half-life
physiologic
p. effect
p. pH
p. regulator
physiologically active calcium
physiological range
physiology
reproductive p.
physiolysis
physique
lean p.
Phyto-EST
phytoestrogen
phytohemagglutinin (PHA)
phytohormone
phytonadione
phytosterolemia
PI
polyphosphoinositide
PIA
purinergic agonist
piarachnoid membrane
pickwickian syndrome
picogram
PICSES
pancreatic islet cell-specific enhancer sequence
PID
primary immune deficiency
Piedmont plateau
piezoelectric effect
PIF
prolactin-inhibiting factor
pigeon
p. breast
p. crop sac-stimulation assay
pigment
age p.
cytochrome p. (CYP)
minocycline-associated p.
p. urochrome
pigmentation
café au lait p.
cutaneous p.
pigmented
p. nodular adrenocortical disease (PPNAD)
pigmentosa
retinitis p.
urticaria p.
xeroderma p.

pigmentosum
PIH
pregnancy-induced hypertension
prolactin-inhibiting hormone
prolactin inhibitory hormone
prolactin release-inhibiting hormone
pIIIp
procollagen-III peptide
PI3′K
phosphoinositide 3′kinase
PI3-K
phosphatidylinositol 3′-kinase
pilaris
keratosis p.
pill
morning-after p.
pilocytic
pilosebaceous dysfunction
Pima
pimagedine
pindolol
pineal
p. antigonadotropin (PAG)
p. dysgerminoma
p. gland
p. hyperplasia
p. recess
p. tumor
pinealectomy
pinealocyte
p. β-receptor
pinealoma
ectopic p.
pinhole
p. collimation
p. collimator
pinocytic vesicle
pinocytosis
pioglitazone
p. HCl
PIP_2
phosphatidylinositol 4,5-bisphosphate
piperazine estrone sulfate
pirbuterol
piriform cortex
piroxicam
Pit-1
pituitary-specific transcription factor-1
Pit-1 gene
prophet of Pit-1 (PROP-1)
pit
clathrin-coated p.
coated p.
Pitocin
pitressin
p. tannate
pitting of nail
pituicyte
p. hormonal phenotype
pituicytoma
pituitaire
tige p.
pituitary
p. adenoma
p. adenoma-adenohypophyseal neuronal choristoma (PANCH)
p. adenoma-neuronal choristoma
p. adenylate cyclase-activating polypeptide
p. adenylate cyclase-activating protein
p. adenylyl cyclase-activating peptide
p. agenesis
p. amyloid
p. aneurysm
anterior p.
p. aplasia
p. carcinoma
p. cell line
p. cell-surface antibody
p. cell-surface receptor
p. corticotrope
p. corticotropinoma
p. craniopharyngioma
p. Cushing disease
p. cyst
p. deficiency
p. diabetes
p. disorder
p. dwarfism
p. dynamic test
p. dysfunction
p. dystopia
p. enlargement
p. fossa
p. function
p. gigantism
p. gland
p. glycoprotein hormone
p. growth hormone

NOTES

pituitary *(continued)*
p. growth hormone-secreting adenoma necrosis
p. growth hormone-secreting macroadenoma
p. hormone deficit
p. hormone function
p. hormone hypofunction
p. hyperplasia
p. hypersecretion
p. hypoplasia
p. hypothyroidism
p. incidentaloma
p. infarction
p. irradiation
p. isolation syndrome
p. lactotroph cell
p. meningioma
p. metastasis
p. microadenoma
p. microsurgery
p. necrosis
p. neurosurgeon
pharyngeal p.
posterior p.
p. resistance to thyroid hormone (PRTH)
p. resistance to thyroid hormone action
p. resistance to thyroid hormone syndrome
p. RTH (PRTH)
p. somatotropinoma
p. stalk
p. stalk interruption syndrome
p. surgery
p. target organ test
p. thyroid hormone resistance (PThHR, PTHR)
p. thyrotropin
p. tumor
p. tumor apoplexy
p. tumor cell growth
p. tumorigenesis
p. tumor lateralization
p. tumor-related acromegaly
pituitary-adrenal function
pituitary-dependent
p.-d. Cushing disease
p.-d. thyrotoxicosis
pituitary-gonadal
p.-g. axis
p.-g. function
pituitary-hypothalamic injury
pituitary-specific transcription factor-1 (Pit-1)
pituitary-thyroid
p.-t. axis
p.-t. function
pituitary-thyroidal axis
pituitrin
pizotifen
PKA
protein kinase A
PKB
protein kinase B
PKC
protein kinase C
PKC-alpha
PKG
protein kinase G
P13-kinase
PKU
phenylketonuria
PLA_2
phospholipase A_2
placenta
definitive p.
hemochorial p.
placental
p. aromatase deficiency
p. blood flow
p. CRH
p. GH
p. hormone deficiency
p. lactogen (PL)
p. septa
p. sulfatase deficiency
p. transfer
p. vasopressinase
placentoma
placode
olfactory p.
planar
P. gamma camera
p. xanthoma
plane
coronal p.
p. radiography
plantar
p. fascia syndrome
p. keratosis
p. surface of hallux
plant stanol ester
planum sphenoidale
planus
hypertrophic lichen p.
plaque
psoriatic p.
Plaquenil
plasma
p. ACTH level
p. aldosterone
p. aldosterone concentration (PAC)

p. aldosterone concentration/plasma renin activity (PAC/PRA)
p. aldosterone-to-plasma renin activity ratio
p. aluminum level
p. appearance rate (PAR)
p. beta-endorphin
p. bone alkaline phosphatase
p. cell dyscrasia with polyneuropathy, organomegaly, endocrinopathy, M protein in plasma, and skin changes syndrome
p. clearance rate (PCR)
p. cortisol
p. endothelin level
p. exchange
p. galanin level
gas chromatography of p.
p. glucose concentration
p. growth hormone-releasing hormone level
p. homocysteine level
p. hormone level
p. hypertonicity
p. insulin
p. insulin level
p. kallikrein
p. ketone level
p. lipid profile
p. membrane fatty acid binding protein ($FABP_{pm}$)
p. osmolality (POSM)
p. osmotic pressure
p. phosphate
p. polymorphonuclear elastase (PMN-3)
p. renin activity (PRA)
p. ristocetin cofactor
p. sex hormone-binding globulin
p. sodium
p. sulfonylurea
p. testosterone
p. testosterone level

plasmacytoma
plasmalemma
plasmapheresis
plasmic islet cell autoantibody
plasmid
plasmin
p. mobilization
p. renin activity (PRA)

plasminogen
p. activator
p. activator inhibitor (PAI)
p. activator inhibitor-1 (PAI-1)

plasminogen-activator stimulation
Plastazote insole
plate
alar p.
basal p.
chorionic p.
cribriform p.
epiphyseal growth p.
pterygoid p.
trabecular p.

plateau
Piedmont p.

platelet
p. activity
p. adhesiveness
p. aggregation
p. antigen genotyping
p. consumption
hemolysis, elevated liver enzymes, and low p.'s (HELLP)
p. lipid peroxide concentration
p. protein
p. stability

platelet-activating factor (PAF)
platelet antigen genotyping
platelet-derived
p.-d. growth factor (PDGF)
p.-d. growth factor A (PDGF-A)
p.-d. growth factor AA
p.-d. growth factor BB
p.-d. growth factor gene

platinum electrode
platybasia
platysma muscle
PLC
phospholipase C

PLD
phospholipase D

pleckstrin homology domain
Plegine
pleiotrophin/midkine growth enhancer (PTN/MK)
pleiotropic
p. domain
p. function
p. gene
p. nature

NOTES

P

pleomorphic
p. carcinoma
pleomorphism
plethora
facial p.
plethoric facies
plethysmography
pleuropericardial cyst
plexus
brachial p.
celiac p.
choroid p.
pampiniform p.
p. pancreaticus capitalis
primary capillary p.
subependymal p.
subtunical venous p.
sympathetic p.
vertebral venous p.
plicamycin
plongeont
goiter p.
plot
Scatchard p.
plug
cervical mucous p.
protein p.
Plummer
P. disease
P. nail
pluriglandular endocrine deficiency
plurihormonal
p. adenoma
p. Cushing disease
p. deficiency
p. neuroendocrine neoplasm
plurimorphous
pluripotent
p. hematopoietic cell
p. pituitary macroadenoma
p. stem cell
pluripotential
p. precursor cell
p. stromal cell
Plus
DHC P.
GrowTrak P.
Lorcet P.
Maalox P.
Riopan P.
Tri-Tannate P.
Vicon P.
plutonium
PM
Midol P.
P.M.
Excedrin P.
PMDD
premenstrual dysphoric disorder
PMN
polymorphonuclear
PMN cell
PMN-3
plasma polymorphonuclear elastase
PMS
premenstrual syndrome
PMS-Cyproheptadine
PMS-Levothyroxine Sodium
PMS-Progesterone
PNEE
pulmonary neuroepithelial endocrine
pneumocephalus
pneumococcus
Pneumocystis
P. carinii
P. carinii pneumonia
P. carinii thyroiditis
pneumoencephalography
Pneumomist
pneumonia
Legionella pneumophila p.
Pneumocystis carinii p.
pneumoniae
Diplococcus p.
Klebsiella p.
Staphylococcus p.
Streptococcus p.
PNMT
phenylethanolamine N-methyltransferase
PNP
purine nucleoside phosphorylase
PNP deficiency
PNS
peripheral nervous system
POA
preoptic area of the hypothalamus
POEMS
polyneuropathy, organomegaly, endocrinopathy, monoclonal component, skin changes
polyneuropathy, organomegaly, endocrinopathy, M proteins, skin changes
POEMS syndrome
poikilothermia
point
abnormal set p.
altered set p.
p. mutation
Point of Change weight management program
pointes
torsades de p.

poisoning
heavy metal p.
polyvinyl chloride p.
polar
p. body
p. triiodothyronine syndrome
p. T_3 syndrome
polarizability
polarization
fluorescence p.
polarized
p. cell
p. light microscopy
pole
anterior p.
posterior p.
Pol II
poliomyelitis
polyacrylamide gel electrophoresis
polyadenylation
polyalcohol
polyaromatic hydrocarbon
polyarteritis nodosa
polyarthritis
polybrominated biphenyl (PBB)
polycaryon
polychlorinated biphenyl (PCB)
Polycitra
Polycitra-K
polyclonal
p. anti-T-cell antibody
p. B cell
p. T cell
Polycose
polycystic
p. kidney disease
p. ovarian disease
p. ovarian syndrome (PCOS)
p. ovary (PCO)
p. ovary disease (PCOD)
p. ovary syndrome (PCOS)
polycythemia
p. vera
polydactyly
polydipsia
primary p.
secondary p.
polydystrophy
pseudo-Hurler p.
polyendocrine
p. deficiency syndrome
p. failure type I syndrome
polyendocrinoma
polyendocrinopathy
polyestradiol
polyethylene glycol-adenosine deaminase (PEG-ADA)
polygalactia
polygenic
p. hypercholesterolemia
polyglandular
p. autoimmune syndrome
p. autoimmune syndrome type I (PGA-I)
p. autoimmune syndrome type II (PGA-II)
p. autoimmunity
p. autoimmunity type 1
p. endocrine deficiency
p. endocrine failure
polygonal cell
polyhedral
p. cell
polyhydramnios
polykaryon
polymannose
polymastia
polymenorrhea
polymer
glucose p.
polymerase
p. chain reaction (PCR)
ribonucleic acid p.
RNA p. II
polymerization
polymerize
polymorphism
genetic p.
restriction fragment length p. (RFLP)
simple tandem repeat p. (STRP)
single nucleotide p. (SNP)
single-strand conformation p. (SSCP)
polymorphonuclear (PMN)
p. cell
p. leukocytosis
polyneuropathy
autonomic p.
distal sensory p.
distal symmetric sensorimotor p.
familial amyloid p. (FAP)
familial amyloidotic p.
hypothyroid p.
mixed sensorimotor p.

NOTES

P

polyneuropathy *(continued)*
p., organomegaly, endocrinopathy, monoclonal component, skin changes (POEMS)
p., organomegaly, endocrinopathy, M proteins, skin changes (POEMS)
proximal diabetic p.
sensory ataxic p.
small fiber p.
symmetrical peripheral p.
polyol pathway
polyostotic
p. fibrous dysplasia (PFD)
p. form
p. lesion
p. Paget disease
polypeptide
beta cell p.
gastric inhibitory p. (GIP)
glicentin-related pancreatic p. (GRPP)
p. hormone
p. hormone gene
islet amyloid p. (IAPP)
p. ligand
pancreatic p. (PP)
parathyroid hormonelike p. (PTH-LP)
pituitary adenylate cyclase-activating p.
relaxin p.
single-chain p.
vasoactive intestinal p. (VIP)
polypeptide-1
apo B mRNA-editing catalytic p. (apobec-1)
polypeptide-producing cell
polyphagia
polypharmacy
polyphosphatidylinositide
polyphosphoinositide (PI)
polyploidic cell
polypoid lesion
polyposis
adenomatous p.
familial adenomatous p.
gastrointestinal p.
polypropylene stent
polyradiculopathy
polysaccharide-iron complex
polyspermy
polysulfated glycosaminoglycan
polythelia
polythiazide
polytomogram
polytomography
polyuria
persistent p.
polyuric syndrome
Poly-Vi-Flor
polyvinyl
p. chloride poisoning
p. sponge
polyvinylpyrrolidone iodine
Poly-Vi-Sol
POMC
proopiomelanocortin
POMC 8-kb gene
Pompase
Pompe
P. disease
P. glycogen storage disease, type II
pona reticularis
Ponaris nasal emollient
ponderal
p. index
pons
medulla p.
Ponstel
pontomesencephalic sulcus
pool
extracellular iodide p.
steroidogenic cytoplasmic p.
total body iodide p.
poorly
p. processed POMC molecule
p. processed proopiomelanocortin molecule
poor wound healing
popcorn calcification
population
iodine-replete goitrous p.
porcine
p. heart valve
p. insulin
porin
mitochondrial p.
pork
Iletin II P.
p. insulin
P. NPH
P. Regular Iletin II
porous
p. calcium phosphate cube
p. collagen matrix
porphobilinogen synthase
porphyria
congenital erythropoietic p.
p. cutanea tarda
cyclic p.
toxic p.
porphyrin
portable endocrine system

portacaval
p. H-graft
p. shunt
portal
p. circulation
p. insulin delivery
p. system
p. vein
portasystemic shunt
Porter-Silber reaction
portion
clival p.
portio vaginalis
portohepatic
p. denervation
p. glucose
positional cloning strategy
positive feedback
positron emission tomography (PET)
POSM
plasma osmolality
POST
peritoneal oocyte and sperm transfer
post
p.-therapeutic hypothyroidism
p. thyroidectomy
postablative hypothyroidism
postabsorptive
p. hypoglycemia
p. state
postadenomectomy hypocortisolism
postchallenge glucose level
postcoital
p. contraception
p. contraceptive
p. test
postcosyntropin plasma cortisol
posterior
p. cerebral artery
p. clinoid process
p. communicating artery
p. cricoarytenoid
p. cricoarytenoid muscle
p. gastric diverticulum
p. hypothalamic area (PHA)
p. lobe hormone
pars p.
p. pituitary
p. pituitary gland
p. pole
p. skull flattening
postfixed
postgadolinium study
postganglionic
sympathetic p.
p. sympathetic fiber
p. sympathetic neuron
postgastrectomy
postimplantation embryofetal loss
postinflammatory testicular atrophy
postischemic acute tubular necrosis
postmeiotic spermatocyte
Postmenopausal Estrogen/Progestin Interventions Trial (PEPI)
postmenopausal osteoporosis
postmortem pancreatic angiography
postpartum
p. blues
p. depression
p. hyperthyroidism
p. hypopituitarism
p. lymphocytic thyroiditis
p. painless thyroiditis
p. pituitary infarction
p. pituitary necrosis
p. silent thyroiditis
p. thyroid disease (PPTD)
p. thyroid dysfunction
postpill amenorrhea
postprandial
p. glucose (PG)
p. glucose concentration
p. glucose excursion
p. glucose-mediated toxicity
p. hyperglycemia
p. hypoglycemia
p. hypotension
p. insulin concentration
p. lipemia
p. state
p. symptom
p. syndrome
postpubertal
p. mumps
p. testicular atrophy
postradioiodine
postreceptor
p. desensitization
p. inhibitor
p. marker
p. pyruvate dehydrogenase activity
p. signaling intermediate
postrema
area p. (AP)

NOTES

postsupraventricular tachycardia
postsurgical hypoparathyroidism
postsynaptic
p. membrane
posttesticular defect
postthyrotropin scan
posttranslational modification
posttransplantation
p. lymphoproliferative disorder (PTLD)
p. osteopenia
posttransplant diabetes mellitus (PTDM)
posttraumatic
p. osteoporosis
p. stress disorder
postural hypotension
posture stimulation test
postvoid residual urine volume
potassium (K)
p.-32
p. chloride
p. citrate
p. citrate and citric acid
p. depletion
p. homeostasis
p. inwardly-rectifying channel, subfamily J, member 1 (KCNJ1)
p. inwardly-rectifying channel, subfamily J, member 1 gene
p. iodide
p. ion (K^+)
p. leak channel
penicillin v p.
p. phosphate
p.-sparing diuretic
p. spectroscopy
total body p.
potency
uterine-stimulating p. (USP)
potential
action p.
redox p.
resting membrane p.
stress-generated p. (SGP)
visual-evoked p.
potentiation
potomania
beer p.
pouch
branchial p.
cleft of the Rathke p.
Heidenhain p.
infundibular p.
pharyngeal p.
Rathke p.
stomodeal hypophysial p.
Pou1F1 gene
POU-homeodomain transcription factor
povidone-iodine
powder
Genotropin p.
Goody's Headache P.'s
Secretin-Ferring P.
PP
pancreatic polypeptide
pyrophosphate
vitamin PP
PPAR
peroxisome proliferator-activated receptor
PPAR ligand
PPHP
pseudoPHP
pseudopseudohypoparathyroidism
PPI
purified pork insulin
PPJ
pure pancreatic juice
PPJ cytologic examination
PPNAD
pigmented nodular adrenocortical disease
PPoma
pancreatic polypeptide-secreting tumor
PPPD
pylorus-preserving pancreatoduodenectomy
PPTD
postpartum thyroid disease
pQCT
computer tomographic methods of peripheral skeleton
PR
progesterone receptor
PRA
plasma renin activity
plasmin renin activity
Prader
P. calipers
P. orchidometer
Prader-Labhart-Willi syndrome
Prader-Willi syndrome (PWS)
Pramet FA
Pramilet FA
pramlintide
p. acetate
Prandase
prandial
Prandin
pravastatin
prazosin
preadipocyte
p. factor-1 (Pref-1)
prealbumin
thyroid-binding p. (TBPA)

thyronine-binding p. (TBPA)
thyroxine-binding p.
prealbumin-associated hyperthyroxinemia (PAH)
preantral follicle
prechondrocyte differentiation
precipitin reaction
Precision
P. QID
P. Xtra Advanced Diabetes Management System
preclinical
p. hypothyroidism
p. myxedema
precocious
p. adrenarche
p. emotional menopause
p. maturation
p. pseudopuberty
p. pubarche
p. puberty
precocity
contrasexual p.
familial male-limited gonadotrophin-independent sexual p.
heterosexual p.
idiopathic sexual p.
incomplete isosexual p.
isosexual p.
sexual p.
precolloid stage
preconception counseling
Precose
precursor
adrenal steroid p.
arginine vasopressor p.
erythroid p.
glycogenic p.
hematopoietic stem cell p.
high-mannose p.
myeloid p.
osteoclast p.
protein p.
precursor/product ratio
Pred
Liquid P.
prediabetes
Predicort-50
prediction
Roche, Wainer, and Thissen method of height p. (RWT)
predictive
p. growth model
p. value
p. value test
predisposing factor
Prednicen-M
prednisolone
Prednisol TBA Injection
prednisone
predominant hyperparathyroid bone disease
preduodenal lipase
preeclampsia
Pref-1
preadipocyte factor-1
prefixed
pregadolinium study
pregananediol-20-glucuronide
preganglionic
p. sympathetic nerve
p. sympathetic nerve fiber
p. sympathetic neuron
pregestational diabetes
pregnancy
acute fatty liver of p.
p. cell
ectopic p.
luteoma of p.
toxemia of p.
pregnancy-induced hypertension (PIH)
pregnane derivative
pregnanediol
pregnanetriol
pregnenolone
Pregnyl
prehormone
preinfusion level
prekallikrein
preleptotene primary spermatocyte
Prelone Oral
Prelu-2
Premack-C
premammillary nucleus
Premarin
P. with methyltestosterone
premature
p. adrenarche
p. ejaculation
p. epiphyseal fusion
p. gonadal failure
p. luteinization
p. menopause

NOTES

premature *(continued)*
- p. ovarian failure
- p. thelarche
- p. top codon (TAA)
- p. ventricular contraction

prematurity
- hypothyroxinemia of p.

Pre-Meal
- Dexatrim P.-M.

premenstrual
- p. dysphoric disorder (PMDD)
- p. molimina
- p. syndrome (PMS)

premixed insulin
Prempak-C
Premphase
Prempro
prenatal
- p. diagnosis
- p. multiple vitamin
- Stuart P.

Prenavite
preoptic
- p. area of the hypothalamus (POA)
- p. region

preosseous cartilage
preosteoblast
preosteoclast
preovulatory follicle
preparation
- acid resistant/coated p.
- insulin p.

preprandially
preprandial recurrent symptom
preprocalcitonin
preproendothelin
preprogastrin
preproglucagone gene
preprohormone
- insulin p.

preprohypocretin
preproinsulin
- p. gene

preproPTH
- p. gene

preprosomatostatin
preprotachykinin A gene
prepubertal
preputial gland
preradial myxedema
prereceptor
- p. inhibitor
- p. metabolism

prerenal azotemia
preseminal fluid
pressor response
pressure
- ankle p.
- atmospheric p.
- basal sphincter p.
- blood p. (BP)
- brachial p.
- colloid osmotic p.
- continuous positive airway p. (CPAP)
- p. diuresis
- elevated intracranial p.
- hydrostatic p.
- intraadrenal p.
- intrahypophyseal p.
- intraocular p.
- intrasellar p.
- p. natriuresis
- p. necrosis
- oncotic p.
- plasma osmotic p.
- pulmonary capillary wedge p.
- toe p.
- transcutaneous oxygen p.
- widened pulse p.

pressure-flow study
Pressyn
PresTab
- Glynase P.

presubunit
presymptomatic diagnosis
presynaptic
- p. nerve terminal

prethyroid
prethyroidal fascia
pretibial
- p. dermopathy
- p. myxedema

Pretz-D
Prevacid
Preven
preventative hormone therapy
previtamin
- p. D
- p. D_3

PRF
prolactin-releasing factor

PRH
prolactin-releasing hormone

priapism
Prilosec
primary
- p. adjuvant treatment
- p. adrenal failure
- p. adrenal hyperfunction
- p. adrenal medullary hormone
- p. adrenocortical insufficiency
- p. afferent nociceptor neuron (PAN)

p. aldosteronism
p. amenorrhea
p. antibody
p. antiphospholipid syndrome
p. biliary cirrhosis
p. capillary plexus
p. central nervous system (PCNS)
p. central nervous system lymphoma
p. cortisol resistance
p. craniosynostosis
p. empty sella syndrome
extrathyroidal p.
p. follicle
p. gonadal failure
p. hyperparathyroidism (PHPT)
p. hyperthyroidism
p. hypertrophic osteoarthropathy
p. hypoadrenalism
p. hypocitraturia
p. hypogonadism
p. hypoparathyroidism
p. immune deficiency (PID)
p. immunoregulatory abnormality
p. infertility
intrathyroidal p.
p. macronodular hyperplasia
p. myxedema
p. oocyte
p. orthostatic hypotension
p. ovarian carcinoid
p. ovarian choriocarcinoma
p. pigmental nodular adrenal dysplasia
p. pigmented nodular adrenal dysplasia
p. polydipsia
p. spermatocyte
p. spongiosa
p. suprasellar dysgerminoma
p. sympathetic neurotransmitter
p. therapy
p. thyroidal hypothyroidism
p. thyroid lymphoma
p. villus

Primobolan

primordial
p. follicle
p. germ cell (PGC)
p. ova

Principen

prion
p. protein

prior distant metastasis

priori
a p.

PRISM
Prospective Record of the Impact and Severity of Menstrual Symptoms
PRISM calendar

PRL
prolactin
PRL-cell adenoma
PRL-secreting adenoma

proadrenomedullin N-20 terminal peptide (PAMP)

proalbumin

proamnion

Pro-Banthine

probe
hybridization histochemistry p.
microdialysis p.
oligodeoxynucleotide antisense p.
oligonucleotide p.
thyroid uptake p.

probenecid

probe-tissue hybridization protocol

Probolin

probucol
p. antioxidant

procalcitonin

procarbazine

procarboxypeptidase B (PCPB)

procedure
antrum-sparing modified Whipple p.
Cushing p.
electroosmotic sampling p.
Fontana-Masson p.
iontophoretic sampling p.
needlescopic p.
neuroradiologic imaging p.
Sistrunk p.

process
anterior clinoid p.
clinoid p.
extrathyroidal immunological p.
gustatory neurosensory p.
infundibular p.
intracellular metabolic p.
microfilament-mediated p.
posterior clinoid p.
pterygoid p.
zygomatic p.

NOTES

processor
signal p.
processus vaginalis
prochlorperazine
procollagen
p. gene
p.-III peptide (pIIIp)
p. level
p. molecule
type I p.
proconceptive
Procrit
product
advanced glycation end p.
advanced glycosylation end p. (AGEP)
Amadori p.
calcium times phosphorus p.
cleavage p.
glycation end p.
Maillard p.
matrix-dissolution p.
production
autoantibody p.
cytokine p.
ectopic hormone p.
ectopic paraneoplastic ACTH p.
endogenous glucose p. (EGP)
hepatic glucose p. (HGP)
theca cell androgen p.
thyroid hormone p.
prodynorphin
proenkephalin
p. A
p. B
p. gene
Profasi HP
profile
lipid p.
Nottingham Health P.
One Touch P.
plasma lipid p.
profunda penis artery
progenitor
bone marrow-derived myogenic p.
p. cell
mesenchymal p.
multipotential p.
progeria
progestagen
Progestasert
P. intrauterine device
P. IUD
progesterone (P)
p. challenge test
micronized p.
p. oil
p. receptor (PR)
p. resistance
p. suppository
venous ovarian plasma p.
progestin
C-19 p.
C-21 p.
p. dienogest
p. ethynodiol diacetate
nonandrogenic p.
nor-derivative p.
progestogen
progestogenic
proglucagon
Proglycem Oral
prognathism
Prograf
program
Diabetes Prevention P. (DPP)
National Cholesterol Evaluation P. (NCEP)
Point of Change weight management p.
split mixed insulin p.
University Group Diabetes P. (UGDP)
XeniCare p.
programmed theory of aging
programming
neuroendocrine p.
progressiva
fibrodysplasia ossificans p. (FOP)
progressive
p. depigmentation
p. diaphyseal dysplasia
p. multifocal axonal neuropathy
p. osteopenia
Progynon
Progynon-B
prohormone
p. convertase
p. convertase 1 (PC1)
p. convertase 2 (PC2)
p. convertase 3 (PC3)
steroid p.
Pro-Indo
proinflammatory cytokine
proinsulin
p. insulin ratio
p. level
proinsulin-like molecule
Project
Human Genome P.
projection
GABAergic p.
gamma-aminobutyric acidergic p.
left temporal p.
maximum intensity p. (MIP)
papillary tumor p.

retinohypothalamic p.
right temporal p.
serotonergic p.
prokaryote
prokaryotic cell
prolactin (PRL)
p. biosynthesis
p. cell adenoma
p. cell hyperplasia
p. deficiency
p. excess
extrapituitary p.
p. hormone-expressing cell
p. inhibitory factor
p. inhibitory hormone (PIH)
p. inhibitory mechanism
iso-B p.
p. pulse amplitude
p. release-inhibiting hormone (PIH)
p. secretion
p. secretion during menstrual cycle
serum p.
p. synthesis
p. transcription
prolactinemia
prolactin-inhibiting
p.-i. factor (PIF)
p.-i. hormone (PIH)
prolactinoma
giant p.
giant invasive p.
p. growth
invasive p.
prolactin-producing
p.-p. pituitary adenoma
p.-p. pituitary tumor
prolactin-releasing
p.-r. factor (PRF)
p.-r. hormone (PRH)
prolactin-secreting
p.-s. adenoma
p.-s. pituitary macroadenoma
p.-s. pituitary tumor
p.-s. pituitary tumor
ProLease encapsulated sustained-release growth hormone
prolidase
proliferating cell nuclear antigen (PCNA)
proliferation
A p.-inducing ligand (APRIL)
appositional crystal p.
p. assay
autonomous parathyroid chief cell p.
chondrocyte p.
epitaxial crystal p.
osteoblast p.
osteoblast progenitor p.
proliferative diabetic retinopathy (PDR)
proline
p. oxidase
prolonged diabetes insipidus
Proluton
prolyl hydroxylase enzyme
promegestone
Promensil
Prometa
Prometrium
prominence
frontooccipital p.
prominent supraorbital ridge
promoter
c-*fos* p.
c-*jun* p.
core p.
Pronestyl
pronuclei
proopiomelanocortin (POMC)
p. gene
p. molecule
proopiomelanocortin derivative
proopiomelanocortin-derived peptide
PROP-1
prophet of Pit-1
PROP-1 transcription factor
Prop1 gene
Propacet
propantheline
propeptide
C-terminal p.
properdin
property
antigenic p.
antirachitic p.
prophet
p. of Pit-1 (PROP-1)
p. of Pit-1 transcription factor
prophylactic pituitary radiotherapy
propionate
testosterone p.
propionic
p. acidemia
p. aciduria

NOTES

P

propionyl-coenzyme A
p.-C. carboxylase
propofol
proportion
eunuchoidal body p.
propoxyphene
p. and acetaminophen
p. and aspirin
propranolol
propressophysin
propria
lamina p.
proprioception
proprotein
p. convertase (PC)
proPTH
proptosis
insidious p.
Propulsid
propylthiouracil (PTU)
Propyl-Thyracil
proreceptor
prorenin
Prorex Injection
Proscar
prosencephaly
prospective
P. Record of the Impact and Severity of Menstrual Symptoms (PRISM)
prostacyclin (PGI2, PGI_2)
prostaglandin
p. A
p. B_2
p. D_2 (PGD_2)
p. E_2 (PGE_2)
p. E_3
p. E_1 (PGE_1)
p. E_2 release
p. $F_{2\alpha}$ ($PGF_{2\alpha}$)
p. $F_{1\alpha}$
p. F_{2a} (PGF_{2a})
p. F receptor
p. G_2 (PGG_2)
p. H_2 (PGH_2)
p. H synthase (PGHS)
p. I_2 (PGI_2)
p. J (PGJ)
vasodilator p.
prostanoid
ProstaScint scan
prostate
electrovaporization of the p.
p. gland
microwave hyperthermia of the p.
transurethral incision of the p. (TUIP)
transurethral resection of the p. (TURP)
prostatectomy
laser p.
prostate-specific
p.-s. antigen (PSA)
p.-s. membrane antigen (PSMA)
prostatic
p. concretion
p. duct
p. urethra
p. utricle
prostatitis
prostatropin
ProStep Patch
prosthesis
penile p.
Prostigmin
protamine zinc insulin
protean
protease
insulin p.
insulinlike growth factor-binding protein p.
kallikrein p.
protease-sensitive site
proteasome
20S p.
26S p.
protector
LATS p.
protein
acid-stable p.
actin-binding p.
adaptor p.
adenovirus E1A p.
adipose tissue-uncoupling p.
agouti p.
albuminoid p.
androgen-binding p. (ABP)
beta-arrestin p.
BGP p.
p. binding
BMAL1 p.
bone G1a p. (BGP)
bone morphogenetic p. (BMP)
bone morphogenic p. (BMP)
bone-related p.
bone-specific p.
brain/muscle AhR nuclear translocator-like p. 1
brain/muscle ARNT-like p. 1 (BMAL1)
calcium-binding p.
calmodulin p.
carrier p.
catabolite activator p. (CAP)
catabolite regulatory p.

CCAAT/enhancer binding p. (C/EBP)
CGI p.
channel-forming integral p. (CHIP)
chimeric p.
cholesterol ester transfer p.
cholesteryl ester transfer p.
chromogranin A, B, C p.
chromogranin-secretogranin p.
CLOCK p.
cloned steroid acute respiratory p.
c-myc p.
coactivator p.
cold-inducible ribonucleic acid-binding p. (CIRP)
cold-inducible RNA-binding p. (CIRP)
cold-shock p.
connexin p.
contractile p.
contraction-associated p. (CAP)
corticotropin-releasing hormone-binding p. (CRH-BP)
COUP-TF thyroid hormone receptor auxillary p.
C-reactive p. (CRP)
CREB-binding p. (CBP)
CRH-binding p. (CRH-BP)
Crk p.
CrkI p.
CrkII p.
CrkL p.
cyclic AMP response-element binding p.
cyclin D1 p.
cytochrome p. (CYP)
cytokinin-regulated p. I (CrkI)
cytokinin-regulated kinase p.
cytokinin-regulated kinase I p.
cytokinin-regulated kinase II p.
cytokinin-regulated kinase L p.
dietary p.
p. disulfide isomerase (PDI)
p. disulfide isomerase-mediated disulfide bond reduction
docking p.
EAAT2 p.
E-cadherin p.
p. efficiency ratio
fatty acid-binding p. (FABP)
fatty acid-binding p. 2 (FABP2)
fatty acid transport p. (FATP)
FK-binding p. (FKBP)
FK-binding p. 12 (FKBP12)
FKBP-rapamycin-associated p. (FRAP)
Fyn p.
G p.
gamma-carboxyglutamic acid p.
gene regulatory p.
G inhibiting p. (G_i)
Gla p.
globulin-vitamin D binding p.
glucocorticoid receptor-interacting p. 1 (GRIP 1)
glucose-transport p. 1 (GLUT-1)
glucose-transport p. 2 (GLUT-2)
glucose-transport p. 3 (GLUT-3)
glucose-transport p. 4 (GLUT-4)
glucose-transport p. 5 (GLUT-5)
glucose-transport p. 6 (GLUT-6)
glucose-transport p. 7 (GLUT-7)
glycine-rich RNA-binding p. (GRP)
glycoprotein crystal growth-inhibitor p.
glycosylated serum p.
Grb-2 p.
green birefringent amyloid p.
growth hormone-binding p. (GHBP)
G-stimulating p. (G_s)
GTPase-activating p. (GAP)
GTP-binding p.
guanine nucleotide binding p.
guanine nucleotide regulatory p. (GNRP)
guanosine triphosphate-activating p. (GAP)
guanosine triphosphate binding p.
heat shock p. (HSP, Hsp)
heat-stable p.
heme-binding p.
heterotrimeric p.
histidine-rich calcium-binding p. (HRC)
hormone-binding p.
human pancreas-specific p. (hPASP)
hydrophobic p.
IGF-binding p. (IGFBP)
inhibitory guanine nucleotide binding regulatory p.
insulin growth factor-binding p.
insulinlike growth factor-binding p. (IGFBP)

NOTES

P

protein *(continued)*
insulin receptor substrate p. (IRS-protein)
iron-binding p.
8-kDa p.
37-kDa p.
p. 70-kDa S6 ribosomal subunit kinase (p70S6k)
p. kinase A (PKA)
p. kinase B (PKB)
p. kinase B/Akt
p. kinase C (PKC)
p. kinase C cascade
p. kinase G (PKG)
p. kinase/phosphatase cascade
LDL receptor-related p. (LRP)
lipocalin p.
5-lipoxygenase activating p. (FLAP)
liver-enriched activating p. (LAP)
liver-enriched inhibiting p. (LIP)
low-density lipoprotein receptor-related p. (LRP)
macrophage inflammatory p.-1-alpha (MIP-1-alpha)
macrophage inflammatory p.-1-beta (MIP-1-beta)
p. mass
matrix Gla p. (MGP)
membrane cofactor p. (MCP)
membrane integral p. (MIP)
p. metabolism
misfolded p.
mitogen-activated p. (MAP)
multidrug resistance p. (MDR)
myelin basic p. (MBP)
nascent p.
Nck p.
NESP55 p.
neuroendocrine secretory p. 55 (NESP55)
neurophysin p.
noncollagenous p.
nonhistone p.
p75 p.
pancreatitis-associated p. (PAP)
parathyroid hormonelike p.
parathyroid hormone-related p.
PDGF p.
pendrin p.
PER p.
period p.
p. phosphatase 2B
phosphorylate membrane p.
photoactive yellow p.
pituitary adenylate cyclase-activating p.
plasma membrane fatty acid binding p. ($FABP_{pm}$)
platelet p.
p. plug
p. precursor
prion p.
protein kinase regulator p.
Rab p.
Rac p.
Rap p.
ras p.
ras-like p.
receptor-coupled membrane p.
ret-fused p. (RFP)
retinol-binding p.
Rho p.
S-100 p.
S-14 p.
serpin p.
serum thyroid hormone-binding p.
single-pass transmembrane p.
soluble *N*-ethylmaleimide-sensitive factor attachment p.
somatomedin C p.
soy p.
soybean p.
Src p.
StAR p.
steroid acute regulatory p. (StAR)
steroid acute respiratory p. (StAR)
steroidogenic acute regulatory p. (StAR)
sterol regulatory element binding p. (SREBP)
stimulatory G p.
surfactant-associated p.
p. synthesis
Syp p.
Tamm-Horsfall p.
tax p.
thyroid hormone receptor auxiliary antibody p.
thyroid hormone transport p.
TIM p.
transport p.
triose isomerase p.
troponin C p.
p. tyrosine kinase (PTK)
p. tyrosine phosphorylation
ubiquitinylated p.
uncoupling p. (UCP)
uncoupling p. 1 (UCP1)
vascular endocrine p.
vitamin D-binding p. (DBP)
v-mpl p.
XL-alpha p.
Yes p.
zinc finger p. (ZFP)
ZOG p.
zona glomerulosa p. (ZOG)

protein-1
activator p. (AP-1)
endothelial PAS-domain p. (EPAS1)
IGF-binding p.
insulinlike growth factor-binding p. (IGFBP-1)
insulinlike growth factor-binding p. (IGFBP-1)
monocyte chemoattractant p.
monocyte chemotactic p. (MCP-1)
protein-2
bone morphogenetic p.
insulinlike growth factor-binding p. (IGFBP-2)
mammalian achaete-scute homologous p. (Mash-2)
osteogenic p.
sterol carrier p. (SCP-2)
protein-3
insulinlike growth factor-binding p. (IGFBP-3)
protein-4
bone morphogenetic p.
insulinlike growth factor-binding p. (IGFBP-4)
protein-5
insulinlike growth factor-binding p. (IGFBP-5)
protein-6
insulinlike growth factor-binding p. (IGFBP-6)
protein-7
bone morphogenetic p.
protein-1alpha
proteinase
protein-1beta
protein-calorie malnutrition
protein-deficient pancreatic diabetes
protein-dimerizing activity
protein-energy malnutrition (PEM)
protein kinase B/Akt
protein-sparing modified fast
proteinuria
proteoglycan
glycosylphosphatidylinositol-anchored heparan sulfate p. (HSPG)
heparan sulfate p.
p. molecule
proteolipid
proteolysis
limited fragment p.
p. of pancreatic zymogen
proteolytic
p. activity
p. cleavage
p. enzyme
p. pathway
proteomics
Proteus
Prothazine-DC
prothoracotropic hormone (PTTH)
Protilase
protirelin
protocol
biotinylated-nucleotide p.
Edmonton P.
probe-tissue hybridization p.
tolerogenic p.
proton
p. beam radiation
p. beam therapy
p. buffer
p. diffusion
proton-pump
protooncogene
p. c-erbA
p. c-*fos*
c-myc p.
p. c-*src*
p. expression
MOS p.
p. TRK
protooncogene TRK
Protostat Oral
Protrophin II
Protropin
Proventil
P. HFA
Provera
P. Oral
provisional calcification
provitamin D
provocation test
provocative testing
Provocholine
proximal
p. convoluted tubule (PCT)
p. diabetic neuropathy
p. diabetic polyneuropathy
p. Golgi apparatus
p. motor neuropathy
p. muscle weakness
Prozac

NOTES

PRPP
phosphoribosylpyrophosphate
PRPP synthase
PRTH
pituitary resistance to thyroid hormone
pituitary RTH
selective pituitary resistance to thyroid hormone
selective PRTH
PRTH syndrome
prurigo
Besnier p.
pruritus
uremic p.
Prussian
P. blue stain
P. blue stain for iron
PS
pancreozymin secretin
PS test
PSA
prostate-specific antigen
psammoma body
P450SCC
P450 side chain cleavage
P-selectin level
pseudoachondroplasia
pseudoacromegaly
pseudoadrenal mass
pseudoaldosteronism
pseudoaneurysm
peripancreatic p.
pseudoatrophic islet
pseudoautosomal region
pseudocapsule
pseudocholinesterase deficiency
pseudoclubbing
pseudocorpus luteum insufficiency
pseudo-Cushing
p.-C. state
p.-C. syndrome
p.-C. syndrome of alcoholism
pseudocyst
pseudodementia
pseudodiabetes
uremic p.
pseudofracture
Looser p.
pseudogene
chimeric p.
glucose-transport protein 6 p.
GLUT-6 p.
homologous p.
pseudogiant cell
pseudogoiter
pseudogout
pseudogranulomatous thyroiditis
pseudohermaphrodism
pseudohermaphrodite
female p.
male p.
pseudohermaphroditism
female p.
male p.
pseudo-Hurler polydystrophy
pseudohyperaldosteronism
pseudohypercortisoluria
pseudohypoaldosteronism (PHA)
type p.
p. type I (PHA I)
p. type II (PHA II)
pseudohypoglycemia
pseudohyponatremia
pseudohypoparathyroidism (PHP)
Aurbach p.
p. type Ia
p. type Ib
pseudohypoxia
Pseudomonas
P. aeruginosa
pseudomotor cerebri
pseudomyotonia
pseudopapillary formation
pseudoparalysis
pseudoperiodic biorhythm
pseudoPHP (PPHP)
pseudopseudohypoparathyroidism
pseudopod
cytoplasmic p.
pseudoprecocious puberty
pseudopregnancy
pseudoprolactinoma
pseudopseudohypoparathyroidism (PPHP, pseudoPHP)
pseudopuberty
precocious p.
pseudorosette
pseudoscleroderma
pseudostratified stereociliated columnar epithelium
pseudothrombocytopenia
pseudotuberculous thyroiditis
pseudotumor
adrenal p.
p. cerebri
pseudotumorous
pseudo-Turner syndrome
pseudovagina
pseudovitamin D deficiency rickets (VDDR)
p70S6k
protein 70-kDa S6 ribosomal subunit kinase
PSMA
prostate-specific membrane antigen
psoriasiform arthritis

psoriasis
psoriatic
p. arthritis
p. plaque
PSP
persephin
***Pst*I restriction enzyme**
psychogenic
p. amenorrhea
p. impotence
Psychological Well Being Index
psychoneuroimmunology
psychosexual
psychosocial dwarfism
psychosurgery
PTA
pancreas transplantation alone
PTB
phosphotyrosine-binding domain
PTC
papillary thyroid carcinoma
PTDM
posttransplant diabetes mellitus
P.T.E.-4
P.T.E.-5
PTEN
phosphatase and tensin homologue deleted on chromosome
pterion
pterional approach
pterygium colli
pterygoid
p. plate
p. process
PTH
parathormone
parathyroid hormone
C-terminal assay for PTH
PThHR
pituitary thyroid hormone resistance
PTH-LP
parathyroid hormonelike polypeptide
PTH-mediated calcium efflux
PTHR
pituitary thyroid hormone resistance
PTHrP, PTH-RP
parathyroid hormone-related peptide
PTHrP-transfected RIN-141 cell
PTK
protein tyrosine kinase
PTLD
posttransplantation lymphoproliferative disorder
PTN/MK
pleiotrophin/midkine growth enhancer
ptosis
PTRTH
peripheral tissue resistance to thyroid hormone
PTTH
prothoracotropic hormone
PTU
propylthiouracil
PTX
parathyroidectomy
pubarche
precocious p.
pubertal
p. development
p. growth spurt
puberty
central precocious p. (CPP)
complete precocious p.
constitutional precocious p.
delayed p.
familial male precocious p.
idiopathic complete precocious p.
idiopathic true precocious p.
incomplete precocious p.
isosexual precocious p.
male-limited familial precocious p.
male precocious p.
neurogenic precocious p.
precocious p.
pseudoprecocious p.
stalled p.
true precocious p.
pubic
p. hair
p. ramus
pubis
mons p.
pubis-to-crown measurement
pudendal nerve
pudendum, pl. **pudenda**
puffiness
periorbital p.
pulmonary
p. angiotensin I converting enzyme (PACE)
p. aspiration
p. capillary wedge pressure

NOTES

P

pulmonary *(continued)*
p. chondroma
p. edema
p. mucormycosis
p. neuroepithelial endocrine (PNEE)
p. osteoarthropathy
Pulmozyme
Pulsar analysis
pulsatile
p. gonadotropin-releasing hormone therapy
p. pituitary hormone release
p. secretion
pulse
p. amplitude
p. dosing
p. frequency
full p.
p. generator
p. incubation
pulsed
p. administration
p. Doppler ultrasound
p. progestin hormone replacement therapy
pulse-height analyzer
Pulvules
Becotin P.
Co-Pyronil 2 P.
Darvon Compound-65 P.
pump
Animas R-1000 insulin p.
Ca^{2+} p.
calcium p.
Dana Diabecare insulin p.
Disetronic Diaport p.
Disetronic Dihedi 25 insulin p.
Disetronic D-Tron insulin p.
Disetronic H-Tron p.
external subcutaneous insulin infusion p.
Felig insulin p.
H-TRON plus V100 insulin infusion p.
implantable intraperitoneal p.
implantable programmable insulin infusion p.
internal intraperitoneal insulin infusion p.
iodide p.
microinfusion p.
MiniMed 508 insulin p.
MiniMed 511 insulin p.
Panomat microinfusion p.
sodium-potassium p.
Versaflow peristatic p.
Pump-N-Shorts pump holder
punctata
chondrodysplasia p.
chondrodystrophia p.
pupillary
p. abnormality
p. defect
p. reaction
pure
p. pancreatic juice (PPJ)
p. pancreatic juice cytologic examination
purified pork insulin (PPI)
purine
p. metabolism
p. nucleoside phosphorylase (PNP)
p. nucleoside phosphorylase deficiency
purinergic
p. activation
p. agonist (PIA)
Purkinje
P. cell
P. cell dendrite
puromycin
purple stria
purplish stria
purpura
idiopathic thrombocytopenic p. (ITP)
purulent hypophysitis
pus
black p.
putative
p. neural axis
p. physiologic role
p. regulatory sequence DNA
p. satiety
p. tumor-suppressor gene
putative-binding site
PVN
paraventricular nucleus
PVN of the hypothalamus
PVT
paraventricular thalamic nucleus
PWS
Prader-Willi syndrome
PYD
pyridinoline
pyelogram
intravenous p.
pyelography
retrograde p.
pyelolithotomy
pyelonephritis
ascending p.
emphysematous p.
pygmy
pyknodysostosis

pyknotic nucleus
Pyle disease
pylori
Helicobacter p.
pylorus-preserving pancreatoduodenectomy (PPPD)
pyogenes
Staphylococcus p.
Streptococcus p.
pyogenic thyroiditis
pyomyositis
pyramidal
p. lobe
p. tract
p. tract sign
pyrexic
pyridinium
p. cross-link
pyridinoline (PYD)
p. cross-link
pyridoglutethimide
pyridostigmine
pyridoxal phosphate
pyridoxine
Pyrilinks-D
P.-D. deoxypyridinoline crosslinks urine assay
P.-D. immunoassay
pyro-Glu-His-Pro-amide
pyroglutamyl-histidyl-prolineamide
pyroglutamic
p. acid
p. aciduria
pyroglutamyl-histidyl-prolineamide (pyro-Glu-His-Pro-amide)
pyroglutamyl peptidase II
pyrophosphatase
pyrophosphate (PP)
p. arthropathy
calcium p.
inorganic p.
technetium p.
pyrophosphoric acid
pyrroline-5-carboxylate dehydrogenase
pyruvate
p. carboxylase
p. dehydrogenase (PDH)
p. kinase

NOTES

P

Q

5q31
chromosome 5q31
QAFT
quantitative autonomic functioning testing
QALYs
quality-adjusted life-years
Q band
QCT
quantified computed tomography
axial QCT
computer tomographic methods of axial skeleton
QID
Precision QID
QKd interval
QST
quantitative sensory testing
QT interval
QTL
quantitative trait locus
quadrantanopia
quadrantanopsia
quadriceps fatigue
Quadrinal
quality-adjusted life-years (QALYs)
quantified computed tomography (QCT)
quantitative
q. autonomic functioning testing (QAFT)
Q. Autonomic Function Test
q. bone histomorphometry
q. insulin sensitivity check index (QUICKI)
q. radiography
Q. Sensory Test
q. sensory testing (QST)
q. trait locus (QTL)
quantum
bone q.
questionnaire
Fibromyalgia Impact Q. (FIQ)
Florida Sexual Q.
Questran
Quibron
Quibron-T
Quibron-T/SR
QUICKI
quantitative insulin sensitivity check index
QuickVue UrinChek urine test strip
quiescence
quiescent
Quiess Injection
quin-2 fluorescent Ca^{2+} chelator
quinagolide
quinidine
quotient
respiratory q. (RQ)

R
Humulin R
R_i
inhibitory receptor
R_s
stimulatory receptor
R257X mutation
5α-RA
5-alpha-reductase activity
RAAS
renin-angiotensin-aldosterone system
rabeprazole
Rab protein
Rabson-Mendenhall syndrome
RAC3
receptor-associated coactivator 3
racemic mixture
racemization
rachitic
r. bone
r. change
r. child
r. deformity
r. disease
r. rosary
rachitic-like
r.-l. lesion
r.-l. skeletal defect
rachitis
Rac protein
Rad gene
radial scar breast lesion
radiata
corona r.
zona r.
radiation
external beam r.
r. injury
ionizing r.
optic r.
r. optic neuropathy
proton beam r.
r. therapy (XRT)
r. thyroiditis
radiation-associated papillary thyroid carcinoma
radiation-damaged thyroid gland
radiation-induced
r.-i. hyperprolactinemia
r.-i. leukemia
r.-i. thyroiditis
radical
free r.
hydroxyl r.
oxygen free r.
radicular dentin
radiculomyelopathy
radiculopathy
radioablation therapy
radioactive
r. iodine (^{131}I, RAI)
r. iodine-induced carcinogenesis
r. iodine uptake (RAIU)
r. ligand
radioautographic study
radiodense striation
radiofluoride uptake
radiofrequency (RF)
r. capacitive heating
r. signal
radiogallium
radiography
bone-age r.
nonionic contrast r.
plane r.
quantitative r.
radioimmunoassay (RIA)
radioimmunology
radioiodinated iodotyrosine
radioiodine
r. ablation therapy
r. thyroid imaging
r. trapping
r. uptake (RAIU)
r. uptake test
radioiodine-induced exacerbation of ophthalmopathy
radioisotope
radiolabeled
r. analogue of norepinephrine
r. breath test
r. octreotide scintigraphy
radiology
radiolucency
radiolucent
radionecrosis
delayed brain r.
radionuclide
r. gastric emptying study
r. imaging
r. scintigraphy
radiopaque
r. dye
r. iodinated radiographic contrast media
r. silastic catheter
radiopharmaceutical
radioreceptor assay (RRA)
radiosensitivity
Radiostol

R

radiostrontium uptake
radiosurgery
cobalt-knife r.
stereotactic r.
radiotherapy
conventional r.
Gamma Knife beam r.
hyperfractionated r.
intracystic r.
intraoperative r.
Lineac particle beam r.
prophylactic pituitary r.
stereotactic r.
radiotherapy-induced hypopituitarism
radiothyroidectomy
radiotracer
radium
radius Z score
RAI
radioactive iodine
RAI-induced carcinogenesis
RAIU
radioactive iodine uptake
radioiodine uptake
thyroidal radioactive iodine uptake test
elevated RAIU
rake
r. defect
Senn r.
ralaxifene
Raleigh
hemoglobin R.
RALES
Randomized Aldactone Evaluation Study
raloxifene
ramipril
ramus, pl. **rami**
pubic r.
white r.
Randle
R. cycle
R. mechanism
random
r. cortisol
r. cortisol level
Randomized Aldactone Evaluation Study (RALES)
range
physiological r.
ranitidine
r. bismuth citrate
r. hydrochloride
RANK
receptor activator of NF-κB
RANKL
RANK-ligand
RANK-ligand (RANKL)
Ranson score
RANTES
regulated on activation, normal T-cell expressed and secreted
rapalimus
rapamycin
mammalian target of r. (mTOR)
Raphe nucleus
Rap protein
RAR
retinoic acid receptor
trans-retinoic acid
RAS
RAS oncogene
ras gene protooncogene expression
rash
mucocutaneous r.
***ras*-like protein**
***ras* protein**
rate
absolute thyroidal uptake r.
aldosterone secretory r.
basal metabolic r. (BMR)
bone formation r. (BFR)
decreased mineral apposition r.
erythrocyte sedimentation r. (ESR)
glomerular filtration r. (GFR)
glucose infusion r.
insulin infusion r.
maximal urinary flow r.
metabolic clearance r.
mineral apposition r. (MAR)
plasma appearance r. (PAR)
plasma clearance r. (PCR)
sedimentation r.
somatotroph cell proliferative r.
ultrafiltration r.
urinary paraaminobutyric acid excretion r.
Rathke
R. cleft cyst
R. pouch
R. pouch cyst
R. pouch homeobox transcription factor (Rpx)
ratio
adrenal vein aldosterone r.
aldosterone-to-renin r.
baseline aldosterone/plasma renin activity r.
brachial-to-penile Doppler blood pressure r.
calcium/creatinine r.
calcium-to-creatinine r.
elevated waist-to-hip r.
epinephrine-to-norepinephrine r.
estradiol/testosterone r.
insulin/C-peptide molar r.
lecithin/sphingomyelin r.

L/S r.
MIT:DIT r.
muscle:fat r.
neck-to-thigh r. (N/T)
N/T r.
PAC lateralization r.
PAC/PRA r.
plasma aldosterone-to-plasma renin activity r.
precursor/product r.
proinsulin insulin r.
protein efficiency r.
renin activity-to-aldosterone r.
thyroid hormone-binding r. (THBR)
triiodothyronine/thyroxine r.
TSH:T_4 r.
T_3:T_4 r.
urinary iodine/thiocyanate r.
VLDL cholesterol/total triglyceride r.
waist-to-hip circumference r. (WHR)
WHR r.
X:A r.
X chromosome to autosome ratio
X chromosome to autosome r. (X:A ratio)

Ravnikar

Raxar

Rb
retinoblastoma gene
Rb gene

RBC
red blood cell

RBG
retinol-binding globulin

RBM
ribonucleic acid-binding motif
RNA-binding motif

RDA
recommended daily allowance
recommended dietary allowance

RDS
respiratory distress syndrome

Reabilan

reabsorption
phosphate r.
renal tubular r.

reactant
acute phase r.

reaction
acid-Schiff r.
acrosomal r.
acrosome r.
argentaffin r.
decreased flare r.
dystonic r.
glial r.
graft versus host r.
GVH r.
intrathyroglobulin iodotyrosine coupling r.
leukemoid r.
Maillard r.
peritumor glial r.
photosensitization r.
polymerase chain r. (PCR)
Porter-Silber r.
precipitin r.
pupillary r.
reverse transcription-polymerase chain r. (RT-PCR)

reactive hypoglycemia

reagent
chemiluminescent r.

Rea-Lo

rearranged
r. during transfection (RET)
r. during transformation oncogene

rearrangement
Amadori-type r.

Reaven syndrome

rebaudiana
Stevia r.

rebound hyperglycemia

receptor
acetylcholine r. (AChR)
r. activator of NF-κB (RANK)
activin r. (ActR)
activin r. I (ActRI)
activin r. IB (ActRIB)
activin r. II (ActRII)
activin r. IIB (ActRIIB)
adrenergic r.
Ah r.
aldosterone r.
$alpha_2$ r.
alpha-adrenergic r.
$alpha_1$-adrenergic r.
$alpha_2$-adrenergic r.
androgen r. (AR)
arylhydrocarbon r. (AhR)
asialoglycoprotein r.
r. autoantibody

NOTES

receptor *(continued)*
r. autoradiography
B-cell antigen r. (BCR)
$beta_1$-adrenergic r.
$beta_2$-adrenergic r.
beta-adrenergic r.
bone cell r.
calcitonin r.
calcium-sensing r. (CaR)
CCK-A and CCK-B r.
c-erbA-beta r.
chemokine r.
chimeric r.
cholecystokinin A and cholecystokinin B r.
cholinergic nicotinic r.
compensatory ligand-induced upregulation of tissue r.
corticosteroid r.
CRH-R1 r.
cytoplasmic r.
r. degradation
r. desensitization
dioxin r.
dopamine r.
dopaminergic r.
E_2 r.
ecdysone r.
ectopic hormone r.
EGF r.
endothelin r.
epidermal growth factor r.
estrogen r. (ER)
r. expression
extracellular r.
Fas r.
fibroblast growth factor r. (FGFR)
follicle-stimulating hormone r.
FSH r.
G_s-alpha-coupled r.
gastrin r.
GH-releasing hormone r. (GHRH-R)
GH-releasing peptide r.
GHRP r.
GlcNAc r.
glucagon r.
glucocorticoid r. (GR)
glucose r.
glycoprotein hormone r.
GnRH r.
gonadotropin r.
gonadotropin-releasing hormone r. (GnRH-R)
G protein-coupled r. (GPCR)
G protein-linked r.
growth hormone secretagogue r. (GHSR)
guanylyl cyclase-linked r.
Hcrtr1 r.
Hcrtr2 r.
hepatoma cell insulin r.
hormone r.
human thyroid hormone r. (hTR)
illicit hormone r.
inappropriate hormone r.
inhibitory r. (R_i)
insulin r. (IR)
insulinlike growth factor-II r. (IGF-IIR)
insulin receptor-related r. (IRR)
interleukin type 2 r.
intracellular r.
isoform-specific thyroid hormone r.
juxtaglomerular stretch r.
kinase-deficient activin r.
r. ligand binding
ligand-dependent action of thyroid hormone r.
ligand-independent action of thyroid hormone r.
r. loss
low-density lipoprotein r.
luteinizing hormone r.
luteinizing hormone/chorionic gonadotropin (LH/CG) r.
macula densa r.
mannose-6-phosphate/IGF-2 r. (M6P/IGF-2R)
Mel1a melatonin r.
melanocortin-2 r. (MC2-R)
melanocortin-3 r. (MC3-R)
melanocortin-4 r. (MC4-R)
Mel1b melatonin r.
membrane-associated estrogen r.
membrane-bound r.
mineralocorticoid r. (MR)
MIS II r.
r. mRNA
müllerian-inhibiting substance r.
muscarinic cholinergic r.
myometrial oxytocin r.
N-acetylglucosamine r.
natriuretic peptide r. (NPR)
nicotinic r.
nicotinic cholinergic r.
nicotinic-type r.
NK1 r.
NK2 r.
NK3 r.
noradrenergic r.
nuclear r. (NR)
nuclear hormone r.
r. occupancy
ORL-1 r.
orphan r.

parathyroid extracellular calcium-sensing r.
peripheral-type benzodiazepine r. (PBR)
peroxisome proliferator-activated r. (PPAR)
pituitary cell-surface r.
progesterone r. (PR)
prostaglandin F r.
retinoic acid r. (RAR)
retinoic acid-related orphan r. (ROR)
retinoid X r. (RXR)
retinoid Z r. (RZR)
ryanodine r.
scavenger r.
serotoninergic r.
serpentine r.
seven-transmembrane-domain r.
signal recognition particle r.
silencing mediator of retinoic acid and thyroid hormone r. (SMRT)
single-transmembrane-domain r.
soluble complement r. (sCR1)
soluble *N*-ethylmaleimide-sensitive factor attachment protein r. (SNARE)
somatostatin r.
spare r.
steroid r.
steroid hormone r.
steroid/thyroid hormone r.
stimulatory r. (R_s)
stretch r.
sulfonylurea r. (SUR)
T_3 r. (TR)
taste r.
T-cell r. (TCR)
tethered ligand thrombin r.
thermolabile r.
thyroid hormone r. (TR)
thyroid hormone receptor-retinoid X r. (TR-RXR)
thyroid-stimulating hormone r. (TSH-R, TSHR)
thyrotropin r. (TSH-R)
thyrotropin-releasing hormone r. (TRH-R)
transferrin r.
TSH r. (TSH-R)
tumor necrosis factor r. (TNFR)
r. tyrosine kinase (RTK)
r. tyrosine kinase activity
unmutated r.
V1 r.
V_{1a} r.
V_{1b} r.
V_2 r.
vasoactive intestinal peptide r.
vasopressin r. (V2R)
VIP r.
vitamin D r. (VDR)
vitronectin r.
volume r.
wild-type r.

receptor-associated coactivator 3 (RAC3)
receptor-binding abnormality
receptor-coupled membrane protein
receptor-effector coupling
receptor-ligand complex
receptor-mediated endocytosis
recess
infundibular r.
optic r.
pineal r.
suprapineal r.
recessive
r. abetalipoproteinemia
r. adrenoleukodystrophy
rechallenge
reciprocal peptidergic fiber
reciprocating saw
Recklinghausen
R. disease
osteitis fibrosa cystica generalisata of von R.
R. syndrome
recognition domain
recombinant
r. adenovirus
r. DNA technique
r. enzyme replacement therapy
r. erythropoietin
r. human growth hormone (RHGH, rhGH)
r. human insulin
r. human insulinlike growth factor (rhIGF)
r. human thyroid-stimulating hormone (rhTSH)
r. human TSH (rhTSH)
r. insulinlike growth factor I
r. interferon-alpha (rIFN-α)

NOTES

recombination
homologous r.
intrahistocompatibility locus antigen r.
intra-HLA r.
nonhomologous r.
recommended
r. daily allowance (RDA)
r. dietary allowance (RDA)
reconstruction
bone r.
Suzuki duodenopancreatobiliary r.
recovery
short T1 inversion r. (STIR)
recta
pars r.
vasa r.
Rectal
Phenergan R.
RMS R.
rectal administration of insulin
rectilinear scanner
rectouterine recess of Douglas
rectus
tubulus r.
recumbent
r. aldosterone
r. dyspnea
recurrent
r. adenoma
r. blepharoptosis
r. laryngeal nerve
r. pituitary tumor
recycling
urea r.
red
r. blood cell (RBC)
r. bone marrow
r. cell coagulability
r. cell coagulation
r. cell mass
r. lochia
vital r.
red-green
r.-g. color blindness
r.-g. deficiency
Redisol
redox
r. potential
r. state
reduced
r. exercise capacity
r. glutathione (GSH)
r. thyroid reserve
reductase
adrenodoxin r.
aldo-keto r. (AKR)
aldose r.
r. deficiency
dihydropteridine r.
flavoprotein NADPH-cytochrome P450 r.
flavoprotein nicotinamide adenine dinucleotide phosphate-cytochrome P450 r.
glutathione r.
17-ketosteroid r. (17-KR)
methylenetetrahydrofolate r.
NADPH-cytochrome P450 r.
renal ferredoxin r.
5-reductase
-r. deficiency
reduction
goiter r.
PDI-mediated disulfide bond r.
protein disulfide isomerase-mediated disulfide bond r.
Redutemp
REE
resting energy expenditure
reesterification
refeeding edema
Refetoff
R. patient
R. syndrome
reflector
parabolic r.
reflex
Achilles r.
Bruchner r.
deep tendon r.
Ferguson r.
glucoregulatory neural r.
milk let-down r.
neuroendocrine r.
slow relaxation phase of deep tendon r.
suckling r.
r. sympathetic dystrophy
refraction
cycloplegic r.
refractoriness
secretory r.
thyrotropin-releasing hormone-induced r.
TRH-induced r.
regeneration
adrenocortical r.
myogenic r.
skeletal r.
tissue r.
regimen
add-back r.
block-replace r.
glucocorticoid-free immunosuppressive r.

insulin-combination r.
multiple-injection r.

region
carboxyl-terminal r.
epithalamic r.
infundibulohypophysial r.
mammillary r.
medial basal hypothalamic r. (MBH)
parasellar r.
perifornical r.
preoptic r.
pseudoautosomal r.
retrochiasmatic r.
sellar r.
suprachiasmatic r.
supraoptic r.
suprasellar r.
third complementarity determining r. (CDR3)
tuberal r.
untranslated r. (UTR)
5′-untranslated r. (UTR)
ventricular r.

Regitine

Regl alpha gene

Reglan

Regranex
R. gel

regrowth
goiter r.

regular
R. (Concentrated) Iletin II U-500
R. Iletin I
R. Insulin
R. Purified Pork Insulin
r. spin-echo technique

regulated
r. on activation, normal T-cell expressed and secreted (RANTES)
r. secretion

regulation
abnormal r. of calcium-dependent parathyroid hormone secretion
adipose tissue r.
hypothalamic neuroendocrine r.
negative feedback r.
osmotic r.
paracrine r.

regulator
autoimmune r. (AIRE)
cystic fibrosis transmembrane r. (CFTR)
hormonal r.
intraovarian r.
nonhormonal r.
physiologic r.

regulatory
r. failure
r. gene defect
r. homodimer
r. lymphocyte
r. peptide

regurgitation
tricuspid r.

Reidel thyroiditis

Reifenstein
R. phenotype
R. syndrome

reinfusion
intraperitoneal r.

Reinke
R. crystal
R. crystalloid
R. edema

Reiter syndrome

rejection
clonal r.

Relafen

RelA-p50 heterodimer

relationship
genotype-phenotype r.
log dose-response r.
neural r.

relative
r. hypoinsulinemia
r. leptin deficiency
r. leptin resistance
r. osteoid volume

relaxation
myometrial r.

relaxin
r. polypeptide

release
calcium r.
endothelin r.
first-phase insulin r.
iodine r.
long-acting r. (LAR)
nocturnal vasopressin r.
octreotide long-acting r.
prostaglandin E_2 r.
pulsatile pituitary hormone r.

NOTES

release *(continued)*
renal glucose r.
tethered cord r.
release-inhibiting hormone
releasing hormone
Relefact TRH
Relief
Diabetic Tussin Allergy R.
relocatable stereotactic frame
Remeron
remethylation
remifentanil
remission
biochemical r.
endocrine r.
remnant
r. hyperplastic tissue
hypertrophied thyroglossal duct r.
lipoprotein r.
r. pancreas
thyroglossal duct r.
thyroid r.
remodeling
adrenal r.
bone r.
r. cycle
vascular r.
removal
tumor r.
RenaGel
renal
r. aplasia
r. artery
r. calcium wasting
r. calculus
r. carcinoma cell
r. colic
r. diabetes
r. erythropoietic factor
r. excretion
r. failure
r. Fanconi syndrome
r. ferredoxin
r. ferredoxin reductase
r. form of diabetes insipidus
r. function
r. gluconeogenesis
r. glucose release
r. insufficiency
r. lithiasis
r. medullary interstitium
r. mucormycosis
r. nephron
r. osteodystrophy
r. papilla
r. pelvis
r. phosphate wasting
r. plasma flow (RPF)
r. pupillary necrosis
r. rickets
r. sodium retention
r. sodium wasting
r. threshold
r. transplant
r. transplantation
r. tubular acidosis (RTA)
r. tubular reabsorption
Renese
renin
active r.
r. activity-to-aldosterone ratio
total r.
upright plasma r.
renin-aldosterone axis
renin-angiotensin-aldosterone
r.-a.-a. axis
r.-a.-a. system (RAAS)
renin-angiotensin system
renin-independent hypermineralocorticoidism
renocortin
Renografin-76
renotropic
renotropin
renovascular
r. disease
r. hypertension
Rentamine
repaglinide
repair
tissue r.
reparative granuloma
repeat
leucine rich r. (LRR)
short tandem r. (STR)
variable number of tandem r. (VNTR)
repertoire
B-cell r.
T-cell r.
repetitive stress of walking
replacement
beta cell r.
glucocorticoid r.
gonadal steroid r.
growth hormone r.
r. therapy
thyroid hormone r.
thyroxine r.
Replens
Repliderm
reporter
r. gene
r. molecule
repression
apoT3R-mediated r.

repressor
bacteriophage lambda r.
inducible cAMP early r. (ICER)
inducible cyclic adenosine monophosphate early r. (ICER)
reproductive
r. milieu
r. physiology
Repronex
RER, rER
rough endoplasmic reticulum
resection
abdominoperineal r.
duodenum-preserving pancreatic head r. (DPRHP)
gastric r.
microsurgical r.
partial r.
Resectisol irrigation solution
reserpine
reserve
adrenal r.
r. capacity
decreased thyroid r.
diminished ovarian r.
ovary r. (OR)
reduced thyroid r.
thyroid r.
reservoir
bony r.
fuel r.
r. transdermal system
residual
r. adenoma
r. lumen
r. pituitary tumor
residue
tyrosyl r.
resin
bile acid r.
bile-binding r.
cholestyramine r.
r. hemoperfusion
ion-exchange r.
nonresorbable r.
r. uptake
resin-embedded semithin section
resistance
absolute leptin r.
acquired end-organ r.
ACTH r.
activated protein C r.
aldosterone r.
androgen r.
end-organ r.
extreme insulin r.
familial glucocorticoid r.
generalized thyroid hormone r. (GTHR)
glucocorticoid r.
growth hormone r.
hereditary end-organ r.
hereditary vitamin D r.
hormone r.
incomplete androgen r.
insulin r.
partial insulin r.
pituitary thyroid hormone r. (PThHR, PTHR)
primary cortisol r.
progesterone r.
relative leptin r.
selective pituitary r.
severe insulin r.
skeletal r.
r. state
syndrome of complete androgen r.
syndrome of generalized thyroid hormone r.
syndrome of incomplete androgen r.
syndrome of insulin r.
systemic vascular r. (SVR)
target organ r.
temporary end-organ r.
r. to thyroid hormone (RTH)
thyroid hormone r.
total peripheral r.
type A syndrome of insulin r.
type B syndrome of insulin r.
type C syndrome of insulin r.
vitamin D end-organ r.
resistant
r. hyperhomocystinemia
r. ovary
r. ovary syndrome
PAS r.
periodic acid-Schiff r.
resistant ovary
resonance
nuclear magnetic r. (NMR)
spin-echo magnetic r.
resorcinol
resorcyclic acid

NOTES

resorption
bone r.
calcium r.
cyclosporine A-induced r.
r. lacuna
osteoblastic r.
osteoclast-activated bone r.
osteoclast-driven bone r.
osteoclastic bone r.
osteoclast-mediated bone r.
paracellular calcium r.
r. trench
Respa-DM
Respa-GF
Respbid
respiration
respiratory
r. acidosis
r. alkalosis
r. compensation
r. distress syndrome (RDS)
r. quotient (RQ)
r. syncytial virus
response
acute insulin r. (AIR)
acute phase r. (APR)
adaptational r.
anamnestic antibody r.
antibody r.
axon r. of Lewis
calcemic r.
catecholamine r.
r. curve decline
r. element
end-organ r.
exocrine r.
first-phase insulin r. (FPIR)
first-year growth velocity r.
glucose r.
growth hormone r.
hormone receptor-mediated r.
humoral immune r.
hypersensitivity r.
hypothalamic-pituitary r.
insulin secretory r. (ISR)
intrinsic r.
lymphocyte adenylate cyclase r.
peak thyroid-stimulating hormone r.
peak TSH r.
phosphaturic r.
pressor r.
secretory r.
T-cell r.
triphasic r.
wheal and flare r.
rest
accessory adrenocortical r.
adrenal r.
intraovarian r.
intratesticular adrenal r.
squamous cell r.
restenosis
resting
r. cell
r. energy expenditure (REE)
r. membrane potential
restricted
HLA r.
human leukocyte antigen r.
restriction
r. enzyme
r. fragment length polymorphism (RFLP)
phosphate-protein r.
phosphorus dietary r.
RET
rearranged during transfection
RET oncogene
ret
r. protooncogene
retardation
growth r.
intrauterine growth r. (IUGR)
mental r.
retention
aluminum r.
r. cyst of the pancreas
nitrogen r.
phosphate r.
renal sodium r.
urinary r.
rete testis
ret-fused protein (RFP)
reticular erythematous mucinosis
reticularis
fasciculata r.
livedo r.
pona r.
zona r.
zone r.
reticulin
r. stain
reticulocytosis
reticuloendothelial system
reticuloendotheliosis
reticulohistiocytosis
multicentric r.
reticulum
endoplasmic r. (ER)
rough endoplasmic r. (RER, rER)
smooth endoplasmic r. (SER, sER)
retina
neovascularization elsewhere in r. (NVE)
retinal
r. angioid streak

r. capillary angioma
r. cerebellar hemangioblastomatosis
r. coloboma
r. detachment
r. hamartoma
r. hemangioblastoma
retinalis
lipemia r.
retinitis pigmentosa
retinoblastoma
r. gene (Rb)
r. tumor
retinohypothalamic
r. projection
r. tract
retinoic
r. acid
r. acid receptor (RAR)
r. acid-related orphan receptor (ROR)
r. acid X receptor beta
9-*cis* r. acid (RXR)
13-*cis* r. acid
retinoid
r. X receptor (RXR)
r. Z receptor (RZR)
retinol-binding
r.-b. globulin (RBG)
r.-b. protein
retinopathy
diabetic r.
nonproliferative diabetic r.
proliferative diabetic r. (PDR)
van Heuven anatomic classification of diabetic r.
Wisconsin Epidemiologic Study of Diabetic R. (WESDR)
retinyl fatty acid ester
retractor
Finochietto r.
malleable brain r.
Richardson r.
retrobulbar tissue expansion
retrochiasmatic
r. area
r. region
retroclavicular
retroendocytosis
retrograde
r. amnesia
r. ejaculation
r. instrumentation
r. menstruation
r. pyelography
retroocular tissue
retroorbital
r. adipose tissue
r. connective tissue
r. fat deposition
retroperitoneal lipomatosis
retrosternal goiter
retrotracheal
retrovirus
reuptake
serotonin r.
reversal
dosage-sensitive sex r.
DSS r.
r. phase
reverse
r. cholesterol transport
r. hemolytic plaque assay
r. hemolytic plaque assay system
r. T3
r. T_3 (rT_3)
r. transcription-polymerase chain reaction (RT-PCR)
r. triiodothyronine
Rexigen Forte
Rezulin
RF
radiofrequency
RFLP
restriction fragment length polymorphism
RFP
ret-fused protein
rFSH
R-Gel
R-Gene
Rh
Rhesus
Rh blood group antigen
Rh C, D, E genotyping
rhabdomyolysis
hypothyroid r.
rhabdomyosarcoma
pelvic r.
rhenium-186
rhenium-188 DMSA
rheologic agent
Rhesus (Rh)
R. factor blood group antigen (Rh blood group antigen)

NOTES

rheumatic
r. fever
r. syndrome
rheumatism
rheumatoid
r. arthritis
r. factor
RHGH, rhGH
recombinant human growth hormone
RHGH treatment
rhIGF
recombinant human insulinlike growth factor
rhinitis medicamentosa
rhinocerebral mucormycosis
rhinorrhea
cerebrospinal fluid r.
CSF r.
Rhinosyn-DMX
Rhizobium meliloti
rhizomelic shortening
Rhizomucor
Rhizopus
rhodamine
rhodopsin
r. kinase
Rho protein
rhTSH
recombinant human thyroid-stimulating hormone
recombinant human TSH
rhythm
activity r.
behavioral r.
circadian/diurnal hormonal r.
circadian hormonal r.
circannual r.
dehydroandrosterone sulfate r.
diurnal r.
endocrine r.
endogenous r.
fetal endocrine r.
fetal hormone r.
fetal/neonatal r.
fetal steroid r.
hormone r.
infradian r.
maternal estradiol r.
melatonin r.
night-day r.
nocturnal r.
nyctohemeral r.
seasonal r.
ultradian r.
uterine activity r.
uterine contractile r.
rhythmicity
uterine r.
RI
type I regulatory dimer
RI regulatory component
RIA
radioimmunoassay
ribavirin
Ribbing disease
riboflavin
ribonuclease A cleavage method
ribonucleic
r. acid (RNA)
r. acid-binding motif (RBM)
r. acid polymerase
ribonucleoprotein
ribose-5-phosphate
riboside
aminoimidazole carboximide r. (AICAR)
ribosome
ribosome-membrane junction
ribosylated
ribosylation
adenosine diphosphate r.
Rich
Rolaids Calcium R.
Richardson retractor
Richner-Hanhart syndrome
ricinoleate
rickets
adult r.
autosomal recessive hypophosphatemic r.
calciopenic r.
familial hypophosphatemic r.
familial X-linked hypophosphatemic r.
hereditary pseudovitamin D deficiency r.
hypercalciuric hypophosphatemic r.
hypophosphatemic r.
nutritional r.
oncogenic r.
phosphopenic r.
pseudovitamin D deficiency r. (VDDR)
renal r.
r. type II
type II vitamin D dependency r.
vitamin D-dependent r. type II
vitamin D-resistant r.
XLH r.
X-linked recessive hypophosphatemic r.
Ridenol
ridge
gonadal r.
mammary r.
prominent supraorbital r.
urogenital r.

Riedel
R. disease
R. disorder
R. struma
rifampicin
rifampin
rIFN-α
recombinant interferon-alpha
right
r. frontal osteoplastic flap
r. hormone growth hormone treatment
r. temporal projection
rigidity
decorticate r.
rigid sinonasal endoscope
Rigi-Scan monitor
RII
type II regulatory dimer
RII regulatory component
Riley-Day syndrome
Riley-Smith syndrome
ring
bromophenolic r.
chromosome r.
iodothyronine r.
Silastic r.
vaginal r.
ring-substitution effect
Riobin
Riopan
R. Plus
rioprostil
risedronate
r. sodium
ristocetin
factor VIII r. cofactor antigen
ritanserin
ritanserine
RMS Rectal
RNA
ribonucleic acid
messenger RNA (mRNA)
RNA polymerase II
RNA-binding motif (RBM)
Robafen
R. AC
Robinul
R. Forte
Robitet Oral
Rocaltrol
Roche, Wainer, and Thissen method of height prediction (RWT)
rod
Silastic r.
rodenticide
roentgenography
rofecoxib
Rogaine Topical
Rokitansky-Küster syndrome
Rolaids
R. Calcium Rich
role
putative physiologic r.
roll
absorbable gelatin film r.
Romozin
rongeur
ethmoidal r.
Kerrison r.
micropituitary r.
straight ethmoidal r.
root
dilatation of aortic r.
ROR
retinoic acid-related orphan receptor
rosary
acromegalic r.
rachitic r.
rose bengal drops
rosiglitazone
r. maleate
***ros* oncogene**
rostral
r. area
r. hypothalamus
r. ventrolateral medulla
rostrum
rotation
injection site r.
Rotocaps
Ventolin R.
rotundum
foramen r.
rough endoplasmic reticulum (RER, rER)
round ligament
Roux stasis syndrome
roving nystagmus
Roxanol SR Oral
Roxicet 5/500
Roxicodone
Roxilox

NOTES

Roxiprin
RPD
Pepcid RPD
RPF
renal plasma flow
Rpx
Rathke pouch homeobox transcription factor
RQ
respiratory quotient
RRA
radioreceptor assay
rT_3
reverse T_3
RTA
renal tubular acidosis
type 4 RTA
RTH
resistance to thyroid hormone
pituitary RTH (PRTH)
RTK
receptor tyrosine kinase
RT-PCR
reverse transcription-polymerase chain reaction
RU2858
RU486
RU5020
RU9115
rubella virus
rubeosis
Rubinstein-Taybi syndrome
rubra
lochia r.
Rubramin-PC
ruffled border
rugger jersey appearance of vertebra
rugger-jersey spine
rule
1500 r.
Bayes r.
Nägele r.
r. of 10s
runt disease
Russ
hemoglobin R.
Russell-Silver syndrome
RWT
Roche, Wainer, and Thissen method of height prediction
Rx
Natabec Rx
Natalins Rx
RXR
9-*cis* retinoic acid
retinoid X receptor
ryanodine receptor
Ryna-CX
RZR
retinoid Z receptor

S
cathepsin S
compound S
hemoglobin S
streptolysin S
S test
4S
Scandinavian Simvastatin Survival Study
10s
rule of 10s
S-100 protein
S-14 protein
SAB
spontaneous abortion
saber shin
sac
chorionic s.
saccharin
sacral autonomic area
sacrococcygeal chordoma
sacrosidase
SAD
seasonal affective disorder
saddle
Turkish s.
S-adenosyl-L-methionine (SAM)
Saethre-Chotzen syndrome
Saizen
Sakamoto
carcinoma of S.
salbutamol
Saleto-200
Saleto-400
Salflex
Salgesic
salicylate
choline s.
sodium s.
salicylic acid and propylene glycol
saline
BES buffered s. (BBS)
hypotonic s.
s. suppression study
s. suppression test
salivary
s. cortisol
s. cortisol concentration
s. cortisol level
s. gland
s. ultrafiltrate
salivatory nucleus
Salla disease
salmeterol
salmon calcitonin
Salmonella
S. brandenberg
S. enteritidis
S. typhi
Salmonine
salpingitis
salpingo-oophorectomy
bilateral s.-o. (BSO)
unilateral s.-o.
salpinx
salsalate
Salsitab
salt
s. absorption
aluminum s.
s. appetite
calcium s.
s. craving
s. delivery
s. loading
magnesium s.
magnesium-lipid s.
s. and pepper appearance of skull
trifluoroacetate s.
urate s.
s. wasting
salt-losing
s.-l. crisis
s.-l. deficiency
salt-wasting
s.-w. crisis
s.-w. hydroxylase deficiency variant
saluresis
Saluron
salvage therapy
SAM
S-adenosyl-L-methionine
sampling
adrenal vein s.
adrenal venous s. (AVS)
arterial stimulation and venous s. (ASVS)
blood s.
cavernous sinus s. (CSS)
chorionic villus s. (CVS)
frequent blood s.
high jugular vein s.
IJV s.
inferior petrosal sinus s. (IPSS)
internal jugular vein s.
petrosal sinus s.
transhepatic portal venous s.
venous s.
Sandhoff disease
Sandimmune

S

Sandostatin
S. LAR
S. LAR Depot
sandwich
s. enzyme immunoassay method
s. immunoassay
Sanfilippo syndrome
SangCya
Sanger dideoxy sequencing method
Sangstat
Sanorex
Santorini
S. duct system
fissure of S.
Santyl
SAP
severe acute pancreatitis
saponification
sarafotoxin
saralasin
sarcoid
sarcoidlike noncaseating granulomatous inflammation
sarcoidosis
granulomatous s.
sarcoma
Kaposi s.
undifferentiated s.
sarcomatous
s. bone
s. degeneration
sarcopenia
sarcoplasma
sarcoplasmic/endoplasmic reticulum calcium ATPase (SERCA)
sarcosine
s. dehydrogenase
sarcosinemia
SARM
selective androgen-receptor modulator
SAT
spontaneous autoimmune thyroiditis
Satietrol
satiety
early s.
easy s.
s. factor
putative s.
saturated solution of potassium iodide (SSKI)
sauvagine
frog skin s.
Savage syndrome
saw
Gigli s.
reciprocating s.
SBGM
self-blood glucose monitoring
SC
sickle cell
SC disease
SCAD
short chain acyl-CoA dehydrogenase deficiency
scale
Attache food s.
Clyde mood s.
Magnum food s.
sliding s.
scalenus anticus
scalloping
peripheral s.
scalpel
#11 bayonet-handled s.
scan
bone s.
color Doppler s.
DEXA s.
genome s.
^{131}I-metaiodobenzylguanidine s.
^{131}I-MIBG s.
iodine-131 total body s. (^{131}I-TBS)
iodocholesterol s.
MIBG s.
NP-59 iodonocholesterol s.
octreotide s.
pertechnetate thyroid s.
postthyrotropin s.
subtraction thyroid s.
technetium bone s.
technetium pertechnetate s.
Thyrogen radioiodine s.
thyroid s.
total body s. (TBS)
whole-body radioiodine s.
Scandinavian Simvastatin Survival Study (4S)
scanner
rectilinear s.
UltraSure DTU-one ultrasound s.
scanning
isotope s.
technetium/thallium subtraction nuclear s.
scaphocephalic skull
scaphocephaly
scapulae
winged s.
Scatchard plot
scavenger
free-radical s.
s. receptor
SCC
side chain cleavage
SCC enzyme

SCF
stem cell factor
Scheie syndrome
scheme
dosimetric s.
Sillence classification s.
schenckii
Sporothrix s.
Schiff
S. base
Schilling test
Schindler disease
Schirmer test
schizophreniform
Schmidt syndrome
Schmid-type
S.-t. metaphyseal chondrodysplasia
S.-t. metaphyseal dysplasia
Schultze sign
Schumann body
Schwabing Insulin Prophylaxis Trial
Schwann
S. cell
S. cell origin
S. cell system
S. envelope
schwannoma
trigeminal s.
schwannoma-derived growth factor
Schwartz-Bartter syndrome
SCID
severe combined immunodeficiency disease
scintigram
scintigraphy
adrenal s.
11-C-hydroxyephedrine s.
$[^{131}I]$-19-iodocholesterol s.
NP-59 s.
nuclear s.
parathyroid s.
pertechnetate s.
radiolabeled octreotide s.
radionuclide s.
sestamibi-pertechnetate subtraction s.
skeletal s.
somatostatin-receptor s.
Tc-99m sestamibi s.
^{99m}Tc sestamibi s.
technetium sestamibi s.
thallium-pertechnetate subtraction s.
thallium-technetium dual isotope s.
thyroid s.
whole-body s.
scintillation camera
scintiscan
thyroid s.
scissors
ethmoidal s.
Mayo s.
SciTojet needle-free injector for human growth hormone
sclera
blue tinge s.
scleredema diabeticorum
scleroderma
scleroderma-like syndrome (SLS)
sclerosing
s. adenosis
s. mediastinitis
sclerosis
amyotrophic lateral s. (ALS)
cranial s.
diaphyseal s.
metaphyseal s.
Monckeberg s.
multiple s.
seminiferous tubule s.
skeletal s.
tuberous s.
sclerostenosis
sclerosus
lichen s.
SCN
suprachiasmatic nucleus
SCN of the hypothalamus
SCO
subcommissural organ
Scop
Transderm S.
scopolamine
score
American Urologic Association symptom s.
APACHE II s.
AUA symptom s.
Ferriman-Gallwey s.
Michigan Diabetic Neuropathy S.
Nerve Disability S.
Nerve Symptom S.
radius Z s.
Ranson s.
Z s.

NOTES

scotoma
cecocentral s.
central s.
hemianopic s.
junctional s.
SCP-2
sterol carrier protein-2
sCR1
soluble complement receptor
scrapie
scratch
Means-Lerman s.
screening
universal s.
scrotal matrix patch
scrotum
bifid s.
SCT
solid cystic tumor
SCTAT
sex cord tumor with annular tubule
scurvy
5-S-cysteinyldopa
seam
osteoid s.
wide osteoid s.
seasonal
s. affective disorder (SAD)
s. rhythm
seasonality
integrative model of s.
sebaceous sweat gland
seborrhea
excessive s.
sebum
Seckel
S. bird-headed dwarfism
S. syndrome
second
s. attack theory
s. hormone syndrome
s. messenger
S. National Health and Nutrition Examination Survey (NHANES II)
secondary
s. adrenal hyperfunction
s. adrenal insufficiency
s. amenorrhea
s. antibody
s. arteritis
s. empty sella
s. empty sella syndrome
s. endocrinopathy
s. follicle
s. gonadal failure
s. hyperaldosteronism
s. hyperparathyroidism
s. hyperprolactinemia
s. hyperthyroidism
s. hypertrophic osteoarthropathy
s. hypoadrenalism
s. hypocitraturia
s. hypogonadism
s. hypoparathyroidism
s. hypothyroidism
s. immunodeficiency
s. infertility
s. interstitial cell
s. malignancy
s. oocyte
s. orthostatic hypotension
s. polydipsia
s. spermatocyte
s. villus
second-generation agent
secosteroid
secosterol
Secran
secretagogue
growth hormone s. (GHS)
insulin s.
secreted
regulated on activation, normal T-cell expressed and s. (RANTES)
secrete lymphokine
secretin
pancreozymin s. (PS)
s. stimulation test
s. test
Secretin-Ferring Powder
secreting pituitary adenoma
secretion
abnormal regulation of calcium-dependent parathyroid hormone s.
apocrine s.
autocrine s.
basal catecholamine s.
basal insulin s.
circadian rhythm of hormone s.
constitutive s.
cortisol s.
ectopic ACTH s.
ectopic adrenocorticotropic hormone s.
ectopic growth hormone-releasing hormone s.
gastric acid s.
glucose-induced insulin s.
glucose-stimulated insulin s. (GSIS)
gonadotropin s.
growth hormone s.
hormone s.
insulin s.
Osteocalcin s.
oxytocin s.
paracrine s.

parathyroid hormone s.
prolactin s.
pulsatile s.
regulated s.
semiautonomous basal insulin s.
serotonin s.
set point for insulin s.
spontaneous s.
sterol s.
syndrome of inappropriate antidiuretic hormone s.
syndrome of inappropriate somatotropin s.
thyroglobulin s.
thyroidal autoantibody s.

secretomotor fiber

secretory
s. burst of growth hormone
s. granule
s. refractoriness
s. response
s. vacuole
s. vesicle

section
paraffin-embedded semithin s.
resin-embedded semithin s.
silver-impregnated semithin s.

sectioning
s. microtome

SED
spondyloepiphyseal dysplasia

sedentary lifestyle

sedimentation rate

see-saw nystagmus

segmental pancreas donation

segmental transplantation

seizure
gelastic s.

Select GT blood glucose system

selectin

selective
s. aldosterone antagonist
s. androgen-receptor modulator (SARM)
s. arterial calcium stimulation study
s. estrogen-receptor modulator (SERM)
s. estrogen response modifier (SERM)
s. $5HT_2$ receptor antagonist
s. hypopituitarism
s. peripheral resistance to thyroid hormone
s. pituitary resistance
s. pituitary resistance to thyroid hormone (PRTH)
s. PRTH
s. serotonin reuptake inhibitor (SSRI)

Select-Lite lancing device

selegiline

selenium

selenoenzyme
type III s.

selenoprotein
s. metabolism

selenosulfide bond

Sele-Pak

Selepen

Selestoject

self-blood glucose monitoring (SBGM)

self-injection
penile s.-i.

self-management
diabetes s.-m.

self-test
Gluco-Protein OTC s.-t.
Gluco-Protein over-the-counter s.-t.

self-tolerance

sella
diaphragma s.
dorsum s.
empty s.
gourd-shaped s.
J-shaped s.
secondary empty s.
s. turcica

sellar
s. cyst
s. disease
s. metastasis
s. region
s. tumor
s. volume

Selye
stress response of S.

semen
s. analysis
s. culture
s. fructose test

semenogelin
s. I
s. II

S

NOTES

semiautonomous basal insulin secretion
seminalis
colliculus s.
seminal vesicle
seminiferous
s. epithelium
s. tubule
s. tubule dysgenesis
s. tubule sclerosis
seminoma
semisynthetic
s. ergot alkaloid
s. insulin
Semmes-Weinstein 5.07 monofilament
senescence
cell s.
tissue s.
senile
s. purpura
s. systemic amyloidosis
senilis
arcus s.
Senior
Phenadex S.
Senn rake
sensate focus exercise
sensation
sexual s.
vibratory s.
sense
time s.
sensing
glucose s.
sensitivity
analytical s.
androgen s.
clinical insulin s.
complete androgen s.
functional s.
hepatic insulin s.
insulin s.
partial androgen s.
peripheral insulin s.
s. test
sensitizer
insulin s.
sensor
Animas R-1000 s.
calcium s.
Diasensor 1000 s.
electrochemical glucose s.
GlucoNIR glucose s.
GlucoWatch Biographer transdermal s.
implantable glucose s.
MiniMed continuous glucose s.
Therasense subcutaneous glucose s.
TouchTrak glucose s.
sensorineural
s. deafness
s. hearing loss
sensorium
clouded s.
sensory
s. ataxic polyneuropathy
s. nerve conduction velocity
sentinel lymph node
Sentry
Sleep S.
sepsis
meningococcal s.
septa
intraglandular fibrous s.
placental s.
septicemia
fungal s.
septicum
Clostridium s.
septooptic dysplasia
septum
s. pellucidum
sphenoid s.
transverse vaginal s.
sequence
adenoma-carcinoma s.
amino acid s.
consensus s.
DQ alpha s.
FASE s.
fast asymmetric spin echo s.
gene-activating s. (GAS)
gradient-echo s.
Kozak consensus translation initiation s.
melanocyte-stimulating hormone s.
pancreatic islet cell-specific enhancer s. (PICSES)
short time inversion recovery s.
SPGR pulse s.
spoiled gradient-recalled acquisition pulse s.
STIR s.
sequential
s. deiodination
s. hormone replacement therapy
sequestered
s. goiter
s. vesicle
sequestrant
bile s.
bile acid s.
sequestration
SER, sER
smooth endoplasmic reticulum

SERCA
sarcoplasmic/endoplasmic reticulum calcium ATPase
Serevent
S. Diskus
series
amine precursor uptake and decarboxylation s.
anion of the Hofmeister s.
APUD s.
erythroid s.
serine
phosphorylated s. 137
s. phosphorylation pathway
s. protease inhibitor (SERPIN)
SERM
selective estrogen-receptor modulator
selective estrogen response modifier
sermorelin acetate
Serophene
Serostim
serotherapy
percutaneous alcohol s.
serotonergic
s. agent
s. axis
s. projection
s. system
serotonin
monoamine s. (5-HT)
s. *N*-acetyltransferase
s. reuptake
s. secretion
s. syndrome
serotoninergic
s. receptor
serous
s. cystadenoma of the pancreas
s. tumor
Serpalan
serpentine receptor
SERPIN
serine protease inhibitor
serpin
s. protein
Serratia marcescens
Ser/Thr-Tyr-Ser
Sertoli
S. cell
S. cell-only syndrome
S. cell testicular tumor
Sertoli-Leydig
S.-L. cell
S.-L. cell tumor
sertraline
serum
s. acid phosphatase test
s. alanine aminotransferase
s. albumin
s. albumin concentration
s. aldosterone
s. alkaline phosphatase
s. antiinsulin antibody
antilymphocytic s. (ALS)
s. bicarbonate
s. cholesterol concentration
s. corticosterone
s. C-peptide level
s. creatine phosphokinase
s. dehydroepiandrosterone sulfate level
s. endoprotease
s. erythropoietin
s. estradiol
s. estrogen-receptor modulator
s. estrone
s. fibronectin
s. fluoride
s. free T_4
s. free testosterone
s. fructosamine level
s. glutamic-oxaloacetic transaminase (SGOT)
s. glutamic-pyruvic transaminase (SGPT)
s. growth hormone level
s. 18-hydroxycorticosterone concentration
s. IGFBP-3 concentration
s. IGF-1 concentration
s. inorganic phosphorus
s. insulinlike growth factor-1
s. insulinlike growth factor binding protein-3 concentration
s. insulinlike growth factor-1 concentration
s. ionized calcium
s. ionized calcium concentration
s. leptin concentration
s. microsomal antibody
s. osmolality
s. osteocalcin
s. parathyroid hormone level

NOTES

serum *(continued)*
s. phosphorus goal
s. prolactin
s. sodium
s. thrombomodulin
s. thymic factor
s. thyroglobulin
s. thyroid hormone-binding protein
s. thyroxine-binding globulin
s. total T_4
s. total testosterone
s. vasopressinase activity
serum tartrate resistant acid phosphatase
serum-to-ascitic albumin gradient
SES
socioeconomic status
sestamibi
99m-technetium s.
technetium-99m s.
sestamibi-pertechnetate subtraction scintigraphy
set
s. point abnormality
s. point for insulin secretion
SETTLE
spindled and epithelial tumor with thymus-like differentiation
sevalemer
sevenless
son of s. (SOS)
seven-transmembrane-domain receptor
severe
s. acute pancreatitis (SAP)
s. combined immunodeficiency
s. combined immunodeficiency disease (SCID)
s. insulin resistance
Sevier-Munger stain technique
sex
s. chromatin
s. chromosome aneuploidy
s. cord stromal tumor
s. cord tumor with annular tubule (SCTAT)
dosage-sensitive s. (DSS)
s. hormone-binding globulin (SHBG)
s. steroid
s. steroid-binding globulin (SSBG)
s. steroid hormone
s. steroid level
sex-binding globulin
sex-determining
s.-d. region of the Y chromosome (SRY)
s.-d. region Y gene (SRY)
s.-d. region Y gene detection
sex-linked
s.-l. adrenoleukodystrophy
s.-l. inheritance
sexual
s. differentiation
s. dimorphic physical change
s. dimorphism
s. infantilism
s. infantility
s. precocity
s. sensation
sexually
s. dimorphic
s. dimorphic nucleus
s. transmitted infection (STI)
SF-1
steroidogenic factor-1
SFO
subfornical organ
SGA
small for gestational age
SGLT
sodium glucose cotransporter
SGLT1
SGLT2
SGOT
serum glutamic-oxaloacetic transaminase
SGP
stress-generated potential
SGPT
serum glutamic-pyruvic transaminase
SH
sulfhydryl
SH2
SH compound
shaft
endoscope s.
SHBG
sex hormone-binding globulin
Sheehan syndrome
sheet
arachnoidal s.
shell
trophoblastic s.
SHH
syndrome of hyporeninemic hypoaldosteronism
shin
saber s.
s. spot
shivering thermogenesis
shock
circulatory s.
hypoglycemic s.
hypovolemic s.
insulin s.
neuronal s.

s. syndrome
s. wave lithotripsy
Shohl solution
short
s. chain acyl-CoA dehydrogenase deficiency (SCAD)
s. luteal phase
s. stature
s. tandem repeat (STR)
s. tandem repeat marker
s. time inversion recovery sequence
s. T1 inversion recovery (STIR)
short-acting insulin
shortened luteal phase
shortening
acromelic s.
fractional s.
mesomelic s.
rhizomelic s.
short-limbed dwarfism
short-loop
s.-l. feedback
s.-l. inhibition
shoulder-hand syndrome
shunt
Denver s.
glandulocavernosal s.
LeVeen s.
peritoneovenous s.
portacaval s.
portasystemic s.
transjugular intrahepatic portosystemic stent s. (TIPS)
ventriculoperitoneal s.
shuttle
carnitine s.
Shwachman syndrome
Shy-Drager syndrome
SIADH
syndrome of inappropriate secretion of antidiuretic hormone
sialadenitis
sialic
s. acid
s. acid content
s. acid storage disease
sialidosis
sialoadenectomy
sialoadenitis
sialoglycolipid
sialography
parotid s.
sialoprotein
biglycan bone s.
bone s. (BSP)
sialylated
s. hCG
s. human chorionic gonadotropin
sialylation
sialyl LewisA
Sibley-Lehninger test
sibship
sibutramine
s. hydrochloride monohydrate
sick
euthyroid s.
s. euthyroid syndrome
sickle
s. cell (SC)
s. cell anemia
s. cell disease
side
s. chain cleavage (SCC)
s. chain cleavage deficiency
s. chain cleavage enzyme
side-chain composition
side-effect profile of use
sideroblastic anemia
side-to-side pancreaticojejunostomy
sign
Chvostek s.
Collier s.
Cullen s.
Dalrymple s.
Darier s.
double-duct s.
Graefe s.
Grey Turner s.
infiltrative eye s.
Joffroy s.
mask s.
Pemberton s.
pyramidal tract s.
Schultze s.
Stellwag s.
Trousseau s.
Unschuld s.
von Graefe s.
signal
afferent s.
autoimmune s.
gastrointestinal s.
hormonal s.
humoral s.

NOTES

signal *(continued)*
long-loop feedback s.
metabolic s.
s. patch
s. peptid
s. peptidase
s. peptide
phosphatidylinositol s.
s. processor
radiofrequency s.
s. recognition particle receptor
stomach-derived paracrine s.
SV40 polyadenylation s.
s. transducer
s. transducer and activator of transcription (STAT)
s. transducer and activator of transcription-4 (Stat4)
s. transducer and activator of transcription-5 (Stat5)
s. transducer and activator of transcription-4 transcription factor
s. transducer and activator of transcription-5 transcription factor
s. transducers and activators of transcription (STATS)
signaling
activin s.
cell s.
s. pheromone
suppressor of cytokine s. 3 (SOCS-3)
signal-transduction pathway
signet-ring appearance
Silain
Silapap
Silastic
S. ring
S. rod
sildenafil
s. citrate
silencer
silencing
s. mediator of retinoic acid and thyroid hormone receptor (SMRT)
transcriptional s.
silent
s. ACTH adenoma
s. autoimmune thyroiditis
s. corticotrope adenoma subtype I
s. corticotrope adenoma subtype II
s. corticotrope adenoma subtype III
s. corticotroph cell adenoma
s. gonadotroph cell adenoma
s. microadenoma
s. somatotroph adenoma
silicon
Sillence
S. classification scheme
S. type I, II, III, IV
silver-impregnated semithin section
simethicone
aluminum hydroxide, magnesium hydroxide, and s.
calcium carbonate and s.
magaldrate and s.
simian sarcoma virus genome
Simmonds disease
simple
s. nonendemic goiter
s. tandem repeat polymorphism (STRP)
s. virilizer
s. virilizing hydroxylase deficiency variant
simplex
thyroiditis akuta s.
SimpleXx
Norditropin S.
Simron
Sims-Huhner test
Simulect
simultaneous
s. pancreas-kidney (SPK)
s. pancreas-kidney transplant
s. pancreas-kidney transplantation
simvastatin
Sindh
dwarfism of S.
sine
s. qua non
s. qua nonsuppressed thyroid-stimulating hormone
sinensis
Clonorchis s.
single
s. gateway hypothesis
s. hormone deficiency
s. nucleotide polymorphism (SNP)
s. thyroid nodule
single-bladed Kurze microscissors
single-chain polypeptide
single-pass transmembrane protein
single-photon
s.-p. absorptiometry (SPA)
s.-p. emission computed tomography (SPECT)
s.-p. emission tomography (SPET)
single-serum dehydroepiandrosterone sulfate value
single-strand conformation polymorphism (SSCP)
single-stranded conformation polymorphism analysis
singlet oxygen

single-transmembrane-domain receptor
sinonasal
s. complication
s. surgery
sinugram
sinus
basilar s.
carotid s.
cavernous s.
conchal type sphenoid s.
incompletely pneumatized sphenoid s.
inferior petrosal s.
lactiferous s.
petrosal s.
sphenoid s.
superior petrosal s.
urogenital s.
sinusoid
sinusoidal pattern
Sipple syndrome
sirolimus
SIRS
systemic inflammatory response syndrome
sister
s. chromatid
S. Mary Joseph node
Sistrunk
S. operation
S. procedure
site
extragonadal s.
extrahypothalamic s.
injection s.
Maillard s.
protease-sensitive s.
putative-binding s.
thyroid hormone-binding s.
tyrosine phosphorylation s.
Zal s.
zona pellucide recognition s.
site-directed mutagenesis
site-specific ovarian cancer syndrome
sitosterolemia
sitotherapy
situs
s. inversus
s. inversus viscerum totalis
sivelestat
size
age, metastases, extent and s. (AMES)
phallic s.
Sjögren syndrome
skeletal
s. abnormality
s. deformity
s. fluoride
s. homeostasis
s. mass
s. muscle
s. muscle ischemia
s. muscle spontaneous infarction
s. regeneration
s. resistance
s. scintigraphy
s. sclerosis
skeleton
appendicular s.
axial s.
computer tomographic methods of axial s. (axial QCT)
computer tomographic methods of peripheral s. (pQCT)
Skelid
Skene
S. paraurethral gland
S. periurethral gland
skin
Composite Cultured S.
s. fold measurement
s. fold thickness
hyperpigmented s.
s. thinning
yellow s.
skull
s. base
salt and pepper appearance of s.
scaphocephalic s.
S/L
A-Spas S.
SLC12A1 gene
SLC12A3 gene
SLE
systemic lupus erythematosus
sleep
s. apnea
slow-wave s.
SW s.
sleep-associated penile tumescence
Sleep Sentry

NOTES

sleep-wake
s.-w. cycle
s.-w. homeostasis
slice
coronal s.
sliding scale
slipped
Slo-bid
Slo-Niacin
Slo-Phyllin
S.-P. GG
sloppy pacemaker
Slow
S. Fe
slow relaxation phase of deep tendon reflex
slow-release
Bontril S.-r.
s.-r. lanreotide
slow-twitch oxidative fiber
slow-wave (SW)
s.-w. sleep
SLS
scleroderma-like syndrome
sludge
biliary s.
Sly syndrome
Sm-A
somatomedin A
Smad
small
s. bowel diabetes
s. cell carcinoma
s. cleaved lymphoma
s. fiber polyneuropathy
s. for gestational age (SGA)
s. goiter
s. noncleaved lymphoma
s. nuclear ribonucleic acid (snRNA)
small-volume pituitary tumor
Sm-C
somatomedin C
smear
buccal s.
Pap s.
Papanicolaou s.
vaginal s.
Smith-Lemli-Opitz syndrome
Smith-Magenis syndrome
smooth endoplasmic reticulum (SER, sER)
SMRT
silencing mediator of retinoic acid and thyroid hormone receptor
SMS
stiff man syndrome
Snaplets-FR Granule
SNARE
soluble *N*-ethylmaleimide-sensitive factor attachment protein receptor
SNARE hypothesis
Snell dwarf mice
SNP
single nucleotide polymorphism
Snp5
S. c/c
S. t/c
S. t/t
snRNA
small nuclear ribonucleic acid
SNS
sympathetic nervous system
socioeconomic status (SES)
socks
Thorlo padded s.
SOCS-3
suppressor of cytokine signaling 3
sodium
s. acetate
alendronate s.
s. ascorbate
s. azide
s. bicarbonate
s. chloride tablet
cromolyn s.
s. excess
s. fluoride
s. glucose cotransporter (SGLT)
s. glucose transporter
s. homeostasis
s. ipodate
s. lactate
levothyroxine s.
liothyronine s.
s. nitrite
phenytoin s.
s. phosphate
plasma s.
PMS-Levothyroxine S.
s. polystyrene sulfonate
risedronate s.
s. salicylate
serum s.
thiopental s.
s. valproate
s. wasting
sodium bicarbonate therapy
sodium-iodide symporter (NIS)
sodium/iodine cotransporter gene
sodium-lactate cotransporter
sodium-potassium
s.-p.-2 chloride cotransporter (NKCC2)
s.-p. adenosine triphosphatase
s.-p. pump

Soehendra dilating catheter
SOFA
stromal osteoclast-forming activity
soft
s. tissue nodule
s. tissue swelling
Softgels
Vita-Plus E S.
soft-tissue calcification
software
Accutility S.
Gammaplan s.
solid
s. cell nest
s. cystic tumor (SCT)
s. phase support
s. pseudopapillary tumor
solid-phase minisequencing
solitarius
nucleus of the tractus s. (NTS)
nucleus tractus s. (NTS)
tractus s.
solitary
s. adenoma
s. nontoxic nodule
s. unilateral macroadenoma
solium
Taenia s.
solochrome
acid s. azurin
s. azurin stain
soluble
s. complement receptor (sCR1)
s. fiber
s. *N*-ethylmaleimide-sensitive factor attachment protein
s. *N*-ethylmaleimide-sensitive factor attachment protein receptor (SNARE)
Solu-Cortef
S.-C. Injection
Solu-Medrol Injection
Solurex L.A.
Soluspan
Celestone S.
solute
s. diuresis
intracellular s.
solution
albumin s.
aqueous s.
balanced electrolyte s. (BES)
Euro-Ficoll s.
Krebs-Ringer s.
Los Angeles preservation s. 1 (LAP-1)
modified University of Wisconsin s.
mUW s.
original University of Wisconsin s. (UW solution)
oUW s.
Resectisol irrigation s.
Shohl s.
University of Wisconsin s.
UW s.
original University of Wisconsin solution
solvent drag
somatic
s. amplification
s. deletion
s. mutation
s. phenotype
s. PTEN mutation
somatocrinin
SomatoKine
somatoliberin
somatomammotropic hormone
somatomammotropin
chorionic s. (CS)
human chorionic s. (hCS)
somatomedin
s. A (Sm-A)
s. C (Sm-C)
s. C level
s. C protein
hepatic s.
s. hypothesis
s. level
somatomegaly
somatopause
somatosensory-evoked potential recovery period
somatostatin (SS, SST)
s.-14
s.-18
s.-28
s. analog
s. analogue octreotide
s. gene
s. infusion
s. receptor

NOTES

S

somatostatinergic
s. innervation
somatostatinoma
somatostatin-producing delta cell
somatostatin-receptor scintigraphy
somatotrope
somatotroph
s. acidophil
s. adenoma of pituitary gland
s. cell
s. cell adenoma
s. cell proliferative rate
s. hormone (STH)
s. hypoplasia
s. tumor
somatotrophinoma
somatotropic
s. axis
s. cell
s. hormone
somatotropin (hGH)
s. deficiency
s. release factor (SRF)
s. release-inhibiting factor (SRIF)
s. release-inhibiting hormone (SRIH)
somatotropinoma
isolated familial s.
pituitary s.
somatrem
somatropin
s. of rDNA origin
Somatulin
Somavert
somnolence
daytime s.
Somogyi
S. effect
S. hypothesis
S. phenomenon
somostatin
SON
supraoptic nucleus of the hypothalamus
sonographic halo
sonorous voice
son of sevenless (SOS)
sorbent dialysis cartridge
sorbinil
S. Retinopathy Trial
sorbitol
SOS
son of sevenless
Soto syndrome
sound
Korotkoff s.
South American blastomycosis
Southern
S. blot
S. blot analysis
soy
s. isoflavone
s. phytoestrogen extract (SPE)
s. protein
soybean protein
SoySelect
SPA
single-photon absorptiometry
space
anterior incisural s.
extradural s.
intertrabecular s.
intervillous s.
periosteocytic s.
perivitelline s.
subarachnoid s.
suprasellar s.
Virchow-Robin s.
spacing
interdental s.
Span-FF
spare receptor
sparse body fat
spasm
carpopedal s.
tonic s.
spasmodic dysphonia
Spasmolin
spasmus nutans
spastic paraplegia
SPE
soy phytoestrogen extract
specialist
insulin infusion s.
specialization
ectoplasmic s.
specific gravity
specificity
s. test
tissue s.
SPECT
single-photon emission computed tomography
spectrometer
spectrometry
mass s.
spectrophotometry
atomic absorption s.
spectroscopy
affinity attenuated total reflectance s.
affinity evanescent wave s.
affinity fluorescence s.
affinity surface plasmon s.
fluorescence quencing s.

magnetic resonance s. (MRS)
potassium s.
SpectRx glucose monitor
speculum
Cushing-Landolt s.
nasal s.
speech dyspraxia
sperm
artificial insemination with donor s.
s. autoantibody
female s.
s. function test
s. granuloma
s. kinematics
male s.
s. transport disorder
s. velocity
spermacrasia
spermarche
spermatic cord leiomyoma
spermatid
spermatocyte
postmeiotic s.
preleptotene primary s.
primary s.
secondary s.
spermatocytogenesis
spermatogenesis
spermatogonia
type A s.
type Ad s.
type A dark s.
type Ap s.
type B s.
spermatogonium
stem s.
spermatogram
spermatozoa
capacitation of the s.
sperm-cervical mucus interaction
spermiation
spermicide
spermiogenesis
SpermMar test
SPET
single-photon emission tomography
SPGR
spoiled gradient-recalled
SPGR pulse sequence
S-phase fraction
sphenoethmoidal encephalocele
sphenoid
s. bone
s. septum
s. sinus
sphenoidale
midline jugum s.
planum s.
sphenoorbital encephalocele
spherocytosis
sphincter
balloon dilation of the pancreatic duct s.
lower esophageal s. (LES)
s. of Oddi dysfunction
s. of Oddi manometry
s. vesicae
sphincteroplasty
sphincterotomy
endoscopic s. (ES)
sphingolipidosis
sphingomyelin
sphygmomanometer
spike
cholesterol s.
spillover
s. syndrome
spinal
s. accessory nerve
s. cord compression
s. muscular atrophy types I, II, III
spindle
s. cell
s. cell carcinoma
spindle cells
spindled and epithelial tumor with thymus-like differentiation (SETTLE)
spindle-shaped fibroplastic morphology
spine
flattened lumbar s.
rugger-jersey s.
spin-echo magnetic resonance
spin-lattice relaxation time
spinnbarkeit
spinobulbar muscular atrophy
spinocerebellar ataxia types I, II, III, VI, VII
spinosum
foramen s.
stratum s.
spinothalamic tract
spin-spin relaxation time

NOTES

S

spiral
s. computed tomography
s. CT
spirit
aromatic ammonia s.
spirometry
flow-volume loop s.
spironolactone
SPK
simultaneous pancreas-kidney
SPK transplant
splanchine glucose uptake
splanchnic
s. bed
s. nerve
spleen
upper pole of s.
s. volume
splenic
s. artery
s. involution
splenomegaly
spliceosome
split mixed insulin program
spoiled
s. gradient-recalled (SPGR)
s. gradient-recalled acquisition pulse sequence
spondylitis
spondylodysplastic
spondyloepiphyseal dysplasia (SED)
spondylolisthesis
spondylometaphyseal dysplasia
sponge
Gelfoam s.
polyvinyl s.
spongiform encephalopathy
spongiosa
primary s.
spongiosum
corpus s.
spongy bone
spontaneous
s. abortion (SAB)
s. autoimmune anti-insulin antibody syndrome
s. autoimmune thyroiditis (SAT)
s. bacterial peritonitis
s. diuresis
s. hypokalemia
s. pituitary necrosis
s. primary hypothyroidism
s. secretion
sporadic
s. carcinoid
s. congenital hypothyroidism
s. goiter
s. silent thyroiditis
s. testitoxicosis
s. thyroid tumor
Sporothrix schenckii
sporotrichosis
lymphocutaneous s.
spot
café au lait s.
G s.
Graefenberg s.
hot s.
shin s.
spotted bone
spotting
midcycle s.
SP-PVC
superior mesenteric-portal vein confluence
spring
arcing s.
coil s.
flat s.
Sprinkle
Humibid S.
sprue
celiac s.
nontropic s.
nontropical s.
SP-1 transcription factor
spurious elevation
spuriously elevated hemoglobin A1c
spurt
growth s.
pubertal growth s.
squamous
s. cell nest
s. cell rest
s. follicular epithelium
Src
S. homology 2 domain
S. protein
SRC-1 coactivator
SREBP
sterol regulatory element binding protein
SRF
somatotropin release factor
SRIF
somatotropin release-inhibiting factor
SRIH
somatotropin release-inhibiting hormone
SR-NaF
sustained-release sodium fluoride
SRY
sex-determining region of the Y chromosome
sex-determining region Y gene
SRY detection
SRY gene
SRY transcription factor

SS
somatostatin
SSBG
sex steroid-binding globulin
SSCP
single-strand conformation polymorphism
SSKI
saturated solution of potassium iodide
supersaturated potassium iodide
SSRI
selective serotonin reuptake inhibitor
SST
somatostatin
St.
S. Anthony fire
S. Louis encephalitis
stability
platelet s.
stack
Golgi s.
Stadol
S. NS
stage
colloid s.
follicular s.
precolloid s.
Tanner s. (I–V)
Stagesic
staghorn stone
staging
Tanner s.
stain
acid-Schiff s.
Alcian blue s.
argentaffin s.
argyrophilic s.
aurintricarboxylic acid s.
Congo red s.
eosin s.
Grocott s.
hematoxylin s.
IHC s.
immunohistochemical s.
Luxol fast blue s.
Masson trichrome s.
May-Giemsa-Grünwald s.
Papanicolaou s.
Prussian blue s.
reticulin s.
solochrome azurin s.
Sudan s.
Wright s.
staining
immunocytochemical s.
immunogold s.
immunohistochemical s.
periumbilical s.
thyroglobulin s.
vital s.
stalk
hypophysial s.
infundibular s.
neural s.
neurohypophysial s.
pituitary s.
s. section effect
stalkitis
stalled puberty
stanolone
stanozolol
Staphylococcus
S. aureus
S. epidermidis
S. non-aureus
S. pneumoniae
S. pyogenes
staphylomata
peripapillary s.
StAR
steroid acute regulatory protein
steroid acute respiratory protein
steroidogenic acute regulatory protein
StAR deficiency
StAR protein
starburst artifact
stare
thyroid s.
Starling
S. curve of the pancreas
S. force
Starlix
stasis
urinary s.
STAT
signal transducer and activator of transcription
Stat4
signal transducer and activator of transcription-4
Stat4 transcription factor
Stat5
signal transducer and activator of transcription-5
Stat5 transcription factor

NOTES

state
eumetabolic s.
euthyroid s.
hormone-resistant s.
hyperandrogen s.
hyperandrogenic s.
hypercalciuric hypophosphatemic s.
hypercontractile s.
hyperestrogenic s.
hypergonadotropic s.
hypertrophic s.
hypocorticotropic s.
induced hypermetabolic s.
lampbrush s.
nonketotic hyperosmolar s.
postabsorptive s.
postprandial s.
pseudo-Cushing s.
redox s.
resistance s.
statin catabolism
Statistics
National Center for Health S. (NCHS)
STATS
signal transducers and activators of transcription
stature
excessive s.
idiopathic short s. (ISS)
nongrowth hormone deficient short s.
short s.
status
s. epilepticus
socioeconomic s. (SES)
thyroid hormone s.
thyrometabolic s.
tumor receptor s.
Staub-Traugott effect
staurosporine
steal syndrome
stearic acid
stearoyl acyl-CoA desaturase
steatoma
steatorrhea
pancreatic s.
steatosis
hepatic s.
Stein-Leventhal syndrome
Stellwag sign
stem
s. cell
s. cell factor (SCF)
s. spermatogonium
Stemex
stenbolone
stenosis
papillary s.
stent
Amsterdam-type biliary s.
polypropylene s.
Wall s.
stenting
Evaluation of Platelet IIb-IIIa Inhibitors for S. (EPISTENT)
step 2 diet
stercoralis
Strongyloides s.
stereoisomer
stereotactic
s. hypophysectomy
s. radiosurgery
s. radiotherapy
sterility
sternocleidomastoid muscle
sternohyoid muscle
sternothyroid muscle
sternum
tie s.
steroid
s. acne
s. acute regulatory protein (StAR)
s. acute regulatory protein deficiency
s. acute respiratory protein (StAR)
s. acute respiratory protein deficiency
alkylated androgenic s.
s. 5-alpha-reductase deficiency
anabolic s.
anabolic-androgenic s.
s. analog
s. biosynthesis
C-18 s.
C-19 s.
C-21 s.
circannual rhythmicity of s.
s. dose
estrogen C_{19} s.
gonadal s.
s. hormone
s. hormone receptor
s. hormone receptor activation
s. hormone receptor antihormone
s. hormone-receptor hormone-response element
s. hormone receptor zinc finger
s. hormone resistance syndrome
s. hormone-response element
hybrid s.
s. hydroxylase
intralesional fluorinated s.
ketogenic s.
17-ketogenic s.

s. prohormone
s. receptor
s. replacement therapy
sex s.
s. sulfatase
s. sulfatase deficiency
urine s.
s. withdrawal syndrome
steroid-dependent tumor
steroid-induced
s.-i. diabetes
s.-i. osteoporosis
steroidogenesis
adrenal s.
gonadal s.
ovarian s.
steroidogenic
s. acute regulatory protein (StAR)
s. acute regulatory protein deficiency
s. cytoplasmic pool
s. enzyme
s. enzyme function
s. factor-1 (SF-1)
s. pathway
steroid-releasing intrauterine device
steroid/thyroid hormone receptor
sterol
s. carrier protein-2 (SCP-2)
s. hormone
s. metabolism
s. regulatory element binding protein (SREBP)
s. secretion
s. synthesis
vitamin D s.
stethoscope
esophageal s.
Stevia rebaudiana
steviol
stevioside
Stewart-Treves syndrome
STH
somatotroph hormone
STI
sexually transmitted infection
Stickler syndrome
sticky colloid
stiff
s. hand syndrome
s. man syndrome (SMS)
stigma, pl. **stigmata**
stigmata of Cushing disease
Turner s.
stilbestrol
Stilphostrol
Stimate
stimulant
luteinization s.
stimulation
blunt estrogenic s.
breast s.
bystander s.
dexamethasone-suppressed corticotropin-releasing hormone s.
dexamethasone-suppressed CRH s.
ligand-independent s.
osteoclastic s.
plasminogen-activator s.
s. test
thyrotropin-releasing hormone s.
vagal s.
stimulator
adenylate cyclase s.
allosteric s.
long-acting thyroid s. (LATS)
Triax metabolic s.
stimulator-protector
long-acting thyroid s.-p. (LATS-P)
stimulatory
s. G protein
s. immunoglobulin
s. receptor (R_s)
stimulus, pl. **stimuli**
aversive s.
diabetogenic s.
dipsogenic s.
kaliuretic s.
nonosmotic s.
osmotic s.
stimuli of thirst
stimulus-secretion coupling
stippled
s. epiphysis
STIR
short T1 inversion recovery
STIR sequence
stochastic
s. theory of aging
Stockholm trial
stocking
stomach
thoracic s.
stomach-derived paracrine signal

NOTES

stomatitis
stomodeal
s. ectoderm
s. hypophysial pouch
stomodeum
stone
ampullary s.
calcium oxalate renal s.
cystine renal s.
infection s.
noncalcareous s.
pancreatic s.
staghorn s.
uric acid renal s.
store
glycogen s.
intracellular s.
storm
thyroid s.
thyrotoxic s.
STR
short tandem repeat
STR marker
strabismus
straight
s. bone curette
s. ethmoidal rongeur
strap muscle
strategy
positional cloning s.
stratum
s. basale
s. functionale
periventricular s.
s. spinosum
strawberry lesion
streak
s. gonad
s. ovary
retinal angioid s.
strength
Acutrim II, Maximum S.
double s. (DS)
Excedrin, Extra S.
extra s. (ES)
hand grip s.
ionic s.
isometric knee extensor s.
Streptococcus
group A S.
S. hemolyticus
S. mutans
S. pneumoniae
S. pyogenes
streptokinase
streptolysin
s. O
s. S
streptozocin
streptozotocin
stress
catabolic s.
end-systolic s.
fluid shear s.
s. fracture
s. hormone
s. response of Selye
stress-generated potential (SGP)
stress-relevant amygdalar nucleus
Stresstabs 600 Advanced Formula Tablets
stretched penile length
stretch receptor
stria, pl. **striae**
abdominal s.
striae medullaris thalami
purple s.
purplish s.
s. terminalis
violaceous s.
striata
osteopathia s.
striation
radiodense s.
stridor
strip
Excel GE electrochemical glucose monitoring test s.
fibrillar collagen s.
Microflo glucose monitoring test s.
Microflo test s.
QuickVue UrinChek urine test s.
stroke
alcohol, epilepsy, insulin, overdose, uremia, trauma, infection, psychiatric, s. (AEIOU TIPS)
coronary artery disease, hypertension, adult-onset diabetes, obesity, and s. (CHAOS)
stroma
bone marrow s.
desmoplastic s.
echogenic ovarian s.
endometrial s.
hematopoiesis-supporting s.
interfollicular s.
thyroid s.
stromal
s. cell
s. enlargement
s. hyperplasia
s. hyperthecosis
s. osteoclast-forming activity (SOFA)
stromelysin-1

stromolysin
Strong
S. Heart Study
Thyroid S.
Strongyloides stercoralis
strongyloidosis
disseminated s.
strontium
STRP
simple tandem repeat polymorphism
structural gene defect
structure
axonemal s.
helix-loop-helix s.
heterodimeric s.
mediobasal brain s.
müllerian duct derived s.
pentalaminar tubular s.
tennis racket-shaped pentalaminar tubular s.
widened cranial s.
Strudwick-type spondyloepimetaphyseal dysplasia
struma
s. granulomatosa
s. lymphomatosa
s. ovarii
Riedel s.
substernal s.
struvite
s. crystal
Stuartnatal 1 + 1
Stuart Prenatal
study
CARE s.
cell culture s.
Cholesterol and Recurrent Events s.
contrast dynamic s.
coronal postgadolinium s.
Deutsch Nicotinamide Diabetes Intervention S. (DENIS)
Diabetes in Early Pregnancy S.
Diabetes Mellitus Insulin-Glucose Infusion in Acute Myocardial Infection s.
Diabetes Prevention Trial research s.
Diabetes Retinopathy S. (DRS)
DIAD s.
DIGAMI s.
DPT-1 research s.
Early Treatment Diabetic Retinopathy S. (ETDRS)
FDG-PET s.
^{18}F-fluorodeoxyglucose positron emission tomography s.
Heart and Estrogen/Progestin Replacement S. (HERS)
histomorphometric s.
hormonal s.
Islet Cell Antibody Registry of Users S. (ICARUS)
Kabi International Growth S. (KIGS)
National Cooperative Growth S. (NCGS)
neurodiagnostic s.
neuroimaging s.
North American Pediatric Renal Transplant Cooperative S. (NAPRTCS)
postgadolinium s.
pregadolinium s.
radioautographic s.
Randomized Aldactone Evaluation S. (RALES)
saline suppression s.
Scandinavian Simvastatin Survival S. (4S)
selective arterial calcium stimulation s.
Strong Heart S.
swallow s.
thyrotropin-releasing hormone s.
Toronto Renal Osteodystrophy S.
TRH s.
twin s.
United Kingdom Prospective Diabetes S. (UKPDS)
whole-body ^{131}I-MIBG s.
xenon-133 washout s.
stunning
thyroid s.
stuttering
s. impotence
stylohyoid muscle
styrene
subacute
s. granulomatous thyroiditis
s. hyperthyroidism
s. painful thyroiditis
subarachnoid
s. fluid

NOTES

subarachnoid *(continued)*
- s. space
- s. space of Virchow-Robin

subcapsular
- s. cataract
- s. follicular microcyst

subchondral cyst
subclinical
- s. hyperthyroidism
- s. hypothyroidism
- s. pheochromocytoma
- s. thyrotoxicosis

subcommissural organ (SCO)
subcutaneous fat necrosis
subendothelium
subependymal plexus
subfornical organ (SFO)
subfrontal surgery
sublabial
- s. transseptal approach
- s. transseptal technique

Sublimaze Injection
subluxation
- globe s.

submicromolar
subsalicylate
- bismuth s.

substance
- goitrogenic s.
- ground s.
- s. K
- müllerian-inhibiting s. (MIS)
- Nissl s.
- noncholecystokinin s.
- s. P

substantia nigra
substernal
- s. goiter
- s. struma
- s. thyroid

substitute
- DiabetiSweet sugar s.

substitution
- amino acid s.
- ether bridge s.

substrate
- s.-1
- s. cycle
- insulin receptor s. (IRS)
- insulin receptor s.-1 (IRS-1)
- insulin receptor s.-2 (IRS-2)

subthalamus
subtilisin
- s.-related endoprotease

subtotal
- s. parathyroidectomy
- s. thyroidectomy

subtraction thyroid scan
subtunical venous plexus
subunit
- acid-labile s. (ALS)
- α-thyroid stimulating hormone s.
- α-TSH s.

succinate
- hydrocortisone sodium s.

succinylacetone
succinyl-CoA
sucked-candy appearance
suckling reflex
Sucraid
sucralfate
- s. suspension

sucrase
sucrose
#8 suction monopolar coagulator
sudanophilic leukodystrophy
Sudan stain
Sudeck atrophy
sudomotor system
Sufenta
sufentanil
sugar
- s. alcohol
- capillary blood s. (CBS)
- finger-stick blood s.
- s. watch

sulcus
- chiasmatic s.
- hypothalamic s.
- s. limitans
- pontomesencephalic s.

sulfadiazine
sulfaguanidine
sulfamethoxazole
- trimethoprim s. (TMP-SMX)

sulfasalazine
sulfatase
- steroid s.

sulfate
- cellulose s.
- chondroitin s.
- s. conjugate
- dehydroepiandrosterone s. (DHEAS, DHEA-S)
- dermatan s.
- DHEA s.
- estrone s.
- ferrous s.
- glucosamine s.
- heparan s.
- indoxyl s.
- keratan s.
- magnesium s.
- morphine s.
- piperazine estrone s.

terbutaline s.
zinc s.
sulfatide
sulfatidosis
juvenile Austin-type s.
sulfation
s. factor
sulfhydryl (SH)
s. amino acid
s. compound
sulfisoxazole
sulfoconjugation
sulfocysteine
sulfocysteinuria
sulfonamide
sulfonate
sodium polystyrene s.
sulfonylurea
bedtime insulin, daytime s. (BIDS)
s. hypoglycemic drug
plasma s.
s. receptor (SUR)
s. receptor gene
sulfotransferase
s. enzyme
phenol s.
sulfur
sulindac
sum
vectorial s.
Sumacal
sump syndrome
Sumycin Oral
supercoiled chromatin
superfecundation
superficial
s. dermal perivasculitis
s. fascia
s. perineal muscle
supergene
superior
s. colliculus
s. hypophyseal artery
s. mesenteric artery
s. mesenteric-portal vein confluence (SP-PVC)
s. oblique palsy
s. ophthalmic vein obstruction
s. orbital fissure syndrome
s. orbital fossa
s. pancreaticoduodenal artery
s. parathyroid artery
s. parathyroid gland
s. petrosal sinus
s. vascular pedicle
superotemporal hemianoptic defect
superovulation
superoxide dismutase
supersaturated potassium iodide (SSKI)
supersaturation
superselective microcoil embolization
supersensitive
supplement
Alphabetic multivitamin s.
dehydroepiandrosterone s.
supplementation
cyclical s.
supply
anastomotic blood s.
support
solid phase s.
suppository
Dilaudid s.
progesterone s.
Supprelin
Suppress
suppressant
appetite s.
Suppressant/Expectorant
Diabetic Tussin DM Maximum Strength Cough S.
suppressed plasma renin activity
suppression
gonadal s.
HPA axis s.
hypothalamic-pituitary-adrenal axis s.
suppressive therapy
suppressor
autocrine s.
s. of cytokine signaling 3 (SOCS-3)
s. T cell
tumor s.
suppressor/cytotoxic T-lymphocyte
Supprettes
B&O S.
suppurative
s. hydradenitis
s. thyroiditis
suprachiasmatic
s. nucleus (SCN)
s. nucleus of the hypothalamus
s. region

NOTES

suprachiasmic nucleus
supraclavicular
s. fat pad
s. fullness
supraclinoid
supradiaphragmatic extrusion
suprahyoid
Supranol
supranormal gonadal steroid level
supranumerous mammary glands and nipples
supraoptic
s. nucleus
s. nucleus of the hypothalamus (SON)
s. region
supraopticohypophysial
s. cell
s. tract
supraphysiologic
s. dose
suprapineal recess
suprasellar
s. cistern
s. cystic lesion
s. disease
s. epidermoid cyst
s. extension
s. germ cell tumor
s. germinoma
s. region
s. space
s. vein
Supreme II blood glucose meter
suprofen
Suprol
SUR
sulfonylurea receptor
suramin
Surbex
S.-T Filmtabs
S. With C Filmtabs
SureStep glucose monitor
surface
basal s.
erosion surface per bone s. (ES/BS)
hypocellular bone s.
luminal s.
osteoid s.
surfactant
s.-associated protein
s. protein gene expression
surge
absence of nocturnal TSH s.
blunting of nocturnal thyroid-stimulating hormone s.
blunting of nocturnal TSH s.
catecholamine s.
nocturnal thyroid-stimulating hormone s.
nocturnal TSH s.
surgery
cytoreductive s.
endonasal endoscopic pituitary s.
pituitary s.
sinonasal s.
subfrontal s.
transsphenoidal s.
tumor-reduction s.
surgical
s. adenomectomy
s. andropause
s. extirpation
s. menopause
s. thyroidectomy
Surgicel
surrogate
s. beta cell
insulin s.
survey
National Health and Nutrition Examination S. (NHANES)
pharmacoepidemiologic s.
Second National Health and Nutrition Examination S. (NHANES II)
Whickham s.
suspension
Nephrox S.
sucralfate s.
suspensory ligaments of Cooper
Sus-Phrine
sustained-release sodium fluoride (SR-NaF)
Sustaire
Sustanon
S. 100
S. 250
suture
lambdoidal s.
Suzuki duodenopancreatobiliary reconstruction
SV40
S. large T antigen
S. large T-antigen gene
S. polyadenylation signal
S.-transformed human fibroblast
S. virus
SVR
systemic vascular resistance
SW
slow-wave
SW sleep

swallow
barium s.
s. study
sweating
excessive s.
gustatory s.
swelling
soft tissue s.
Swiss cheese disease
Swyer syndrome
Sylvius
aqueduct of S.
Symlin
symmetrical peripheral polyneuropathy
sympathectomy
sympathetic
s. cell
s. chain
s. ganglia
s. nerve
s. nervous system (SNS)
s. plexus
s. postganglionic
s. preganglionic axon
sympathoadrenal neuroendocrine system
sympathogonia
sympatholytic drug
sympathomimetic
s. amine
s. drug
sympathoneural
symporter
iodide s.
sodium-iodide s. (NIS)
symptom
acromegalic s.
humoral s.
local s.
neuroglycopenic s.
postprandial s.
preprandial recurrent s.
Prospective Record of the Impact and Severity of Menstrual S.'s (PRISM)
systemic s.
symptomatic
s. hypocalcemia
s. hyponatremia
symptothermal rhythm method
Synacthen
S. test
Synalgos-DC
synapse
ganglionic s.
synaptic
s. cleft
s. transmission
s. vesicle
synaptophysin
synaptosome
Synarel
syncytial trophoblast
syncytiotrophoblast
s. cell
s. mass
syndactyly
syndrome
ACL s.
acquired immune deficiency s. (AIDS)
acquired immunodeficiency s. (AIDS)
acromegaly, cutis verticis, leukoma s.
ACTH-dependent Cushing s.
ACTH-independent Cushing s.
acute phase response s.
adiposogenital s.
adrenocorticotropic hormone-dependent Cushing s.
adrenogenital s.
adult respiratory distress s.
Albright hereditary osteodystrophy s.
Allgrove s.
Alstrom s.
amenorrhea-galactorrhea s.
androgen insensitivity s. (AIS)
androgen resistance s.
Angelman s.
antenatal Bartter s.
Apert s.
s. of apparent mineralocorticoid excess
Arnold-Healy-Gordon s.
Asherman s.
aspirin-sensitive asthma s.
Bannayan-Ruvalcaba-Riley s.
Bannayan-Zonana s.
Bardet-Biedl s.
bare lymphocyte s.
Bartter s.
basal cell nevus s.
Bassen-Kornzweig s.

NOTES

syndrome *(continued)*
battered baby s.
Beckwith-Wiedemann s.
Berardinelli-Seip s.
Bercu s.
beta cell dysmaturation s.
s. of bioinactive growth hormone
Blackfan-Diamond s.
blepharophimosis, ptosis, epicanthus inversus s.
blind-loop s.
Bloom s.
blue-diaper s.
blue-toe s.
bowel-associated dermatosis-arthritis s.
breast/ovarian cancer s.
bronchial carcinoid variant s.
BRR s.
Buschke-Ollendorff s.
Caffey s.
candidiasis endocrinopathy s.
capillary leak s.
carbohydrate-deficient glycoprotein s.
carcinoid s.
cardiofaciocutaneous s.
cardiovascular dysmetabolic s.
Carney s.
carpal tunnel s.
cavernous sinus s.
Charcot-Marie-Tooth s.
Chediak-Higashi s.
Chiari-Frommel s.
chiasmal s.
chiasmatic s.
childhood Cushing s.
chronic fatigue s.
chylomicronemia s.
Cockayne s.
Coffin-Lowry s.
s. of complete androgen resistance
congenital GH resistance s.
congenital growth hormone resistance s.
congenital rubella s. (CRS)
Conn s.
contiguous gene s.
Cope s.
Cornelia de Lange s.
corticotropin-dependent Cushing s.
cortisol resistance s.
Cowden s.
cri du chat s.
Crouzon s.
Cushing s.
Dandy-Walker s.
de Lange s.
de Morsier s.
Denys-Drash s.
diabetes associated with certain s.
diabetes-deafness s.
diabetic foot s.
diencephalic s.
DiGeorge s.
DIMOAD s.
Down s.
Dubovitz s.
dumping s.
ectopic ACTH s.
ectopic adrenocorticotropic hormone s.
ectopic corticotropin-releasing hormone s.
ectopic CRH s.
ectopic Cushing s.
ectopic hormone s.
Ehlers-Danlos s. types I, II, III, IV, VII
elfin facies s.
Ellis-van Creveld s.
embryonic testicular regression s.
empty sella s.
endocrine tumor s.
eosinophilia myalgia s.
euthyroid sick s.
familial atypical multiple mole-melanoma s.
familial Down s.
FAMMM s.
Fanconi s.
feminizing adrenal s.
fertile eunuch s.
fetal alcohol s. (FAS)
food-dependent Cushing s.
fragile X s.
fragile X-E s.
Frasier s.
FRAXE s.
Freeman-Sheldon s.
Fröhlich s.
galactorrhea-amenorrhea s.
Gardner s.
gastric carcinoid variant s.
s. of generalized thyroid hormone resistance
genetic hormone resistance s.
Gitelman s.
s. of globus hystericus
glucagonoma s.
goiter-deafness s.
Goltz s.
Goodpasture s.
Gordon s.
Gorlin s.
growth hormone resistance s.

Guillain-Barré s.
HAIRAN s.
hairless woman s.
Hartnup s.
HELLP s.
hemolysis, elevated liver enzymes, and low platelets s.
s. of hereditary hypophosphatemic rickets with hypercalciuria (HHRH)
hereditary nonpolyposis colon cancer/ovarian cancer s.
Hermansky-Pudlak s.
hirsutism-anovulation s.
Hoffmann s.
Holmes-Adie s.
Horner s.
hungry bone s.
Hunter s.
Hurler s.
Hurler-Scheie s.
Hutchinson-Gilford s.
hyperchylomicronemic s.
hyperglycemic hyperosmolar s. (HHS)
hyperinsulinemic polycystic ovary s.
hyperprostaglandin E s.
hypertonic s.
s. of hyporeninemic hypoaldosteronism (SHH)
hypotonic s.
iatrogenic Cushing s.
idiopathic postprandial s.
s. of inappropriate antidiuretic hormone secretion
s. of inappropriate secretion of antidiuretic hormone (SIADH)
s. of inappropriate somatotropin secretion
s. of inappropriate thyroid-stimulating hormone
s. of incomplete androgen resistance
infertile male s.
inherited hormone resistance s.
insulin-autoimmune s.
insulinotropininsulin resistance s.
insulin-resistance s.
s. of insulin resistance
insulin-resistant s. X
Jackson-Weiss s.
Jerusalem s.
Johanson-Blizzard s.
Kahn s.
Kallmann s.
Kartagener s.
Kearns-Sayre s.
Kennedy s.
Kenney-Caffey s.
Kleine-Levin s.
Klinefelter s.
Klippel-Trenaunay-Weber s.
Klüver-Bucy s.
Kobberling-Dunnigan s.
Kocher-Debré-Sémélaigne s.
kwashiorkor s.
Laron s.
late dumping s. (LDS)
Laurence-Moon s.
Laurence-Moon-Biedl s.
Lawrence s.
Lemmel s.
lentiginosis s.
Lenz-Majewski s.
leprechaunism s.
Lesch-Nyhan s.
Liddle s.
Li-Fraumeni s.
linear nevus sebaceous s.
lipodystrophy s.
Louis-Bar and Nijmegen breakage s.
low-bone-turnover s.
Lowe s.
low-T_3 s.
low-triiodothyronine s.
luteinized unruptured follicle s. (LUFS)
Lynch s.
male Turner s.
marasmus s.
Marfan s.
Marine-Lenhart s.
maternal deprivation s.
Maurie s.
McCardle s.
McCune-Albright s. (MAS)
s. of melancholia
MELAS s.
MEN s.
Mendenhall s.
metabolic s.
milk-alkali s.
Milkman s.

NOTES

S

syndrome *(continued)*
Miller s.
Miller-Dicker s.
Möbius s.
Morgagni s.
Morquio s.
Morris s.
müllerian duct s.
multiple hamartoma s.
Münchausen s.
Nager s.
nail-patella s.
Najjar s.
Nelson s.
nephrotic s.
neuroleptic malignant s.
nonthyroidal illness s.
Noonan s.
obesity/type 2 diabetes s.
orbital apex s.
osteomalacia s.
ovarian hyperstimulation s. (OHSS)
overlap s.
Pallister-Hall s.
paraneoplastic s.
parasellar s.
parathyroid hormone resistance s.
Parinaud s.
PCO s. (PCOS)
Pearson s.
Pendred s. (PDS)
penis at twelve s.
Perheentupa s.
Perrault s.
persistent müllerian duct s.
Peutz-Jeghers s.
Pfeiffer s.
pickwickian s.
pituitary isolation s.
pituitary resistance to thyroid hormone s.
pituitary stalk interruption s.
plantar fascia s.
plasma cell dyscrasia with polyneuropathy, organomegaly, endocrinopathy, M protein in plasma, and skin changes s.
POEMS s.
polar T_3 s.
polar triiodothyronine s.
polyglandular autoimmune s. type II (PGA-II)
polycystic ovarian s. (PCOS)
s. of polycystic ovary
polycystic ovary s. (PCOS)
polyendocrine deficiency s.
polyendocrine failure type I s.
polyglandular autoimmune s.
polyuric s.
postprandial s.
Prader-Labhart-Willi s.
Prader-Willi s. (PWS)
premenstrual s. (PMS)
primary antiphospholipid s.
primary empty sella s.
s. of primary hyperaldosteronism
PRTH s.
pseudo-Cushing s.
pseudo-Turner s.
Rabson-Mendenhall s.
Reaven s.
Recklinghausen s.
Refetoff s.
Reifenstein s.
Reiter s.
renal Fanconi s.
resistant ovary s.
respiratory distress s. (RDS)
rheumatic s.
Richner-Hanhart s.
Riley-Day s.
Riley-Smith s.
Rokitansky-Küster s.
Roux stasis s.
Rubinstein-Taybi s.
Russell-Silver s.
Saethre-Chotzen s.
Sanfilippo s.
Savage s.
Scheie s.
Schmidt s.
Schwartz-Bartter s.
scleroderma-like s. (SLS)
Seckel s.
secondary empty sella s.
second hormone s.
serotonin s.
Sertoli cell-only s.
Sheehan s.
shock s.
shoulder-hand s.
Shwachman s.
Shy-Drager s.
sick euthyroid s.
Sipple s.
site-specific ovarian cancer s.
Sjögren s.
Sly s.
Smith-Lemli-Opitz s.
Smith-Magenis s.
Soto s.
spillover s.
spontaneous autoimmune anti-insulin antibody s.
steal s.
Stein-Leventhal s.
steroid hormone resistance s.
steroid withdrawal s.

Stewart-Treves s.
Stickler s.
stiff hand s.
stiff man s. (SMS)
sump s.
superior orbital fissure s.
Swyer s.
systemic inflammatory response s. (SIRS)
Takatsuki s.
testicular regression s.
thyroid hormone adaptation s.
thyroid hormone resistance s.
thyroid storm s.
Tolosa-Hunt s.
toxic shock s.
tumor-induced osteomalacia s.
tumor lysis s.
Turner s.
type A s.
type B extreme insulin resistance s.
type II autoimmune polyglandular s.
type 1 polyglandular s.
Ullrich s.
ulnar-mammary s.
undervirilized fertile male s.
vanishing testis s.
vascular steal s.
vasopressin resistance s.
velocardiofacial s.
Verner-Morrison s.
virilizing adrenal s.
von Hippel-Lindau s.
wasting s.
Waterhouse-Friderichsen s.
s. of water intoxication
watery diarrhea s.
s. of watery diarrhea, hypokalemia, and achlorhydria
WDHA s.
Werdnig-Hoffman s.
Werner s.
Wernicke-Korsakoff s.
Williams s.
Williams-Beuren s.
Wilms tumor-aniridia-genital anomalies-mental retardation s. (WAGR)
Wilson s.
Wiskott-Aldrich s.
Wolcott-Rallison s.
Wolf-Hirschhorn s.
Wolfram s.
xeroderma pigmentosa/Cockayne s.
X-linked immunodeficiency s.
Young s.
Zellweger s.
Zieve s.
Zollinger-Ellison s.

syndrome X

synechia
asymptomatic s.

synergism

synergistic necrotizing cellulitis

synexin

Synflex

synkinesis
bimanual s.

synostosis

synteny

synthase
carbamoyl phosphate s.
citrate s.
cystathionine s.
estrogen s.
fatty acid s.
glycogen s.
lactose s.
nitric oxide s. (NOS)
NO s. (NOS)
phosphoribosylpyrophosphate s.
porphobilinogen s.
prostaglandin H s. (PGHS)
PRPP s.

synthesis
aldosterone s.
calcium-binding protein s.
collagen s.
de novo s.
eicosanoid s.
endothelin-induced protein s.
estrogen s.
glycogen s.
glycosaminoglycan s.
growth hormone s.
hepatic glycogen s.
immunoglobulin s.
prolactin s.
protein s.
sterol s.
testosterone s.
thrombospondin s.

NOTES

S

synthesis *(continued)*
thyroglobulin s.
thyroid hormone s.
thyroid peroxidase s.
thyroid-stimulating hormone s.
synthesis-secretion coupling
synthetase
dihydrobiopterin s.
fatty acid s. (FAS)
synthetic
s. bCgA
s. conjugated estrogen
s. corticotropin-releasing hormone
s. glucocorticoid
s. human insulin
Synthroid
syntrophoblast
syphilis
syphilitic gumma
Syp protein
Syprine
Syracol-CF
system
Accu-Chek Advantage glucose meter s.
Accu-Chek Advantage non-wipe blood glucose monitoring s.
Accu-Chek Complete blood glucose monitoring s.
Accu-Chek Complete glucose meter s.
Accu-Chek II Freedom s.
Accu-Chek Instant glucose meter s.
Accu-Chek InstantPlus s.
Accu-Chek Simplicity blood glucose monitoring s.
actin scavenger s.
Acusyst-Xcell monoclonal antibody culturing s.
adenohypophysial s.
adenylate cyclase s.
ADICOL s.
adrenomedullary hormonal s.
AERx diabetes management s.
afferent s.
amphetamine-related transcript s.
amplification refractory mutation s. (ARMS)
Androderm Transdermal S.
Appraise diabetes monitoring s.
Assure blood glucose monitoring s.
AtLast blood glucose monitoring s.
autocrine s.
autonomic nervous s.
blood glucose buffer s.
cardiac endocrine aldosterone s.
cardiac steroidogenic s.
catecholaminergic s.
central nervous s. (CNS)
CFC BioScanner S.
closed-loop insulin delivery s.
continuous glucose monitoring s. (CGMS)
countertransport s.
diffuse endocrine s.
diffuse neuroendocrine s. (DNES)
dopaminergic s.
dynorphin s.
efferent s.
enkephalin s.
enteric nervous s. (ENS)
excurrent duct s.
extrahypothalamic nervous s.
extraneuronal amine transport s.
FastTake blood glucose monitoring s.
GABA/BZD s.
gamma-aminobutyric acid/benzodiazepine s.
Genotropin s.
Glucocheck Pocketlab II blood glucose s.
Glucometer DEX diabetes care s.
Glucometer II home glucose monitoring s.
Greenberg retractor mounting s.
haversian s.
hematopoietic s.
HemoCue blood glucose s.
hormone-sensitive adenylate cyclase s.
hypophysial-hypothalamic portal s.
hypophysial portal s.
hypophysiotropic s.
hypothalamohypophysial portal s. (HHPS)
immune s.
In Charge Diabetes Control S.
kallikrein-kinin s.
lacrimal s.
LifeGuide S.
limbic s.
magnocellular neurosecretory s.
matrix transdermal s.
Medi-Ject needle-free insulin injection s.
Medi-Jector Choice needle-free insulin injection s.
nonoral estradiol delivery s.
One Touch II hospital blood glucose monitoring s.
osteocytic membrane s.
paracrine s.
parasympathetic nervous s.
peripheral nervous s. (PNS)
portable endocrine s.

portal s.
Precision Xtra Advanced Diabetes Management S.
primary central nervous s. (PCNS)
renin-angiotensin s.
renin-angiotensin-aldosterone s. (RAAS)
reservoir transdermal s.
reticuloendothelial s.
reverse hemolytic plaque assay s.
Santorini duct s.
Schwann cell s.
Select GT blood glucose s.
serotonergic s.
sudomotor s.
sympathetic nervous s. (SNS)
sympathoadrenal neuroendocrine s.
TD Glucose Monitoring s.
Testoderm testosterone transdermal s.
Testoderm Transdermal S.
testosterone transdermal s.
thyrolymphatic s.
tissular hormonal s.
TLX alloantigen s.
transdermal testosterone delivery s.
transscrotal testosterone delivery s.
trophoblast-lymphocyte cross-reactive alloantigen s.
tuberoinfundibular s.
uterine-endocrine s.
vitamin D endocrine s.
WHO classification s.
World Health Organization classification s.

systemic
s. arterial hypertension
s. estrogen
s. inflammatory response syndrome (SIRS)
s. lupus erythematosus (SLE)
s. symptom
s. vascular resistance (SVR)
s. vasculitis
s. virilization

Systen

Sytobex

S

NOTES

T
testosterone
T cell
T helper cell
T helper 1 cell
T helper 2 cell
T lymphocyte
^{201}Tl
thallium-201
T_3
3,5,3′-triiodo-I-thyronine
triiodothyronine
free T_3
T_3 receptor (TR)
T_3 resin uptake test
T_3 responsive element (T_3RE)
reverse T_3 (rT_3)
T_3 suppression test
total T_3 (TT_3)
T_4
thyroxine
fetal T_4
free T_4
peripheral T_4
serum free T_4
serum total T_4
total T_4 (TT_4)
$T\alpha_1$
thymosin $alpha_1$
T_m
tubular transport maximum
T1 relaxation time
T1-weighted image
T2 relaxation time
T2-weighted spin-echo image
TAA
premature top codon
Tab
Meda T.
Tabby gene
tabes dorsalis
tablet
Amaryl glimepiride t.
Brontex T.
Dostinex t.
Ergoset t.
Gaviscon T.
Gaviscon-2 T.
K-Phos Neutral t.
sodium chloride t.
Stresstabs 600 Advanced Formula T.'s
Tums E-X Extra Strength T.
Tac-3 Injection
Tac-40 Injection
TACE
transcatheter arterial chemoembolization
Tace
tachyarrhythmia
atrial t.
tachycardia
ventricular t.
tachygastria
tachykinin
tachyphylaxis
tachysterol
tacrolimus
TAD
thiazolidinedione
trans-activation domain
Taenia solium
TAF
transactivation factor
tag
expressed sequence t. (EST)
Tagamet
Tagamet-HB
tailing
Takatsuki syndrome
TAL
thick ascending limb
Talacen
tall cell
Talwin
T. NX
Tamm-Horsfall protein
tamoxifen
tamsulosin
Tangier disease
tannate
pitressin t.
Tanner
T. stage (I–V)
T. staging
TAO
thyroid-associated ophthalmopathy
TAP
trypsinogen-activating peptide
Tapanol
Tapazole
tape
Deknatel t.
***Taq*I restriction enzyme**
tarda
porphyria cutanea t.
target
accommodative t.
t. cell
t. gland function

T

target *(continued)*
t. organ resistance
t. tissue
Targretin
tarsorrhaphy
tartrate
belladonna, phenobarbital, and ergotamine t.
pentolinium t.
t.-resistant acid phosphatase (TRAP)
taste receptor
TATA box
taurine
tautomycin
tax protein
Tay-Sachs disease
TB
total bound
Tb_4
thymosin b_4
thymosin $beta_4$
TBBMD
total body bone mineral density
TBG
thyroid-binding globulin
thyroid hormone-binding globulin
thyroxine-binding globulin
TBG deficiency
TBG excess
TBIAb
thyroid-stimulating hormone-binding inhibitor antibody
TBII
thyroid-stimulating hormone-binding inhibitor immunoglobulin
thyrotropin-binding inhibitory immunoglobulin
TSH-binding inhibitory immunoglobulin
TBII assay
T-box gene family
TBPA
thyroid-binding prealbumin
thyronine-binding prealbumin
TBS
total body scan
TC
total cholesterol
^{99m}Tc
technetium-99m
t/c
Snp5 t/c
Tc-99m MIBI
TCA
tricarboxylic acid
tricyclic antidepressant
TCDD
2,3,7,8-tetrachlorodibenzo-*p*-dioxin
^{99m}Tc-DMSA
technetium-99m dimercaptosuccinic acid
T-cell
T.-c. antigen
T.-c. epitope
T.-c. growth factor (TCGF)
T.-c. lymphoma
T.-c. receptor (TCR)
T.-c. repertoire
T.-c. response
TCGF
T-cell growth factor
TCL
thyroid T-cell line
Tc-99m sestamibi scintigraphy
Tc-99m-TcO4
pertechnetate
TCP
tropical calcific pancreatitis
^{99m}Tc-pentavalent dimercaptosuccinate
TCR
T-cell receptor
^{99m}Tc sestamibi
^{99m}Tc s. scintigraphy
^{99m}Tc-tetrafosmin
TD
thyroid dysgenesis
TD Glucose meter
TD Glucose Monitoring system
TDA
testis-determining antigen
$T_4$5′-deiodinase type 2 (D2)
TDF
testis-determining factor
TDI
therapeutic donor insemination
TdT
terminal deoxynucleotide transferase
Tebamide
TeBG
testosterone-binding globulin
Techlite lancet
technetium
t. bone scan
99m-t. sestamibi
t. pertechnetate
t. pertechnetate scan
t. pyrophosphate
t. sestamibi scintigraphy
triple-phase scan with t.
technetium-99m (^{99m}Tc)
t. dimercaptosuccinic acid (^{99m}Tc-DMSA)
t. sestamibi
t. tetraforsmin
technetium/thallium subtraction nuclear scanning

technique
aldehyde thionin staining t.
assisted reproduction t.
coupled amplification and sequencing t.
double-labeling t.
dye-diluting t.
endonasal endoscopic t.
endoscopic pituitary surgery t.
euglycemic glucose clamp t.
fast spin-echo t.
Grimelius stain t.
histomorphometric t.
hyperinsulinemic-euglycemic clamp t.
imaging t.
immunogold-labeling t.
immunohistochemical staining t.
immunohistochemistry t.
immunoperoxidase t.
interstitial hyperthermic t.
Ishikawa cytodiagnostic t.
Karydakis t.
neuroanatomic t.
pause and squeeze t.
perimetric t.
recombinant DNA t.
regular spin-echo t.
Sevier-Munger stain t.
sublabial transseptal t.
tetracycline double-labeling t.
thermodilution t.
Uchida t.
technology
assisted reproductive t. (ART)
Kumetrix microneedle t.
Tedral
TEF
thyrotroph embryonic factor
T-effector lymphocyte
Tega-Vert Oral
tegmentum
telachoroidea
telangiectasia
ataxia t.
hereditary hemorrhagic t.
t. macularis eruptiva perstans
venous t.
telencephalon
basal t.
Telepaque
telogen
telomerase enzyme
telopeptide
C-terminal type I collagen t.
type I collagen C-terminal t.
temperature
ambient t.
basal body t. (BBT)
thermoneutrality t.
temporal
t. balding
t. bone osteomyelitis
t. craniotomy
t. fiber
t. horn
temporary end-organ resistance
Tempra
tendinous xanthoma
tendon
t. xanthoma
tennis racket-shaped pentalaminar tubular structure
tenosynovitis
tense
t. ascites
t. tumor capsule
tension
decreased oxygen t.
tentorial incisura
Tenuate
T. Dospan
teratocarcinoma
teratogenic
teratoma
atypical t.
benign cystic t.
mature t.
ovarian t.
terazosin
terbutaline
t. sulfate
terconazole
teriparatide
terminal
autonomic postganglionic nerve t.
t. deoxynucleotide transferase (TdT)
t. hair
t. nerve ending
t. nerve fiber
neurohypophysial nerve t.
t. oxidase
presynaptic nerve t.

NOTES

terminalis
lamina t.
organum vasculosum of the lamina t. (OVLT)
organum vasculosum laminae t. (OVLT)
stria t.
terminus
amino t.
ternary complex
terpin
t. hydrate
t. hydrate and codeine
Terry nail
tertiary
t. adrenal insufficiency
t. chorionic villus
t. follicle
t. hyperaldosteronism
t. hyperparathyroidism
t. hypogonadism
t. hypothyroidism
t. messenger
Tesamone Injection
TESE
testicular sperm extraction
Teslac
Tessalon Perles
test
Access Ostase blood t.
adrenocorticotrophin stimulation t.
alkaline phosphatase antialkaline phosphatase antibody t.
Allen t.
alternate cover t.
antibody-dependent cytotoxicity t.
arginine infusion t.
arginine tolerance t. (ATT)
ascitic fluid t.
Benedict t.
[13C]-acetate t.
calcium stimulation t.
captopril t.
chorionic gonadotropin stimulation t.
Chvostek t.
clomiphene citrate challenge t. (CCCT)
clonidine suppression t.
[13C]-octanoic acid t.
corticotroph stimulation t.
corticotropin-releasing hormone t.
Cortrosyn stimulation t.
cosyntropin stimulation t.
C-peptide suppression t.
CRH stimulation t.
crossed t.
Cytomel suppression t.
deferoxamine t.
dexamethasone suppression t.
DFO t.
2,4-dinitrophenylhydrazine t.
duodenal intubation t.
epinephrine provocation t.
ether-stimulation t.
fecal chymotrypsin t.
ferric chloride t.
fructosamine t.
glucagon stimulation t.
glucose tolerance t. (GTT)
Glycosal diabetes t.
gonadotropin-releasing hormone t.
hCG pregnancy t.
high-dose dexamethasone suppression t.
human zona pellucide binding t.
hydrogen breath t.
insulin tolerance t. (ITT)
intravenous glucose tolerance t. (IVGTT)
iodine-perchlorate discharge t.
KetoSite t.
Kveim t.
LDL direct t.
L-dopa t.
Liddle t.
low-dose dexamethasone t.
low-dose short synacthen t. (LDSST)
methasone-suppressed corticotropin-releasing hormone t.
metrapone stimulation t.
metyrapone t.
Michigan Neuropathy Screening T.
Micral urine dipstick t.
morning corticotropin-releasing hormone t.
morning CRH t.
nitroblue tetrazolium t.
oral glucose tolerance t. (OGTT)
osmolality dehydration t.
overnight high-dose dexamethasone suppression t. (ONDST)
overnight metyrapone t.
overnight 1-mg dexamethasone suppression t.
pancreatic functioning diagnostant t.
pancreolauryl t.
pancreozymin secretin t.
pentagastrin provocation t.
perchlorate discharge t.
PFD t.
pituitary dynamic t.
pituitary target organ t.
postcoital t.
posture stimulation t.

predictive value t.
progesterone challenge t.
provocation t.
PS t.
Quantitative Autonomic Function T.
Quantitative Sensory T.
radioiodine uptake t.
radiolabeled breath t.
S t.
saline suppression t.
Schilling t.
Schirmer t.
secretin t.
secretin stimulation t.
semen fructose t.
sensitivity t.
serum acid phosphatase t.
Sibley-Lehninger t.
Sims-Huhner t.
specificity t.
sperm function t.
SpermMar t.
stimulation t.
Synacthen t.
Thorn t.
Thyrogen serum thyroglobulin t.
thyroidal radioactive iodine uptake t. (RAIU)
thyroid function t.
thyroperoxidase antibody t.
thyrotropin-releasing hormone t.
thyroxine suppression t.
tolbutamide t.
tolbutamide stimulation t.
T_3 resin uptake t.
TRH stimulation t.
triiodothyronine resin uptake t.
triiodothyronine suppression t.
Trousseau t.
T_3RU t.
TSH stimulation t.
T_3 suppression t.
two-day high-dose dexamethasone suppression t.
vagostigmin t.
van den Bergh t.
Wassermann t.
water deprivation t.
water restriction t.

testicular
t. atrophy
t. choriocarcinoma
t. feminization
t. fluid
t. regression syndrome
t. sperm extraction (TESE)
t. volume

testing
acute insulin response t.
blood glucose t.
Cortrosyn stimulation t.
metyrapone t.
Monojector fingerstick device for blood glucose t.
nocturnal penile tumescence t.
NPT t.
provocative t.
quantitative autonomic functioning t. (QAFT)
quantitative sensory t. (QST)
thyroid antibody t.
vibration perception t.
water deprivation t.

testis
canalicular t.
feminizing t.
intraabdominal t.
Leydig cells of the t.
mediastinum t.
rete t.
varicocele t.

testis-determining
t.-d. antigen (TDA)
t.-d. factor (TDF)

testitoxicosis
familial t.
sporadic t.

Testoderm
T. testosterone transdermal system
T. Transdermal System
T. TTS

testolactone
aromatase inhibitor t.

Testopel Pellet

testosterone (T)
buccal t.
t. buciclate
t. cyclodextrin
t. cypionate
t. enanthate
endogenous t.
t. ester
estradiol and t.
t. estradiol-binding globulin

T

NOTES

testosterone *(continued)*
ethinyl t.
free t.
t. implant
intramuscular t.
plasma t.
t. propionate
serum free t.
serum total t.
t. skin patch
t. synthesis
total t.
t. transdermal system
t. undecenoate
testosterone-binding globulin (TeBG)
testosterone-deficient patient
Testoviron
T. Depot 100
T. Depot 50
testoxicosis
Testred
tetany
cerebral t.
hypocalcemic t.
latent t.
uterine t.
tethered
t. cord
t. cord release
t. ligand thrombin receptor
Tetracap Oral
2,3,7,8-tetrachlorodibenzo-*p*-dioxin (TCDD)
tetracycline
t. double-labeling technique
t. labeling
tetradecapeptide
tetraforsmin
technetium-99m t.
tetraglycine hydroperiodide
tetrahydroaldosterone
tetrahydrobiopterin
tetrahydrocortisol (THE)
tetrahydrocortisone (THF)
tetraiodoacetic acid
tetraiodo-L-thyronine
tetraiodothyroacetic acid
tetralogy of Fallot
tetramer
tetrapeptide
texture
inhomogeneous t.
TF5
thymosin fraction 5
TG, Tg
thyroglobulin
turtle TG
TGBI
thyroid growth-blocking immunoglobulin
T-Gen
T-Gesic
TGF
transforming growth factor
tubuloglomerular feedback
TGF system
TGF-A, TGFα
transforming growth factor alpha
TGF-B, TGFβ
transforming growth factor beta
TGI
thyroid growth immunoglobulin
Th1 cell
Th2 cell
thalami
striae medullaris t.
thalamic nucleus
thalamus
nucleus ventralis anterior of t.
α-thalassemia
thalassemia major
thalidomide
Thalitone
thallium-201 (^{201}Tl)
thallium chloride (TI-201)
thallium-pertechnetate subtraction scintigraphy
thallium-technetium dual isotope scintigraphy
THAM
tromethamine
THAM-E
tromethamine E
thanatophoric
t. dysplasia type I
t. dysplasia type II
TH beta-receptor deficiency
THBR
thyroid hormone-binding ratio
THDA
tuberohypophyseal dopaminergic neuron
THE
tetrahydrocortisol
theca
t. cell
t. cell androgen production
t. externa
t. externa cell
t. folliculi
t. interna
t. interna cell
t. interstitial cell
t. interstitial cell dysregulation
t. lutein cell

thecal
t. dysregulation
t. hyperplasia
thecoma
thelarche
premature t.
Theo-24
Theobid
theobromine
Theochron
Theoclear-80
Theoclear L.A.
Theo-Dur
Theolair
theophylline
t. toxicity
theophylline-induced hypercalcemia
theory
second attack t.
Theo-Sav
Theostat-80
Theovent
Theo-X
Therabid
Thera-Combex H-P Kapseals
Theragran
T. Hematinic
Theragran-M
therapeutic
t. donor insemination (TDI)
t. irrigation
therapy
aminoglutethimide t.
anabolic t.
androgen-lowering t.
androgen replacement t. (ART)
antigen-specific preventive t.
antimicrobial t.
antiresorptive t.
antiretroviral t.
basal insulin t.
BIDS t.
blood purification t.
Bragg peak proton irradiation t.
bromocriptine t.
B vitamin t.
calcitriol t.
coherence t.
combined t.
continuous-combined hormone replacement t. (ccHRT)
continuous hormone replacement t.
corticosteroid t.
cyclical hormone replacement t.
deferoxamine t.
desferrioxamine t.
dexamethasone suppression t.
dialytic t.
diuretic t.
D-Modem and insulin pump t.
dopamine agonist t.
electroconvulsive t.
endocrine t.
Enterra t.
estrogen t.
estrogen/androgen t.
estrogen replacement t. (ERT)
exogenous glucocorticoid t.
fludrocortisone replacement t.
foscarnet t.
fractionated radiation t.
gene t.
glucocorticoid replacement t.
gonadotropin-releasing hormone-agonist t.
growth factor t.
growth hormone t.
hemodialysis t.
hormonal add-back t.
hormone replacement t. (HRT)
hydrocortisone replacement t.
^{131}I t.
insulin pump t.
intensive t.
interferon t.
intracystic radiation t.
iodine-131 t.
levothyroxine suppression t.
lipid-lowering t.
metyrapone t.
mineralocorticoid replacement t.
multiport collimated cobalt-60 t.
neurotrophic t.
octreotide t.
pharmacologic t.
preventative hormone t.
primary t.
proton beam t.
pulsatile gonadotropin-releasing hormone t.
pulsed progestin hormone replacement t.
radiation t. (XRT)
radioablation t.

NOTES

therapy *(continued)*
radioiodine ablation t.
recombinant enzyme replacement t.
replacement t.
salvage t.
sequential hormone replacement t.
steroid replacement t.
suppressive t.
thionamide drug t.
thyroid hormone replacement t.
thyrotropin suppressive t.
thyroxine replacement t.
tolerogenic t.
vidarabine t.
warfarin t.
Therasense subcutaneous glucose sensor
thermal
t. cycler
t. injury
t. perception
thermic effect of food
thermocoagulation
thermodilution technique
thermogenesis
facultative t.
nonshivering t.
obligatory t.
shivering t.
thermogenic
thermography
imaging t.
thermolabile receptor
thermolability
thermoneutrality temperature
thermoregulation
thermosensitive neuron
thermostatic hypothesis
THF
tetrahydrocortisone
thiamine
thiazide
t. diuretic
t. diuretic agent
thiazoladinedione
thiazolidinedione (TAD, TZD)
thick ascending limb (TAL)
thickened
t. acral part
t. adrenal limb
thickening
calvarial t.
t. of cortex
thickness
endometrial t.
osteoid seam t.
skin fold t.
thick-walled hypha
thiethylperazine
Thigh Thing pump holder
thinning
t. fat pad
skin t.
trabecular t.
thin-walled simple cyst
thiocyanate
granidinium t.
thioglucoside
thioguanine
thiolase
acetoacetyl-CoA t.
thionamide
t. antithyroid drug
t. drug therapy
thionin
aldehyde t.
thiopental sodium
thiophorase
thioredoxin
thiouracil
thiourea
t. compound
t. drug
ethylene t.
thioureylene group
thioxanthine
third
t. complementarity determining region (CDR3)
t. ventricle
third-generation assay
thirst
impaired t.
intense t.
t. mechanism
stimuli of t.
t. threshold
thoracic stomach
Thorazine
Thorlo padded socks
Thorn test
Thr
threonine
Thr-410
thread
mucus t.
three-compartment model
threonine (Thr)
threshold
osmotic t.
renal t.
thirst t.
vibration t.
thrifty genotype hypothesis
thrive
failure to t. (FTT)

thrombin
t. generation
t. receptor-activating peptide 6 (TRAP-6)
thrombocytopenia
thromboembolic event
thromboembolism
venous t. (VTE)
thrombolytic therapy
thrombomodulin
serum t.
thrombophilia
thrombophlebitis
cavernous sinus t.
thrombopoietin (TPO)
thrombosis
adrenal vein t.
cerebral vein t.
exuberant t.
vascular t.
thrombospondin
t. synthesis
thromboxane (TX)
t. A2 (TXA2, TxA2)
t. analog
t. B2 (TXB2, TxB2)
thrombus formation
thyamidine autoradiography
thymectomy
thymic
t. branch
t. carcinoid
t. hyperplasia
t. involution
t. lymphocyte
thymicolymphaticus
thymidine
t. autoradiography
thymocyte
thymoma
ACTH-producing t.
thymosin
t. $alpha_1$ ($T\alpha_1$)
t. b_4 (Tb_4)
t. peptide
thymosin fraction 5 (TF5)
thymoxamine
thymulin
thymus
t. gland
t. hypertrophy
Thypinone
Thyrar
Thyrel-TRH
thyroacetic acid
thyroarytenoid
Thyro-Block
thyrocalcitonin
thyrocardiac disease
thyrocervical trunk
thyrocyte
Thyrogen
T. radioiodine scan
T. serum thyroglobulin test
thyrogenic carcinoma
thyroglobin synthesis defect
thyroglobulin (TG, Tg)
t. antibody
t. antigen
t. assay
t. autoantibody
t. expression
human t. (hTg)
t. hydrolysis
t. iodination
t. level
t. secretion
serum t.
t. staining
t. synthesis
thyroglobulin-producing tissue
thyroglossal
t. duct
t. duct carcinoma
t. duct cyst
t. duct remnant
thyroglucase
gold t.
thyroid
t. ablation with ^{131}I
t. acropachy
t. adenylate cyclase
t. antibody testing
t. antigen-antibody nephritis
Armour T.
t. axis
t. biopsy
black t.
t. cartilage
t. C cell
t. colloid
t. computed tomography
t. cork phenomenon
t. crisis

NOTES

thyroid *(continued)*
t. deficiency cell
t. dermopathy
desiccated t.
t. diverticulum
t. dysgenesis (TD)
t. dyshormonogenesis
ectopic t.
t. epithelial cell
t. extract
t. eye disease
t. follicle
t. follicular cell
t. function
t. function test
t. gland
t. gland adenoma
t. gland autonomy
t. gland carcinoma
t. growth-blocking immunoglobulin (TGBI)
t. growth immunoglobulin (TGI)
gummata of the t.
t. hemosiderosis
t. hormone
t. hormone action
t. hormone adaptation syndrome
t. hormone-binding globulin (TBG)
t. hormone-binding ratio (THBR)
t. hormone-binding site
t. hormone metabolism
t. hormone nuclear receptor isoform
t. hormone production
t. hormone receptor (TR)
t. hormone receptor auxiliary antibody protein
t. hormone receptor defect
t. hormone receptor homodimer
t. hormone receptor monomer
t. hormone receptor-retinoid X receptor (TR-RXR)
t. hormone receptor-retinoid X receptor heterodimer
t. hormone replacement
t. hormone replacement therapy
t. hormone resistance
t. hormone resistance syndrome
t. hormone-response element (TRE)
t. hormone status
t. hormone synthesis
t. hormone target gene
t. hormone transport protein
t. hormonogenesis
t. hormonogenesis defect IIB
t. hyperplasia
t. ima artery
t. inflammatory disease
t. iodide transporter
t. iodide trap
t. isthmus
lateral aberrant t.
lingual t.
t. magnetic resonance imaging
medullary carcinoma of the t. (MCT)
t. microsomal antibody
t. necrosis
t. nodule
t. ophthalmopathy
t. orbitopathy
t. overactivity
t. papillary carcinoma
t. parafollicular cell
t. parenchyma
t. peroxidase (TPO)
t. peroxidase activity
t. peroxidase antibody
t. peroxidase antigen
t. peroxidase autoantibody
t. peroxidase synthesis
t. radioiodine uptake
t. remnant
t. reserve
t. scan
t. scintigraphy
t. scintiscan
t. stare
t. stimulation-blocking antibody (TSBAb)
t. storm
t. storm hyperthermia
t. storm syndrome
t. stroma
T. Strong
t. stunning
substernal t.
t. symptom checklist
t. T-cell line (TCL)
t. technetium pertechnetate uptake
t. transcription factor (TTF)
t. transcription factor 1 (TTF-1)
t. transcription factor 2 (TTF-2)
t. transport
t. trapping activity
t. ultrasound
t. uptake probe
t. venous effluent

thyroidal
t. ablation
t. autoantibody secretion
t. C cell
t. hypothyroidism

t. radioactive iodine uptake test (RAIU)
thyroid-associated ophthalmopathy (TAO)
thyroid-binding
t.-b. globulin (TBG)
t.-b. prealbumin (TBPA)
thyroidectomy
t. cell
near-total t.
post t.
subtotal t.
surgical t.
thyroiditis
acute lymphocytic t.
acute suppurative t.
agoiterous autoimmune t.
t. akuta simplex
Aspergillus t.
atrophic chronic autoimmune t.
atrophic Hashimoto t.
autoimmune t.
bacterial t.
chronic autoimmune t.
chronic fibrous t.
chronic lymphocytic t.
Coccidioides immitis t.
coccidioidomycosis-induced t.
cytokine-induced t.
de Quervain nonsuppurative t.
experimental autoimmune t. (EAT)
giant cell t.
goitrous chronic autoimmune t.
goitrous Hashimoto t.
granulomatous t.
Hashimoto t.
infectious t.
interferon-alpha-induced t.
invasive fibrous t.
lymphocytic t.
painful t.
painful subacute t.
painless postpartum t.
palpation t.
perineoplastic t.
Pneumocystis carinii t.
postpartum lymphocytic t.
postpartum painless t.
postpartum silent t.
pseudogranulomatous t.
pseudotuberculous t.
pyogenic t.
radiation t.
radiation-induced t.
Reidel t.
silent autoimmune t.
spontaneous autoimmune t. (SAT)
sporadic silent t.
subacute granulomatous t.
subacute painful t.
suppurative t.
thyroidologist
thyroidology
thyroid-releasing hormone-degrading ectoenzyme
thyroid-specific tracer
thyroid-stimulating
t.-s. antibody (TSAb)
t.-s. hormone (TSH)
t.-s. hormone abnormality
t.-s. hormone-binding inhibitor antibody (TBIAb)
t.-s. hormone-binding inhibitor immunoglobulin (TBII)
t.-s. hormone-binding inhibitor immunoglobulin assay
t.-s. hormone deficiency
t.-s. hormone receptor (TSH-R, TSHR)
t.-s. hormone receptor antibody (TSH-RAb)
t.-s. hormone receptor autoantibody (TSH-RAb)
t.-s. hormone receptor expression
t.-s. hormone receptor mutation
t.-s. hormone-releasing hormone
t.-s. hormone-secreting pituitary tumor
t.-s. hormone-secreting tumor
t.-s. hormone synthesis
t.-s. immunoglobulin (TSI)
thyroid-stimulating-blocking antibody (TSBAb)
α-thyroid stimulating hormone subunit
Thyrolar
thyrolymphatic system
thyromegaly
thyrometabolic status
thyromimetic
t. action
t. compound
thyronine-binding prealbumin (TBPA)
thyroparathyroidectomy (TPTX)
thyroperoxidase (TPO)

NOTES

thyroperoxidase *(continued)*
t. antibody (TPO Ab)
t. antibody test
thyroperoxidase-iodide complex
thyropexin
thyrotoxic
t. crisis
t. Graves disease
t. myopathy
t. osteodystrophy
t. periodic paralysis
t. phase
t. storm
thyrotoxicosis
accelerated t.
amiodarone t.
amiodarone-associated t.
amiodarone-induced destructive t.
apathetic t.
autoimmune t.
destruction-induced t.
destructive t.
exogenous t.
t. factitia
gestational transient t. (GTT)
hamburger t.
hereditary t.
t. of hyperemesis gravidarum
iatrogenic t.
iodine-induced t.
lithium-associated t.
t. medicamentosa
mild overt t.
pituitary-dependent t.
subclinical t.
T_3-predominant t.
transient t.
TSH-dependent t.
TSH-induced t.
thyrotrope
t. adenoma
thyrotroph
t. carcinoma
t. cell
t. cell adenoma
t. cell hyperplasia
t. embryonic factor (TEF)
thyrotroph-derived adenoma
thyrotropic cell
thyrotropin
t. alfa
t. alpha
t.-binding inhibitory immunoglobulin (TBII)
chorionic t.
human chorionic t.
nonpituitary t.
pituitary t.
t. receptor (TSH-R)
t. receptor antibody
t. receptor autoantibody (TRAb)
t. receptor-stimulating antibody (TSH-RAb)
t. release factor (TRF)
t. suppressive therapy
thyrotropinoma
thyrotropin-receptor activating mutation
thyrotropin-releasing
t.-r. hormone (TRH)
t.-r. hormone receptor (TRH-R)
t.-r. hormone stimulation
t.-r. hormone study
t.-r. hormone test
thyrotropin-releasing hormone-induced refractoriness
thyrotropin-secreting
t.-s. pituitary adenoma
t.-s. pituitary tumor
thyrotropin-stimulating
t.-s. hormone (TSH)
t.-s. hormone-expressing cell
thyroxine, thyroxin (T_4)
basal t.
blood free t.
free t. (FT_4)
peripheral t.
t. radioisotope assay (T_4RIA)
t. replacement
t. replacement therapy
t. suppression test
thyroxine-binding
t.-b. globulin (TBG)
t.-b. globulin deficiency
t.-b. globulin excess
t.-b. prealbumin
Thytropar
TI-201
thallium chloride
tibiae
tibolone
ticlopidine
Ticon
TIDA
tuberoinfundibular dopaminergic neuron
tie sternum
TIF2
transcriptional intermediary factor 2
TIF2 coactivator
Tigan
tige pituitaire
tight junction
tiglic acid
tilt
gantry t.
tiludronate
t. disodium

TIM
triose isomerase
TIM gene
TIM protein
time
ankle reflex t.
longitudinal relaxation t.
mineralization lag t.
t. sense
spin-lattice relaxation t.
spin-spin relaxation t.
transverse relaxation t.
T1 relaxation t.
T2 relaxation t.
Timecelles
timing
meal t.
timolol
TIMP
tissue inhibitor of metalloproteinase
TIMP-1
tissue inhibitor of metalloproteinases-1
tinctorial feature
tincture
iodine t.
opium t.
tinea versicolor
tiopronin
TIPS
transjugular intrahepatic portosystemic stent shunt
AEIOU TIPS
alcohol, epilepsy, insulin, overdose, uremia, trauma, infection, psychiatric, stroke
tiratricol
tissue
aberrant mediastinal thyroid t.
adipose t.
adrenal rest t.
t. aluminum
t. aluminum toxicity
brown adipose t. (BAT)
chromaffin t.
t. concentration
connective t.
ectopic thyroid t.
endomysial connective t.
erectile t.
excitable t.
fibroglandular t.
goitrous t.
gut-associated lymphoid t. (GALT)
hyperfunctioning t.
t. inhibitor of metalloproteinase (TIMP)
t. inhibitor of metalloproteinases-1 (TIMP-1)
insulin target t.
juxtathyroidal t.
t. kallikrein
lateral aberrant thyroid t.
lean t.
macroalteration in muscle t.
marginal zone/mucosa-associated lymphoid t. (MALT)
microalteration in muscle t.
mucosa-associated lymphoid t. (MALT)
t. necrosis factor (TNF)
t. nonspecific alkaline phosphatase gene
orbital t.
parasellar t.
pathological endocrine t.
pericardial bioprosthetic t.
t. plasminogen activator (TPA)
t. regeneration
remnant hyperplastic t.
t. repair
retroocular t.
retroorbital adipose t.
retroorbital connective t.
t. senescence
t. specificity
target t.
thyroglobulin-producing t.
trophoblastic t.
white adipose t. (WAT)
tissue-type plasminogen activator
tissular hormonal system
Titanic phenomenon
titanium mesh
titer
antibody t.
antithyroid antibody t.
microsomal antibody t.
^{201}Tl-thallous chloride
TLX
trophoblast-lymphocyte cross-reactive
TLX alloantigen system
T-lymphocyte
helper/inducer T.-l.

T

NOTES

T-lymphocyte *(continued)*
T.-l. insulin binding and degradation
suppressor/cytotoxic T.-l.
TMG
toxic multinodular goiter
TMP-SMX
trimethoprim sulfamethoxazole
TNF
tissue necrosis factor
tumor necrosis factor
TNF-alpha
tumor necrosis factor-alpha
TNF-beta
tumor necrosis factor-beta
TNFR
tumor necrosis factor receptor
TNF-related apoptosis inducing ligand (TRAIL)
TNF-weak homologue (TWEAK)
TNG
toxic nodular goiter
TNM
tumor/node/metastases
TNM classification
TOBEC
total body electrical conductivity
tocolysis
tocolytic agent
tocopherol
tocophersolan
toe
t. box
t. pressure
tolazamide
tolbutamide
t. stimulation test
t. test
Tolectin
T. DS
tolerance
glucose t.
impaired glucose t. (IGT)
insulinopenic impaired glucose t.
tolerogenic
t. protocol
t. therapy
Tolinase
tolmetin
Tolosa-Hunt syndrome
tolrestat
tomography
axial quantified computed t.
computed t. (CT)
dual-phase spiral computed t.
dynamic computed t.
^{18}F-fluorodeoxyglucose positron emission t. (FDG-PET)
helical computed t.
parathyroid computed t.
positron emission t. (PET)
quantified computed t. (QCT)
single-photon emission t. (SPET)
single-photon emission computed t. (SPECT)
spiral computed t.
thyroid computed t.
tone
dopaminergic t.
hypothalamic opioidergic t.
peroxide t.
Tongyi Tang Diabetes capsule
tonic
t. muscle contraction
t. spasm
tonicity
tonofilament
Topical
Aquacare T.
Carmol T.
Lanaphilic T.
Nutraplus T.
Rogaine T.
Ultra Mide T.
Ureacin-20 T.
topotecan
Toradol
toremifene
Tornalate
Toronto Renal Osteodystrophy Study
Torpedo californica
torsades de pointes
torsemide
tortuous blood vessel
Tostrex
Totacillin
total
t. alopecia
t. androgen binding
t. blood volume
t. body bone mineral density (D_β, TBBMD)
t. body electrical conductivity (TOBEC)
t. body iodide pool
t. body nitrogen
t. body potassium
t. body scan (TBS)
t. body water
t. bound (TB)
t. Ca^{2+}
t. cholesterol (TC)
t. deoxypyridinoline cross-link
t. hormone
t. intestinal calcium
t. Mg^{2+}

t. pancreatectomy
t. parathyroidectomy
t. parenteral nutrition (TPN)
t. peripheral resistance
t. renin
t. serum calcium concentration
t. T_3 (TT_3)
t. T_4 (TT_4)
t. testosterone
t. thyroidectomy
totalis
situs inversus viscerum t.
TouchTrak
T. glucose sensor
Touro Ex
toxemia of pregnancy
toxic
t. adenoma
t. calcinosis
t. delirium
t. diffuse goiter
t. epidermal necrolysis
t. multinodal goiter
t. multinodular goiter (TMG)
t. nodular goiter (TNG)
t. pemphigus foliaceus
t. porphyria
t. shock syndrome
t. solitary nodule
t. thyroid nodule (TTN)
toxicity
aluminum t.
cell-mediated t.
glucose t.
postprandial glucose-mediated t.
theophylline t.
tissue aluminum t.
T4 toxicosis
toxicosis
T3 t.
triiodothyronine t. (T_3-toxicosis)
toxin
botulinum t.
botulinum A t.
cholera t.
pertussis t.
toxin-induced diarrhea
toxin-sensitive
pertussis t.-s.
Toxoplasma gondii
toxoplasmosis
TPA
tissue plasminogen activator
T-Phyl
TPN
total parenteral nutrition
TPO
thrombopoietin
thyroid peroxidase
thyroperoxidase
TPO Ab
T_3-predominant thyrotoxicosis
TPTX
thyroparathyroidectomy
TR
thyroid hormone receptor
T_3 receptor
TR homodimer
TR monomer
$T_3R\alpha$
$T_3R\beta$
$T_3R\beta2$
T_3Ra1
TRAb
thyrotropin receptor autoantibody
trabecular
t. adenoma
t. bone
t. osteopenia
t. pattern
t. plate
t. thinning
trabecule
Trace-4
trace metal
tracer
T. Blood Glucose Micro-monitor
thyroid-specific t.
t. uptake
tracheomalacia
trachomatis
Chlamydia t.
Tracker catheter
tract
geniculohypothalamic t. (GHT)
hypothalamohypophysial nerve t.
hypothalamoneurohypophysial t.
mammillothalamic t.
optic t.
pyramidal t.
retinohypothalamic t.
spinothalamic t.
supraopticohypophysial t.

NOTES

tract *(continued)*
tuberohypophyseal t.
urinary t.
tractus solitarius
TRAF
tumor necrosis factor receptor-associated factor
TRAIL
TNF-related apoptosis inducing ligand
trait
Fitzgerald t.
Flaujeac t.
Fujiwara t.
Williams t.
TRAM
transverse rectus abdominis muscle
TRAM-1 coactivator
tramadol
TRANCE
tumor necrosis factor-related activation-induced cytokine
Trandate
tranexamine acid
tranquilizer
major t.
minor t.
trans
t. clomiphene citrate
t. mechanism
trans-acting factor
transactivation
t. factor (TAF)
t. function 1
t. function 2
***trans*-activation domain (TAD)**
transaminase
alanine t.
beta-alanine t.
isoleucine t.
ornithine t.
ornithine-ketoacid t. (OKT3)
serum glutamic-oxaloacetic t. (SGOT)
serum glutamic-pyruvic t. (SGPT)
valine t.
transamination
transcallosal-transforaminal approach
transcaltachia
transcarbamylase
ornithine t. (OTC)
transcatheter
t. arterial chemoembolization (TACE)
t. celiac artery embolization
transcellular
t. fluid compartment
t. water
transcortin
transcript
agouti-related t.
cocaine and amphetamine regulated t. (CART)
cocaine and amphetamine-responsive t.
CRH-mRNA t.
GHRH-mRNA t.
X-inactive specific t. (Xist)
transcription
monoallelic t.
parathyroid hormone gene t.
prolactin t.
signal transducer and activator of t. (STAT)
signal transducer and activator of t.-4 (Stat4)
signal transducer and activator of t.-5 (Stat5)
signal transducers and activators of t. (STATS)
transcriptional
t. cross-talk
t. intermediary factor 2 (TIF2)
t. silencing
transcriptome
transcutaneous oxygen pressure
transcytosis
transdermal
Alora t.
Climara t.
Duragesic t.
Esclim t.
Estraderm t.
t. estradiol
t. estrogen
t. 1% hydroalcoholic gel
t. scrotum testosterone patch
t. testosterone delivery system
t. torso testosterone patch
Vivelle t.
Transderm Scop
transducer
signal t.
transducin
transepithelial phosphate transport
transethmoidal basal encephalocele
transfect
transfection
rearranged during t. (RET)
transfer
embryo t. (ET)
gamete intrafallopian t. (GIFT)
gene t.
insulin gene t.
peritoneal oocyte and sperm t. (POST)
placental t.

t. ribonucleic acid (tRNA)
zygote intrafallopian t. (ZIFT)

transferase
chloramphenicol acetyl t. (CAT)
diacylglyceroacyl t. (DGAT)
gamma glutaryl t.
glutamyl t.
3-oxoacid-CoA t.
terminal deoxynucleotide t. (TdT)
UDP-galactosyl t.

transferrin
t. receptor

transforming
t. growth factor (TGF)
t. growth factor alpha (TGF-A, TGFα)
t. growth factor beta (TGF-B, TGFβ)

transfusion
neonatal exchange t.

transgastric endoscopic ultrasound

transgenic mouse model

trans-Golgi network

transhepatic portal venous sampling

transhydrogenase
glutathione-insulin t. (GIT)

transient
t. diabetes insipidus
t. hypoparathyroidism
t. neonatal hypothyroidism
t. neonatal thyroid dysfunction
t. postradioiodine hypothyroidism
t. thyrotoxicosis

transjugular intrahepatic portosystemic stent shunt (TIPS)

transketolase (TRK)

translateral retroperitoneal approach

translation

translocase
adenine nucleotide t.
fatty acid t. (FAT)

translocation
bacterial t.
chromosome t.
glucose transporter t.
nuclear t.

translocator
AhR nuclear t. (ARNT)

transmembrane
t. domain
t. Ser/Total hip replacement kinase activity

transmeridian travel

transmission
synaptic t.
vertical t.

transmitter
excitatory t.
inhibitory t.

transmucosal
Actiq Oral T.
t. calcium flux

transnasal-transseptal approach

transplacental antibody

transplant
beta cell t.
encapsulated islet t.
fetal pancreas t.
islet cell t.
renal t.
simultaneous pancreas-kidney t.
SPK t.

transplantation
bone-forming cell t.
bone marrow t.
cadaveric pancreas t.
Center for Human Islet T.
islet t.
islet cell t.
living segmental donor pancreas t.
orthotopic liver t.
PAK t.
pancreas after kidney t.
renal t.
segmental t.
simultaneous pancreas-kidney t.

transport
active salt t.
calcium t.
cholesterol t.
insulin-stimulated glucose t.
iodide t.
ionic t.
t. protein
reverse cholesterol t.
thyroid t.
transepithelial phosphate t.

transporter
euthyroid brain glucose t.
facilitative glucose t.
glucose t. (GLUT)
norepinephrine t. (NET)
sodium glucose t.
thyroid iodide t.

NOTES

transporter *(continued)*
uptake-1 t.
uptake-2 t.
urea t. (UT)
vesicular monoamine t. (VMAT)
transportors
transrectal
t. biopsy
t. ultrasound measurement
***trans*-retinoic acid (RAR)**
transrhinosphenoidal adenomectomy
transscrotal testosterone delivery system
transsphenoidal
t. approach
t. bipolar forceps
t. debulking
t. encephalocele
t. hypophysectomy
t. microadenomectomy
t. microsurgical adenomectomy
t. pituitary adenomectomy
t. selective adenomectomy
t. surgery
transsulfuration
transthyretin (TTR)
t.-ligand complex
t.-thyroid hormone analogue complex
transudate
transurethral
t. incision of the prostate (TUIP)
t. resection of the prostate (TURP)
t. ultrasound (TRUS)
t. ultrasound-guided biopsy
t. ureterolithotripsy (TUL)
transverse
t. arytenoid
t. rectus abdominis muscle (TRAM)
t. relaxation time
t. vaginal septum
transversus perinei superficialis muscle
TRAP
tartrate-resistant acid phosphatase
TRAP-6
thrombin receptor-activating peptide 6
trap
iodide t.
thyroid iodide t.
trapping
iodide t.
radioiodine t.
trauma
chest wall t.
travel
transmeridian t.
TRE
negative T_3 response element
thyroid hormone-response element
T_3RE
T_3 responsive element
treatment
gestagen t.
gonadal suppression t.
high-dose statin t.
hyperbaric oxygen t.
multidose insulin t.
neuraminidase t.
pharmacologic t.
primary adjuvant t.
recombinant human growth hormone t.
RHGH t.
tree
ackee t.
tremor
intention t.
tremulousness
trenbolone
trench
resorption t.
Trendar
TRF
thyrotropin release factor
TRH
thyrotropin-releasing hormone
TRH mRNA
Relefact TRH
TRH stimulation test
TRH study
TRH-DE
TRH-degrading ectoenzyme
TRH-degrading ectoenzyme (TRH-DE)
TRH-induced refractoriness
TRH-R
thyrotropin-releasing hormone receptor
T_4RIA
thyroxine radioisotope assay
TRIAC
3,5,3′-triiodothyroacetic acid
Triacin-C
triad
Carney t.
t. of Carney
fragile histidine t. (FHIT)
Whipple t.
Trial
Diabetes Control and Complications T. (DCCT)
Diabetes Prevention T. (DPT-1)
European Nicotinamide Diabetes Intervention T. (ENDIT)
Hypertensive Optimal Treatment T. (HOT)

Multiple Risk Factor Intervention T.
Postmenopausal Estrogen/Progestin Interventions T. (PEPI)
Schwabing Insulin Prophylaxis T.
Sorbinil Retinopathy T.
Veterans Administration Cooperative Study on Glycemic Control and Complications in Type 2 Diabetes T.

trial
catch t.
EPILOG t.
EPISTENT t.
Evaluation of Platelet IIb-IIIa Inhibitors for Stenting t.
Evaluation of PTCA to Improve Long-Term Outcome by C7E3 GpIIb/IIIa Receptor Blockade T.
HOPE t.
Kmuna t.
Stockholm t.

Triam-A Injection
triamcinolone
Triam Forte Injection
Triamonide Injection
triamterene
triangle
gastrinoma t.
Ward t.

triangular facies
triantennary
Triax
T. Metabolic Accelerator
T. metabolic stimulator

Triban
Pediatric T.

tricarboxylic acid (TCA)
trichilemmoma
trichlormethiazide
Trichomonas
trichomoniasis
trichorrhexis
t. nodosa

trichothiodystrophy
trichrome
TriCor
tricuspid regurgitation
tricyanoaminopropene
Tri-Cyclen
Ortho T.-C.

tricyclic
t. antidepressant (TCA)
t. dibenzodiazepine

tridihexethyl
trientine
Trifed-C
trifluoroacetate salt
triflupromazine
triflutate
corticorelin ovine t.

trifunctional pyridinium cross-link
trigeminal
t. nerve
t. schwannoma

triglyceride
Trigonella foenum-graecum
triidothyronine
triiodoacetic acid
3,5,3′-triiodo-I-thyronine (T_3)
triiodo-L-thyronine
3,5,3′-triiodothyroacetic acid (TRIAC)
triiodothyroacetic acid
triiodothyronine (T_3)
free t. (FT_3)
t. monomer
t. resin uptake (T_3RU)
t. resin uptake test
reverse t.
t. suppression test
t. toxicosis (T_3-toxicosis)

triiodothyronine/thyroxine ratio
Tri-Kort Injection
Trilafon
Tri-Levlen
Trilisate
Trilog Injection
Trilone Injection
trilostane
Trimazide
trimegestone
trimer
G-protein t.

trimethadione
trimethaphan camsylate
trimethobenzamide
trimethoprim sulfamethoxazole (TMP-SMX)
Trimox
Tri-Norinyl
triopathy

NOTES

T

triose
t. isomerase (TIM)
t. isomerase protein
Triostat
T. Injection
tripeptide
t. amide
triphasic
t. diabetes insipidus
t. response
Triphasil
triphenylethylene
triphosphatase
adenosine t. (ATPase)
guanosine t. (GTPase)
hydrogen adenosine t. (H^+-ATPase)
sodium-potassium adenosine t.
triphosphate
adenosine 5′ t. (ATP)
deoxyinosine t. (dITP)
deoxynucleotide t. (dNTP)
guanosine t. (GTP)
guanosine 5′ t. (GTP)
inositol t. (IP3)
nucleotide t.
1,4,5-triphosphate
inositol 1,4,5-t. (IP3)
triple-phase scan with technetium
triple response of Lewis
tripyrrole
trisalicylate
choline magnesium t.
trisilicate
aluminum hydroxide and magnesium t.
Trisoject Injection
trisomy
t. 21
t. X mosaicism
Tri-Tannate Plus
Tritec
triventricular dilation
Tri-Vi-Flor
Tri-Vi-Sol
TRK
transketolase
protooncogene TRK
TRK-A
TRK-B
tRNA
transfer ribonucleic acid
tRNA mitochondrial myopathy
Trocal
trochlear nerve
troglitazone
t. monotherapy
troleandomycin
tromethamine (THAM)
ketorolac t.
tromethamine E (THAM-E)
trophectoderm
mural t.
trophic
t. factor
t. hormone
trophoblast
t. cell
intermediate t.
syncytial t.
villous t.
trophoblastic
t. cell column
t. disease
t. lesion
t. neoplasm
t. shell
t. tissue
trophoblast-lymphocyte
t.-l. cross-reactive (TLX)
t.-l. cross-reactive alloantigen system
trophoblastoma
trophosphate
guanosine t.
tropical
t. calcific pancreatitis (TCP)
t. diabetes mellitus
tropic anterior pituitary hormone
tropics
chronic calcific pancreatitis of the t. (CCPT)
troponin C protein
Trousseau
T. sign
T. test
trovafloxacin
Trovan
Trovert
Trovett pegvisomant
TR-RXR
thyroid hormone receptor-retinoid X receptor
TR-RXR heterodimer
T_3RU
T_3 resin uptake
triiodothyronine resin uptake
T_3RU test
Tru-Cut needle
true
t. hermaphroditism
t. periodic biorhythm
t. precocious puberty

truncal
t. adiposity
t. obesity
truncus arteriosus
trunk
thyrocervical t.
Truphylline
TRUS
transurethral ultrasound
TRUS-guided biopsy
Trypanosoma brucei
trypanosomiasis
African t.
trypsin
trypsinization
trypsinogen-activating peptide (TAP)
tryptamine
tryptophan
t. hydroxylase
TSA
tumor-specific antigen
TSAb
thyroid-stimulating antibody
TSBAb
thyroid-stimulating-blocking antibody
thyroid stimulation-blocking antibody
TSH stimulation blocking antibody
T-score
tsetse fly
TsF
T-suppressor factor
TSG
tumor-suppressor gene
TSH
thyroid-stimulating hormone
thyrotropin-stimulating hormone
TSH deficiency
inappropriate secretion of TSH
TSH receptor (TSH-R)
TSH receptor antibody measurement
TSH receptor autoantibody
TSH receptor-blocking antibody
TSH receptor expression
TSH receptor mutation
TSH receptor-stimulating antibody
recombinant human TSH (rhTSH)
TSH stimulation blocking antibody (TSBAb)
TSH stimulation test
TSH-binding
T.-b. inhibitory antibody
T.-b. inhibitory immunoglobulin (TBII)
TSH-dependent thyrotoxicosis
TSH-induced thyrotoxicosis
TSH-oma
TSH-secreting pituitary adenoma
TSH-R
thyroid-stimulating hormone receptor
thyrotropin receptor
TSH receptor
TSH-R antibody
TSH-R gene
TSHR
thyroid-stimulating hormone receptor
TSH-RAb
thyroid-stimulating hormone receptor antibody
thyroid-stimulating hormone receptor autoantibody
thyrotropin receptor-stimulating antibody
TSH-secreting
T.-s. pituitary adenoma (TSH-oma)
T.-s. pituitary tumor
α-TSH subunit
TSH:T_4 ratio
TSI
thyroid-stimulating immunoglobulin
TSI assay
T-suppresser lymphocyte
T-suppressor factor (TsF)
TT_4
total T_4
TT_3
total T_3
t/t
Snp5 t.
TTF
thyroid transcription factor
TTF-1
thyroid transcription factor 1
TTF-2
thyroid transcription factor 2
TTN
toxic thyroid nodule
T_3-toxicosis
triiodothyronine toxicosis
TTR
transthyretin
T_3:T_4 ratio
TTR-ligand complex
TTR-thyroid hormone analogue complex

NOTES

TTS
Estracomb TTS
Testoderm TTS
T-type calcium channel
tube
endotracheal t.
fallopian t.
nasogastric t.
nasogastrojejunal t. (NGJT)
neural t.
NG t.
uterine t.
tuber
t. cinereum
t. cinereum hamartoma
tuberalis
pars t.
tuberal region
tubercle bacillus
tuberculoma
intrasellar t.
tuberculosis
adrenal t.
miliary t.
Mycobacterium t.
pancreatic t.
tuberculous
t. endometritis
t. meningitis
t. orchitis
tuberohypophyseal
t. dopaminergic neuron (THDA)
t. neuron
t. tract
tuberoinfundibular
t. dopaminergic neuron (TIDA)
t. neuron
t. system
tuberous
t. sclerosis
t. xanthoma
tubular
t. bulbo complex
t. cristae
t. dialysis membrane
t. transport maximum (T_m)
t. ultrafiltrate
tubule
collecting t.
dentinal t.
distal convoluted t. (DCT)
early collecting t.
t. fluid
late distal t.
proximal convoluted t. (PCT)
seminiferous t.
sex cord tumor with annular t. (SCTAT)
tubulin
tubuli recti coalesce
tubuloalveolar salivary gland
tubuloglomerular feedback (TGF)
tubulointerstitial
t. nephropathy
t. renal disease
tubulovesicular mitochondria
tubulus rectus
TUIP
transurethral incision of the prostate
TUL
transurethral ureterolithotripsy
tumescence
nocturnal penile t. (NPT)
sleep-associated penile t.
tumor
acidophilic t.
activin-nonresponsive pituitary t.
adenomatous t.
alpha subunit-secreting t.
androgen-producing t.
brain t.
breast t.
Brenner t.
brown t.
carcinoid t.
carcinoid-like t.
carcinoma with thymus-like differentiation t.
carotid body t.
CASTLE t.
t. cell
chorionic gonadotropin-secreting t.
chromophobe t.
clinically silent t.
corticotroph t.
debulking of t.
deoxycorticosterone-producing t.
dumbbell-shaped t.
ectopic ACTH-secreting t.
ectopic neuroendocrine t.
endocrine t.
endodermal sinus t.
endo-exocrine t.
endometrioid t.
enterohepatic t.
estrogen-producing t.
t. flare
t. gene
germ-cell t.
GHRH-secreting t.
giant cell t.
glial t.
glioneural t.
glomus jugulare t.
glucagon-producing t.
glucagon-secreting t.

glycoprotein-secreting pituitary t.
gonadotropin-secreting t.
granular cell t.
granulosa cell t.
growth hormone-producing t.
growth hormone-releasing hormone-secreting t.
growth hormone-secreting pituitary t.
gsp-positive somatotroph t.
Hardy classification of pituitary t.
hepatic t.
hepatocellular t.
hormone receptor-negative t.
hormone receptor-positive t.
hormone-secreting adrenal t.
hormone-secreting pituitary t.
Hürthle cell t.
hypothalamic t.
hypovascular islet cell t.
islet cell t.
lactotroph t.
Leydig cell t.
lipid t.
lipid-containing t.
lipoid cell t.
luteinizing hormone-secreting t.
t. lysis syndrome
malignant islet cell t.
mesenchymal t.
t. metastasis
metastatic t.
mixed phenotype t.
Mostofi classification of testicular t.
mucinous cystic t.
t. necrosis factor (TNF)
t. necrosis factor-alpha (TNF-alpha)
t. necrosis factor-beta (TNF-beta)
t. necrosis factor gene
t. necrosis factor receptor (TNFR)
t. necrosis factor receptor-associated factor (TRAF)
t. necrosis factor-related activation-induced cytokine (TRANCE)
neural t.
neuroendocrine t.
nonaggressive t.
nonbeta cell t.
nonfunctioning pituitary t.
nonislet cell t.
nonsecreting pituitary t.
optic tract pituitary t.
osteoblastic t.
ovarian t.
pancreatic alpha-cell t.
pancreatic endocrine t.
pancreatic islet cell t.
pancreatic polypeptide-secreting t. (PPoma)
paraneoplastic t.
parasellar t.
pineal t.
pituitary t.
prolactin-producing pituitary t.
prolactin-secreting pituitary t.
t. receptor status
recurrent pituitary t.
t. removal
residual pituitary t.
retinoblastoma t.
sellar t.
serous t.
Sertoli cell testicular t.
Sertoli-Leydig cell t.
sex cord stromal t.
small-volume pituitary t.
solid cystic t. (SCT)
solid pseudopapillary t.
somatotroph t.
sporadic thyroid t.
steroid-dependent t.
t. suppressor
suprasellar germ cell t.
thyroid-stimulating hormone-secreting t.
thyroid-stimulating hormone-secreting pituitary t.
thyrotropin-secreting pituitary t.
TSH-secreting pituitary t.
urothelial t.
vasoactive intestinal peptide-secreting t. (VIPoma)
vasoactive intestinal polypeptide-secreting t.
VIP-secreting t.
Wilms t.
Wilms t. 1 (WTI)
t. xenograft model
yolk sac t.

tumoral calcinosis

tumor-forming pancreatitis

tumorigenesis
adrenocortical t.

NOTES

T

tumorigenesis *(continued)*
Knudson two-hit model of t.
pituitary t.
tumorigenic
tumorigenicity
tumor-induced osteomalacia syndrome
tumorlet
tumor-like calcification
tumor/node/metastases (TNM)
tumor/node/metastases classification
tumor-reduction surgery
tumors
tumor-specific antigen (TSA)
tumor-suppressor gene (TSG)
Tums
T. E-X Extra Strength Tablet
tunica
t. media
t. vaginalis
turbid fluid
turcica
bridged sella t.
sella t.
Turkish saddle
Turner
T. mosaicism
T. stigma
T. syndrome
turnover
bone t.
iron t.
water t.
TURP
transurethral resection of the prostate
turtle Tg
Tussin
Diabetic T.
TWEAK
TNF-weak homologue
twin
t. study
uniovular t.
twins
dizygotic t.
monozygotic t.
two-day high-dose dexamethasone suppression test
two-site
t.-s. sandwich immunoassay
TX
thromboxane
TXA2, TxA2
thromboxane A2
TXB2, TxB2
thromboxane B2
Tyk-2
tyrosine kinase-2
Tylenol
T. With Codeine
Tylox
Ty-Pap
type
t. A adipsia
achondrogenesis t. II
activin cell-surface receptor t. I
activin cell-surface receptor t. II
t. A dark spermatogonia
t. Ad spermatogonia
t. 1 angioneurotic edema
t. 2 angioneurotic edema
apolipoprotein t. 3
t. Ap spermatogonia
t. A spermatogonia
t. A syndrome
t. A syndrome of insulin resistance
t. II autoimmune polyglandular syndrome
t. 1 autosomal recessive vitamin D dependency (ARVDD-1)
t. B adipsia
11-beta-hydroxysteroid dehydrogenase t. 1 (11-beta-HSD1)
11-beta-hydroxysteroid dehydrogenase t. 2 (11-beta-HSD2)
t. B extreme insulin resistance syndrome
t. B spermatogonia
t. B syndrome of insulin resistance
t. C adipsia
t. I collagen
t. I collagen C-terminal telopeptide
t. I collagen heterotrimer
t. II collagen
t. IX collagen
t. X collagen
t. I congenital adrenal hyperplasia
t. II congenital adrenal hyperplasia
t. IV congenital adrenal hyperplasia
t. V congenital adrenal hyperplasia
t. C syndrome of insulin resistance
t. 1 deiodinase (D1)
t. 2 deiodinase (D2)
t. 3 deiodinase (D3)
t. 1 diabetes
t. 2 diabetes
t. 1 diabetes mellitus
t. 2 diabetes mellitus
differentiated thyroid carcinoma, intermediate t.
distal renal tubular acidosis t. 4
dystonia t. 1
t. 2 energy pathway

familial multiple endocrine neoplasia t. 1
t. 1 fiber
t. 2 fiber
t. 1, 2, and 3 gastric carcinoid
t. IV hyperlipidemia
t. 3 hyperlipoproteinemia
insulin growth factor-binding protein t. 1–6
melanocortin receptor t. 4 (MCAR)
5′-monodeiodinase t. I
t. II multiple endocrine glandular failure
t. II muscle fiber
t. II muscle fiber atrophy
polyglandular autoimmune syndrome t. I (PGA-I)
t. 1 polyglandular syndrome
t. I procollagen
t. 1 procollagen peptide
t. pseudohypoaldosteronism
t. I regulatory dimer (RI)
t. II regulatory dimer (RII)
t. 4 renal tubular acidosis
t. 4 RTA
t. III selenoenzyme
t. II vitamin D dependency rickets
t. I von Willebrand disease
Waardenburg syndrome t. I

typhi
Salmonella t.

tyramine

tyropanoate

tyrosinase

tyrosine
t. aminotransferase
t. aminotransferase enzyme
diiodinated t. (DIT)
t. hydroxylase
t. kinase
t. kinase-2 (Tyk-2)
t. kinase activity
monoiodinated t. (MIT)
t. phosphorylation
t. phosphorylation site

tyrosinemia
t. I
t. II

tyrosinosis

tyrosyl
t. residue

TZD
thiazolidinedione

T- and Z- scores of bone mass

T

NOTES

U
Humulin U
U-500
Regular (Concentrated) Iletin II U.
UB
ultimobranchial body
ubiquinone
ubiquitin
u. fusion degradation 1 gene
u. mechanism
ubiquitin-proteasome pathway
ubiquitinylated protein
Uchida
U. method
U. technique
UCP
uncoupling protein
UCP1
uncoupling protein 1
UDCA
ursodeoxycholic acid
UDP-galactosyl transferase
UFC
urine free cortisol
uFSH
urinary FSH
UGDP
University Group Diabetes Program
UGP
urinary gonadotropin peptide
UICC
Union Internationale Contre le Cancer
UKPDS
United Kingdom Prospective Diabetes Study
ulcer
necrotic palatal u.
neuropathic u.
ulceration
corneal u.
Ulcogant
ulcus cruris
Ullrich syndrome
ulnar-mammary syndrome
ultimobranchial
u. body (UB)
u. gland
u. organ
Ultiva
ultradian
u. oscillation
u. rhythm
ultrafiltrate
salivary u.
tubular u.
ultrafiltration
extracorporeal u.
u. rate
Ultralente insulin
Ultram
Ultra Mide Topical
Ultrase MT
ultrasensitive
ultrashort-loop feedback
ultrasonography
color Doppler u. (CDU)
color duplex u.
ultrasound
endoscopic u. (EUS)
intraductal u. (IDUS)
intraoperative u. (IOUS)
u. mammography
parathyroid u.
pulsed Doppler u.
thyroid u.
transgastric endoscopic u.
transurethral u. (TRUS)
ultrastructural feature
ultrastructure
osteoclast u.
UltraSure DTU-one ultrasound scanner
ultrathin pancreatoscope
ultraviolet (UV)
unawareness
hypoglycemia u.
uncompensated metabolic acidosis
uncoupling
u. protein (UCP)
u. protein 1 (UCP1)
uncus
undecenoate
testosterone u.
undercalcified bone
underpneumatization
undervirilized
u. fertile male syndrome
u. male
underwater body weight
undifferentiated
u. pattern
u. sarcoma
UNE
unopposed estrogen
unesterified arachidonic acid
unexplained microcytic anemia
unformed visual hallucination
Uni-Ace
Unicap
Unicelles
Melfiat-105 U.

Uni-Dur
unilateral
u. adrenal disease
u. adrenalectomy
u. aldosterone excess
u. aldosterone-producing adenoma
u. APA
u. lobectomy
u. renal agenesis
u. salpingo-oophorectomy
uniloculate
uninodular
u. goiter
union
anomalous pancreaticobiliary u.
U. Internationale Contre le Cancer (UICC)
uniovular twin
uniparental disomy
Uniphyl
Uni-Pro
unit
basic multicellular u. (BMU)
bipolar cautery u.
bone structural u.
fetoplacental u.
gamma u.
granulocyte-macrophage colony-forming u. (GM-CFU)
hormone response u. (HRU)
international u. (IU)
United Kingdom Prospective Diabetes Study (UKPDS)
Unithroid
Unitrol
universal
u. gas constant
u. pacemaker
u. salt iodization (USI)
u. screening
universalis
calcinosis u.
University
U. Group Diabetes Program (UGDP)
U. of Wisconsin (UW)
U. of Wisconsin solution
unmineralized lamellar osteoid
unmutated receptor
unmyelinated
u. nerve fiber
unopposed estrogen (UNE)
unresponsiveness
hypoglycemia u.
unsaturated fatty acid
Unschuld sign
unstable Cushing disease
untranslated
u. region (UTR)
5′-u. region (UTR)
upper
u. clivus
u. pole of spleen
u. pretracheal node
upregulate
upregulation
upright plasma renin
Uprima
uptake
bromodeoxyuridine u.
elevated radioactive iodine u.
fluorodeoxyglucose u.
hepatic free fatty acid u.
insulin-mediated glucose u.
L-triiodothyronine u.
net hepatic glucose u. (NHGU)
radioactive iodine u. (RAIU)
radiofluoride u.
radioiodine u. (RAIU)
radiostrontium u.
resin u.
splanchine glucose u.
thyroid radioiodine u.
thyroid technetium pertechnetate u.
tracer u.
T_3 resin u. (T_3RU)
triiodothyronine resin u. (T_3RU)
uptake-1
u. transporter
uptake-2
u. transporter
Urabeth
Uracel
uranium
urate
amorphous u.
u. nephropathy
u. salt
urate-hydroxyl exchanger
urate-lactate exchanger
urea
u. cycle
interstitial u.
u. recycling
u. transporter (UT)
Ureacin-20 Topical
ureagenesis
urealyticum
Ureaplasma u.
Ureaphil Injection
ureaplasm
Ureaplasma urealyticum
urease
enzyme u.
Urecholine

uremia
uremic
u. metabolic acidosis
u. osteodystrophy
u. pruritus
u. pseudodiabetes
ureter
ureterolithotomy
ureterolithotripsy
transurethral u. (TUL)
ureteropelvic junction
ureterosigmoidoscopy
ureterovesical junction
urethra
internal u.
membranous u.
penile u.
prostatic u.
urethral gland
urethritis
urethrocystoscopy
uric
u. acid
u. acid crystal
u. acid renal stone
uricase method
uricemia
uricosuric
u. agent
uridine
u. 5′-diphosphate
u. diphosphate glucose
urinary
u. calcium
u. concentrating mechanism
u. creatinine
u. follicle-stimulating hormone
u. free cortisol
u. FSH (uFSH)
u. genistein excretion
u. gonadotropin peptide (UGP)
u. 17-hydroxycorticosteroid
u. hydroxyproline
u. hydroxyproline excretion
u. iodine/thiocyanate ratio
u. 17-ketosteroid
u. N-telopeptide collagen cross-link
u. paraaminobutyric acid excretion rate
u. phosphoethanolamine
u. potassium wasting
u. pyridinoline cross-link excretion
u. retention
u. stasis
u. tract
urine
u. aldosterone
u. collection
u. concentration
u. free cortisol (UFC)
u. glucose level
u. hydroxyproline level
hypotonic u.
u. osmolality
u. output
u. pH
u. phosphorus excretion
u. steroid
urinometer
Urispas
urochrome
pigment u.
urocortin
u. fiber
urodilatin
uroerythrin
urofollitropin
urogenital
u. diaphragm
u. fold
u. ridge
u. sinus
urogenitogram
urography
intravenous u.
urokinase plasminogen activator
urokinase-type plasminogen activator
Urolen blue
urolithiasis
uropontin
urotensin I–IV
urothelial tumor
ursodeoxycholic acid (UDCA)
urticaria
u. pigmentosa
use
side-effect profile of u.
USI
universal salt iodization
USP
uterine-stimulating potency
UT
urea transporter
uteri (*pl. of* uterus)

NOTES

uterine
u. activity rhythm
u. arcuate artery
u. atony
u. contractile activity
u. contractile rhythm
u. endometrium
u. gland
u. leiomyoma
u. milk
u. rhythmicity
u. tetany
u. tube
uterine-endocrine system
uterine-stimulating potency (USP)
uteroplacental blood flow
uterotonin
uterotropin
uterus, pl. **uteri**
cervix u.
corpus u.
isthmus u.
UTR
untranslated region
5′-untranslated region
utricle
prostatic u.
UV
ultraviolet
uveal coloboma
UW
University of Wisconsin
UW solution

V1 receptor
vaccine
bacillus Calmette-Guérin v.
BCG v.
Heptavax-B v.
7-valent v.
vaccinia virus growth factor
vacor
Vaculance
Microlet V.
vacuole
secretory v.
vacuolization
marrow cell v.
vacuum
v. tumescence device
vagal
v. afferent
v. neural crest
v. nucleus
v. stimulation
Vagifem
V. 17B
vagina
vaginal
v. candidiasis
Cleocin V.
v. fornix
Ogen V.
v. ring
v. smear
vaginalis
Gardnerella v.
portio v.
processus v.
tunica v.
vaginitis
candidal v.
vaginoplasty
vagostigmin test
vagotomy
vagus
v. nerve
valence
7-valent vaccine
valerate
17-beta-estradiol v.
Valertest No. 1
valgum
valgus
cubitus v.
valine
v. transaminase
Valisone
valproate
sodium v.
valproic acid
value
insulin surrogate v.
predictive v.
single-serum dehydroepiandrosterone sulfate v.
valve
bicuspid aortic v.
porcine heart v.
Vamate Oral
van
v. Buchem disease
v. den Bergh test
v. Heuven anatomic classification of diabetic retinopathy
vanadate
vanadium
Vancocin
V. Injection
V. Oral
Vancoled Injection
vancomycin
vanillylmandelic acid (VMA)
VANIQA cream
vanishing testis syndrome
Vaponefrin
vara
cox v.
variable
v. number of tandem repeat (VNTR)
v. number of tandem repeat markers
variance
analysis of v. (ANOVA)
variant
antenatal-hypercalciuric v.
fertile eunuch v.
hypocalciuric-hypomagnesemic v.
oncocytic v.
salt-wasting hydroxylase deficiency v.
simple virilizing hydroxylase deficiency v.
variation
circadian v.
varicella zoster
varices (*pl. of* varix)
varicocele
v. testis

varicosity
neurophysin-positive v.
Varidase
varix, pl. **varices**
varum
vas, pl. **vasa**
ampulla of the v. deferens
v. deferens
vasa nervorum
vasa recta
vascular
v. calcification
v. compliance
v. endocrine protein
v. endothelial cell growth inhibitor (VEGI)
v. endothelial growth factor (VEGF)
v. injury
v. permeability factor (VPF)
v. remodeling
v. smooth muscle cell (VSMC)
v. steal syndrome
v. thrombosis
vasculitis
systemic v.
vasculopathy
diabetic v.
vasculosum
organum v.
vasculosyncytial membrane
vasectomy
vasoactive
v. intestinal peptide (VIP)
v. intestinal peptide receptor
v. intestinal peptide-secreting tumor (VIPoma)
v. intestinal polypeptide (VIP)
v. intestinal polypeptide-secreting tumor
vasoconstriction
vasodilation
beta-adrenergic v.
cutaneous v.
vasodilator
v. peptide
v. prostaglandin
vasomotor flush
vasopressin
arginine v. (AVP)
desamino D-arginine v. (DDAVP)
1-desamino-8-d arginine v.
v. excess
lysine v.
v. neurophysin II
v. receptor (V2R)
v. resistance syndrome
vasopressinase
placental v.
vasopressinergic fiber
vasopressor
vasospasm
digital v.
painless cold-sensitive digital v.
Vasotec
vasotocin
arginine v. (AVT)
Vasoxyl
VDAC
voltage-dependent anion channel
VDDR
pseudovitamin D deficiency rickets
VDDR-II
vitamin D-dependent rickets type II
VDR
vitamin D receptor
VDRE
vitamin D-response element
vector
baculovirus v.
vectorial sum
Veetids
vegan
vegetative
VEGF
vascular endothelial growth factor
VEGI
vascular endothelial cell growth inhibitor
vein
adrenal v.
emissary v.
hepatic v.
innominate v.
internal jugular v. (IJV)
percutaneous femoral v.
portal v.
suprasellar v.
vellus
v. hair
velocardiofacial syndrome
velocity
falling height v.
growth v. (GV)
nerve conduction v. (NCV)
sensory nerve conduction v.
sperm v.
Velosulin
V. BR
V. BR insulin
velum interpositum
venlafaxine
venography
venous
v. digital angiography
v. ovarian plasma progesterone

v. sampling
v. telangiectasia
v. thromboembolic disease
v. thromboembolism (VTE)
Ventolin
V. Rotocaps
ventral adrenergic bundle
ventricle
anteroventral 3rd v. (AV3V)
third v.
ventricular
v. arrhythmia
v. fibrillation
v. myxoma
v. region
v. septal defect (VSD)
v. tachycardia
ventriculoperitoneal shunt
ventrolateral medulla
ventromedial
v. nucleus (VMN)
v. nucleus of the hypothalamus (VMN)
vera
polycythemia v.
Veralipride
verapamil
v-*erb* A oncogene
vermis
cerebellar v.
Verner-Morrison syndrome
vernix
verrucosity
verrucous vulgaris
Versaflow peristatic pump
versicolor
tinea v.
vertebra
codfish v.
rugger jersey appearance of v.
vertebral venous plexus
vertical
v. banded gastroplasty
v. ring gastroplasty
v. transmission
verticis
cutis v.
vertigo
very
v. long chain acyl-CoA dehydrogenase (VLCAD)
v. long chain acyl-CoA dehydrogenase deficiency
v. low birth weight (VLBW)
v. low calorie diet
v. low density lipoprotein (VLDL)
v. low density lipoprotein C (VLDL-C)
v. low density lipoprotein fraction
vesica, pl. **vesicae**
sphincter vesicae
vesicle
acrosomal v.
aldehyde-thionin-positive v.
chromaffin v.
clathrin-coated v.
matrix v.
phospholipid v.
pinocytic v.
secretory v.
seminal v.
sequestered v.
synaptic v.
vesicular
v. follicle
v. monoamine transporter (VMAT)
Vesprin
vessel
endoneurial blood v.
epineurial blood v.
extrahypophyseal portal v.
hypothalamic-hypophyseal portal v.
intrahypophyseal portal v.
neurosecretory v.
tortuous blood v.
vestibule
vestibulum, pl. **vestibuli**
bulbus vestibuli
Veterans Administration Cooperative Study on Glycemic Control and Complications in Type 2 Diabetes Trial
VHL
von Hippel-Lindau
VHL disease
VHL tumor suppressor gene
Viagra
vibration
v. perception testing
v. threshold
vibratory sensation

NOTES

Vibrio
  V. cholerae
  V. vulnificus
vibrios
  marine v.
Vicodin
  V. ES
Vicon
  V. Forte
  V. Plus
Vicon-C
Vicoprofen
vidarabine
  v. therapy
Vi-Daylin
Vi-Daylin/F
vide infra
VII
  clotting factor V.
  spinocerebellar ataxia types I, II, III, VI, V.
villous
  v. cytotrophoblast
  v. hypertrichosis
  v. trophoblast
villus, pl. **villi**
  chorionic v.
  primary v.
  secondary v.
  tertiary chorionic v.
Vim-Silverman needle
vinblastine
vincristine
vinculum
vinpocetine
Vioform
Viokase
violaceous
  v. stria
viosterol
Vioxx
VIP
 vasoactive intestinal peptide
 vasoactive intestinal polypeptide
  VIP receptor
  VIP-secreting tumor
VIPoma
 vasoactive intestinal peptide-secreting tumor
viral
  v. infection
  v. oncogene
  v. orchitis
Virchow-Robin
  V.-R. space
  subarachnoid space of V.-R.
virilism
virilization
  systemic v.
virilized external genitalia
virilizer
  simple v.
virilizing adrenal syndrome
Virilo-IM
Virilon
virulence
virus
  adeno-associated v. (AAV)
  avian myeloblastosis v. (AMV)
  bovine viral diarrhea mucosal disease v.
  BVD-MD v.
  canine distemper v.
  Epstein-Barr v. (EBV)
  hepatitis A v.
  human immunodeficiency v. (HIV)
  lymphadenopathy-associated v. (LAV)
  mammary tumor v. (MTV)
  mumps v.
  myeloproliferative leukemia v. (MPLV)
  respiratory syncytial v.
  rubella v.
  SV40 v.
virus-induced diabetes
viscera (*pl. of* viscus)
visceral
  v. calcification
  v. fat accumulation
visceromegaly
viscous
  v. colloid
  v. dietary fiber
viscus, pl. **viscera**
Visidex
  V. II
vision
  color v.
Vistacon-50 Injection
Vistaquel Injection
Vistaril
  V. Injection
  V. Oral
Vistazine Injection
visual
  v. acuity
  v. examination
  v. field assessment
  v. field defect
  v. field disturbance

v. hallucination
v. loss
v. outcome
visual-evoked potential
visualization
panoramic v.
visuotopic
Vita-C
vital
v. red
v. staining
vitamin
v. A
v. A_1
v. A_2
v. A intoxication
v. B6
v. B_c
v. B complex
v. B complex with vitamin C
v. B complex with vitamin C and folic acid
v. B_x
v. C drops
v. D
v. D_1
v. D_2
v. D_3
v. D analog
v. D-binding globulin
v. D-binding protein (DBP)
v. D-binding protein macrophage-activating factor
v. D-deficiency osteomalacia
v. D-dependent rickets type II (VDDR-II)
v. D effect
v. D endocrine system
v. D end-organ resistance
v. D 24-hydroxylase (24-OHase)
v. D intoxication
v. D metabolite
v. D receptor (VDR)
v. D receptor deficiency
v. D-regulatory element
v. D-replete child
v. D-resistant rickets
v. D-response element (VDRE)
v. D sterol
v. E
v. F
v. G
v. H
injectable multiple v.
v. K_1
v. K_2
v. K_5
v. K_6
v. K_7
v. L
v. L_1
v. L_2
v. M
oral multiple v.
v. P
pediatric multiple v.
v. PP
prenatal multiple v.
v. T
v. U
Vita-Plus E Softgels
Vitec
vitiligo
vitrectomy
vitreous hemorrhage
vitro
in v.
in vitro fertilization (IVF)
vitronectin receptor
Vivelle
V. transdermal
vivo
in v.
VLBW
very low birth weight
VLCAD
very long chain acyl-CoA dehydrogenase
VLDL
very low density lipoprotein
VLDL cholesterol/total triglyceride ratio
VLDL fraction
VLDL-C
very low density lipoprotein C
VMA
vanillylmandelic acid
VMAT
vesicular monoamine transporter
VMN
ventromedial nucleus
ventromedial nucleus of the hypothalamus
v-mpl protein

NOTES

VNTR
variable number of tandem repeat
VNTR markers
vocal
v. cord disorder
v. cord paralysis
voglibose
voice
deepening of v.
sonorous v.
Volkmann canal
Vollman cycle
voltage-dependent anion channel (VDAC)
voltage-gated
v.-g. Ca^{2+} channel
v.-g. K^+ channel
v.-g. Na^+ channel
voltage gradient
voltammetric microelectrode
Voltaren Oral
Voltaren-XR Oral
volume
v. assessment
blood v.
v. depletion
effective circulating v.
end-systolic v.
extracellular fluid v. (EFV)
goiter v.
intravascular v.
liver v.
v. receptor
relative osteoid v.
sellar v.
spleen v.
testicular v.
total blood v.
vomer
vomeronasal organ
vomerosphenoidal articulation
vomiting
intractable v.
von
v. Basedow disease
v. Gierke disease
v. Graefe sign
v. Hippel-Lindau (VHL)
v. Hippel-Lindau disease
v. Hippel-Lindau syndrome
v. Hippel-Lindau tumor-suppressor gene
v. Recklinghausen disease
v. Recklinghausen disease of bone
v. Willebrand disease
v. Willebrand factor (vWF)
VP-16
VPF
vascular permeability factor
V2R
vasopressin receptor
V_{1a} receptor
V_2 receptor
V_{1b} receptor
VSD
ventricular septal defect
v-*sis* transforming gene
VSMC
vascular smooth muscle cell
VTE
venous thromboembolism
vulgaris
pemphigus v.
verrucous v.
vulnificus
Vibrio v.
vulva
hypoplastic v.
vWF
von Willebrand factor
Vytone

Waardenburg syndrome type I
waddling gait
WAGR
Wilms tumor-aniridia-genital anomalies-mental retardation syndrome
WAI
wheat amylase inhibitor
Waist It pump holder
waist-to-hip circumference ratio (WHR)
walking
repetitive stress of w.
wallerian degeneration
Wall stent
Warburg apparatus
Ward triangle
warfarin
w. therapy
warm nodule
Warthin-like papillary carcinoma
Wassermann test
wasting
cerebral salt w.
w. disease
nitrogen w.
renal calcium w.
renal phosphate w.
renal sodium w.
salt w.
sodium w.
w. syndrome
urinary potassium w.
WAT
white adipose tissue
watch
sugar w.
water
w. balance
body w.
w. composition
w. deprivation
w. deprivation test
w. deprivation testing
w. diuresis
w. homeostasis
w. intoxication
w. metabolism
w. restriction test
total body w.
transcellular w.
w. turnover
Waterhouse-Friderichsen syndrome
water-soluble hormone
watery
w. diarrhea, hypokalemia, achlorhydria (WDHA)
w. diarrhea syndrome
wavelength
WBC
white blood cell
w/C
Aprodine w/C
w/Codeine
Allerfrin w.
WDHA
watery diarrhea, hypokalemia, achlorhydria
WDHA syndrome
w/DM
weakness
muscular w.
proximal muscle w.
web
metabolic w.
webbed neck
wedge
mucoid w.
Wegener granulomatosis
weight
body w.
w. gain
w. loss
low birth w. (LBW)
underwater body w.
very low birth w. (VLBW)
weight-loss medicine
Wellbutrin
Werdnig-Hoffman syndrome
Werner syndrome
Wernicke encephalopathy
Wernicke-Korsakoff syndrome
WESDR
Wisconsin Epidemiologic Study of Diabetic Retinopathy
Western
W. blot
W. blot analysis
wet keratin
Wharton jelly
wheal
w. and flare response
wheat amylase inhibitor (WAI)
Whickham survey
Whipple
W. disease
W. triad
W. trial of insulinoma

white
w. adipose tissue (WAT)
w. blood cell (WBC)
W. classification
W. classification of diabetes mellitus
w. muscle
w. ramus
WHO
World Health Organization
WHO class 1, 2 and 3 anovulation
WHO classification system
WHO (type I, II, III)
whole-body
w.-b. ^{131}I-MIBG study
w.-b. radioiodine scan
w.-b. scintigraphy
whole body counter
WHR
waist-to-hip circumference ratio
WHR ratio
widened
w. cranial structure
w. palpebral fissure
w. pulse pressure
wide osteoid seam
widespread xanthoma
width
capillary basement membrane w. (CBMW)
wild-type
w.-t. K-ras gene
w.-t. receptor
Williams
W. syndrome
W. trait
Williams-Beuren syndrome
Willis
circle of W.
Wilms
W. lung
W. tumor
W. tumor 1 (WTI)
W. tumor-aniridia-genital anomalies-mental retardation syndrome (WAGR)
W. tumor 1 gene
W. tumor 1 transcription factor
Wilson
W. disease
W. syndrome
window
winged scapulae
Winpred
Winstrol
Wisconsin
W. Epidemiologic Study of Diabetic Retinopathy (WESDR)
modified University of W. (mUW)
original University of W. (oUW)
University of W. (UW)
Wiskott-Aldrich syndrome
Wolcott-Rallison syndrome
Wolff-Chaikoff effect
wolffian duct
Wolf-Hirschhorn syndrome
Wolfram syndrome
Wolman disease
woman
eumenorrheic hirsute w.
normoprolactinemic w.
Women
Brief Index of Sexual Functioning for W. (BISF-W)
workup
metabolic stone w.
World
W. Health Organization (WHO)
W. Health Organization classification system
W. Health Organization (type I, II, III)
worm
biliary w.
wormian bone
wound
w. dehiscence
w. healing
woven
w. bone
w. osteoid
Wright stain
WTI
Wilms tumor 1
WTI gene
WTI transcription factor
Wygesic
Wymox

X
X body
X chromatin
X chromosome to autosome (X:A)
X chromosome to autosome ratio (X:A ratio)
X chromosome inactivation
clotting factor X
disseminated histiocytosis X
histiocytosis X
X inactivation center (Xic)
X pacemaker
X zone
X:A
X chromosome to autosome
X:A ratio
Xanax
xanthelasma, pl. **xanthelasmata**
xanthine oxidase deficiency
xanthinuria
xanthochromic fluid
xanthogranulomatous cholecystitis
xanthoma, pl. **xanthomata**
achillean x.
x. disseminatum
x. homogenate
planar x.
tendinous x.
tendon x.
tuberous x.
widespread x.
xanthomatosis
aggressive x.
cerebrotendinous x.
xanthomectomy
X-body
X-chromosome
adhesion molecule-like from the X.-c. (ADMLX)
X.-c. linkage
Xe
xenon
^{133}Xe
xenon-133
Xenical
XeniCare program
xenobiotic
x. chemical
xenobiotic-response element (XRE)
xenogeneic
xenogenic
xenograft
islet x.
xenografting
xenon (Xe)
xenon-133 (^{133}Xe)
w. washout study
Xenopus
X. laevis
X. oocyte expression assay
xenorexia
xenotransplantation
xenotropic
xeroderma
x. pigmentosa
x. pigmentosa/Cockayne syndrome
xerophthalmia
xeroradiography
xerostomia
Xic
X inactivation center
X-inactivation
X-inactive specific transcript (Xist)
xiphoid
Xist
X-inactive specific transcript
Xist gene
XL
Glucotrol XL
Lodine XL
XL-alpha protein
XL-alpha-s exon
XLH
X-linked hypophosphatemia
XLH rickets
X-linked
X.-l. diabetes insipidus
X.-l. dominant pedigree
X.-l. hydrocephalus
X.-l. hypohidrotic ectodermal dysplasia
X.-l. hypophosphatemia (XLH)
X.-l. ichthyosis
X.-l. immunodeficiency syndrome
X.-l. inheritance
X.-l. lymphoproliferative disease
X.-l. myotubular myopathy
X.-l. recessive adrenoleukodystrophy
X.-l. recessive hypophosphatemic rickets
Xopenex
XO/XY mosaicism
XP
Cophene XP

XP/CS
x-ray crystallography
XRE
xenobiotic-response element
XRT
radiation therapy
X-Trozine
xylitol

Y
Y. body
Y. chromatin
Y. chromosome detection
Y. chromosome microdeletion
Y. chromosome mosaicism
Y. chromosome RNA recognition motif (YRRM)
Y. hormone
Y. pacemaker
yellow
y. body
y. bone marrow
y. skin
Yersinia enterocolitica
yersiniosis
Yes protein
Yocon
Yodoxin
yohimbine
Yohimex
yolk sac tumor
young
mature-onset diabetes of the y. (MODY)
maturity-onset diabetes in the y. (MODY)
Y. syndrome
youth
maturity-onset diabetes of y. (MODY)
YRRM
Y chromosome RNA recognition motif
yttrium-90
y. radioactive isotope
yttrium-91
colloidal y.
YY
peptide YY

Y

Z
- Z. element
- Z. score

Zadine
Zal site
Zanosar
zanoterone
Zantac
Zaroxolyn
Zartan
Z-disk
zearalanol
zein
zeism
Zeitgeber
- Z. gene

Zellweger syndrome
Zemplar
Zestril
ZFP
zinc finger protein
- ZFP gene

Zhen Qi capsule
zidovudine
Ziehl-Neelsen method
Zieve syndrome
ZIFT
zygote intrafallopian transfer
zimeldine
zinc (Zn)
- z. chloride
- z. finger
- z. finger protein (ZFP)
- z. finger Y gene
- z. metalloproteinase
- z. sulfate

Zinca-Pak
zinc-finger motif
Zinn annulus
zirconium-containing compound
zirconium oxide
Zithromax
ZK98299
ZK 98,734
Zn
zinc
ZNP Bar
ZOG
zona glomerulosa protein
- ZOG protein

Zoladex
- Z. Implant

zoledronic acid for injection
Zollinger-Ellison syndrome
Zoloft
zolpidem
Zometa
zona, pl. **zonae**
- z. fasciculata
- z. fasciculata cell
- z. glomerulosa
- z. glomerulosa cell
- z. glomerulosa protein (ZOG)
- z. incerta
- z. pellucida
- z. pellucida 1 (ZP1)
- z. pellucida 2 (ZP2)
- z. pellucida 3 (ZP3)
- z. pellucida receptor for glycoprotein 3
- z. pellucide recognition site
- z. radiata
- z. reticularis

zona-free hamster oocyte penetration test
zone
- adult z.
- clear z.
- fetal z.
- hole z.
- hypothalamic z.
- z. incerta
- lateral z.
- Looser z.
- lucent z.
- medial z.
- midline z.
- z. occludens
- periventricular z.
- z. of provisional calcification
- z. reticularis
- X z.

zonula
- z. adherens
- z. occludens

zonule
ZORprin
zoster
- herpes z.
- varicella z.

Zostrix
Zostrix-HP
Zovia
ZP1
zona pellucida 1
ZP2
zona pellucida 2
ZP3
zona pellucida 3
Z-score

Zuckerkandl
organ of Z.
Z. peduncle
Zuclomiphene citrate
zwitterion
Zydone
zygoma
hypoplastic z.
zygomatic process
zygomycosis
zygosity
zygote
z. intrafallopian transfer (ZIFT)
Zymase
zymogen
z. granule
pancreatic digestive z.
proteolysis of pancreatic z.

Appendix 1

Anatomical Illustrations

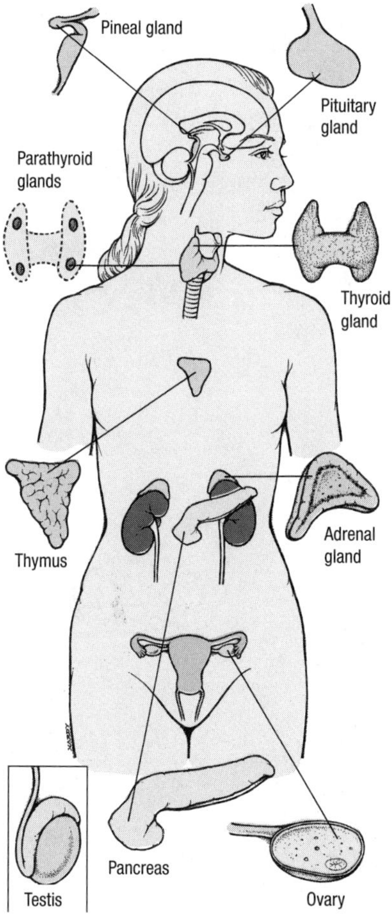

Figure 1. Endocrine system, showing various endocrine glands.

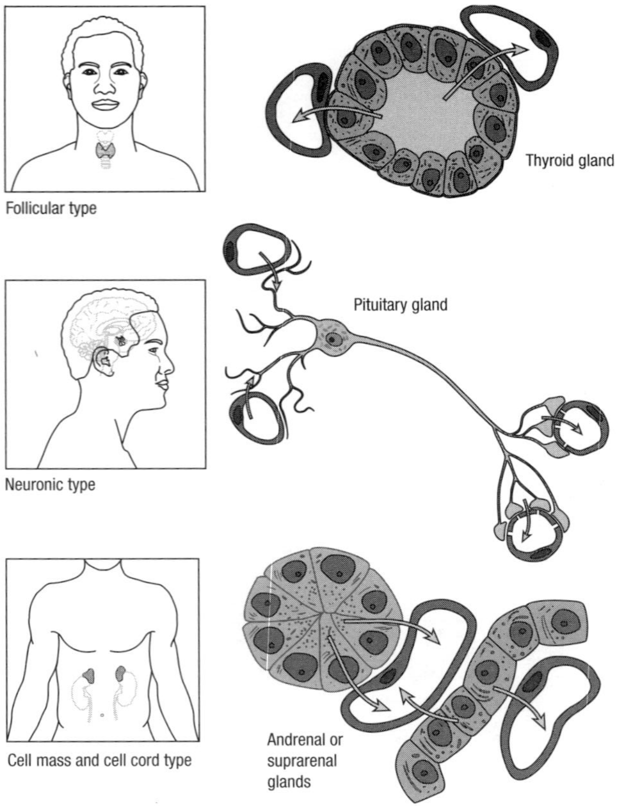

Figure 2. Types of endocrine glands.

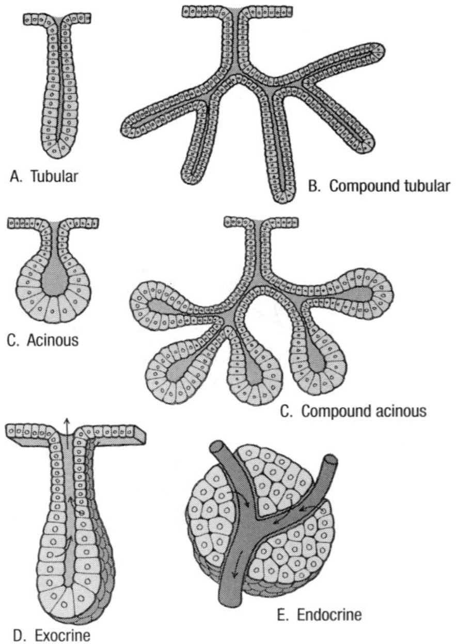

Figure 3. Types of glands. (A) Tubular gland: a gland composed of one or more tubules ending in a blind extremity. (B) Compound tubular gland: a gland whose larger excretory ducts branch repeatedly into smaller ducts, which ultimately drain secretory units. (C) Compound acinous gland: a gland in which the secretory unit(s) has (have) a grapelike shape and a very small lumen. (D) Exocrine gland: a gland from which secretions reach a free surface of the body by ducts. (E) Endocrine gland: a gland that has no ducts; its secretions are absorbed directly into the blood.

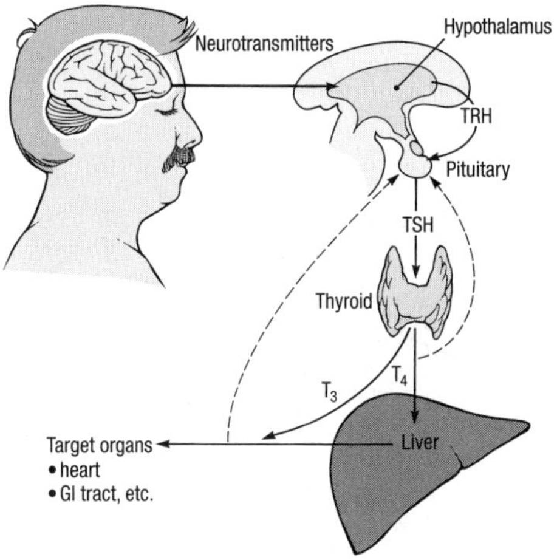

Figure 4. Hypothalamic-pituitary-thyroid axis. Thyroid-releasing hormone (TRH) from the hypothalamus stimulates the pituitary gland to secrete thyroid-stimulating hormone (TSH). TSH acts to produce thyroid hormone (T3 and T4). High circulating levels of T3 and T4 inhibit further TSH secretion and thyroid hormone production through a negative feedback mechanism (dashed lines). This image, created by Mikki Senkarik for *Stedman's Medical Dictionary, 27th Edition,* Baltimore, Lippincott Williams & Wilkins, 2000, p. 865, appears here with permission and courtesy of Lippincott Williams & Wilkins.

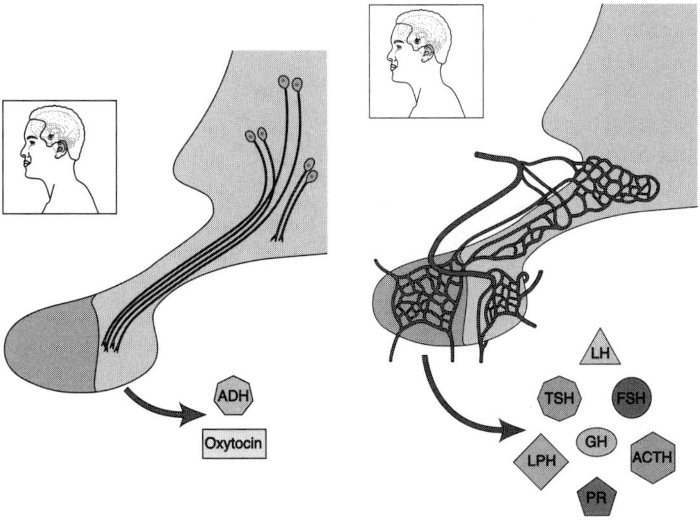

Figure 5. The pituitary gland consists of two major subdivisions: the neurohypophysis (left) and the adenohypophysis (right). ADH = antidiuretic hormone, LH = luteinizing hormone, TSH = thyroid-stimulating hormone, FSH = follicle-stimulating hormone, GH = growth hormone, LPH = lipotropic pituitary hormone, ACTH = adrenocorticotropic hormone, PR = prolactin.

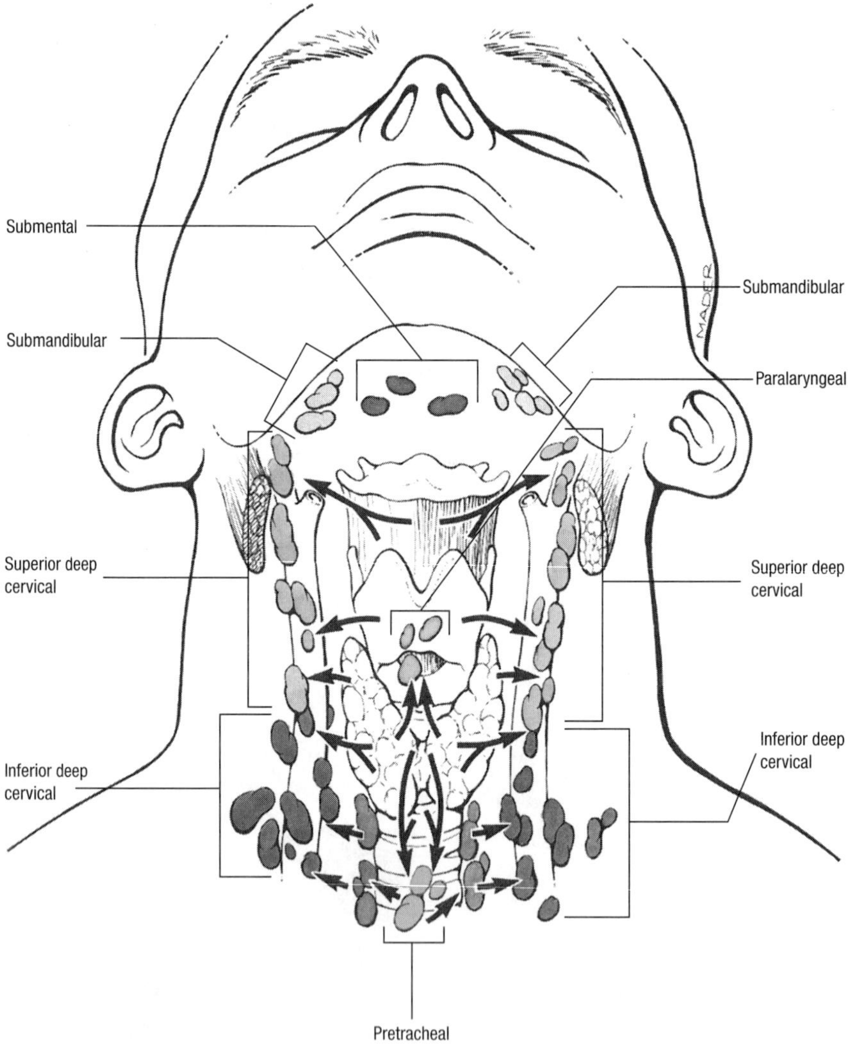

Figure 6. Lymphatic drainage of the thyroid gland, larynx, and trachea.

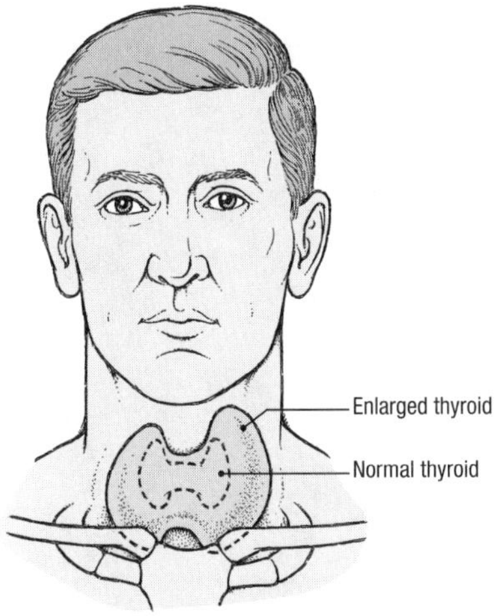

Figure 7. Goiter.

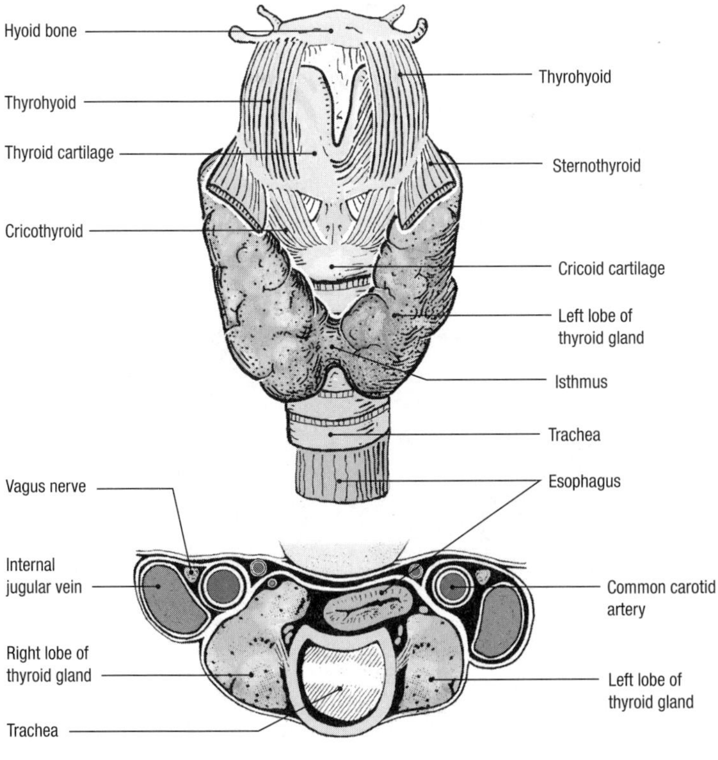

Figure 8. The thyroid gland and its relations in anterior view (top) and transverse section (bottom).

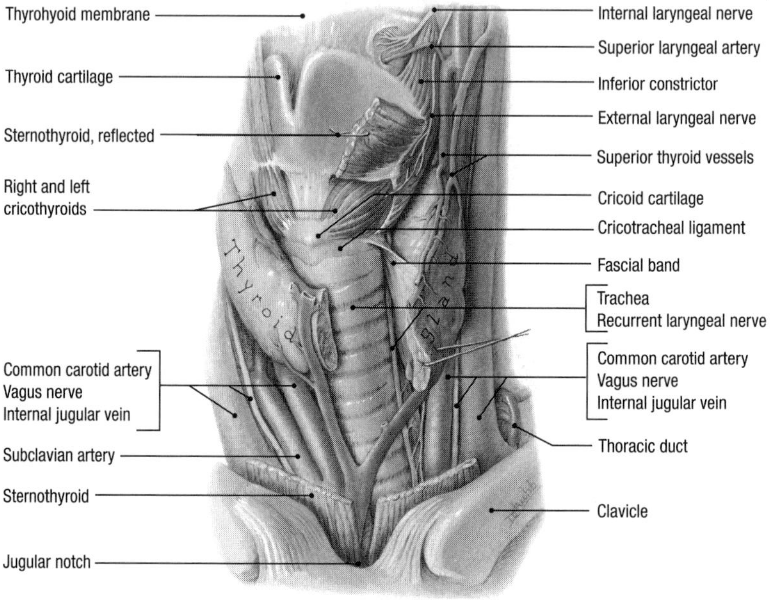

Figure 9. Thyroid gland retracted, anterolateral view of the neck. The isthmus of the thyroid gland is divided, and the left lobe is retracted.

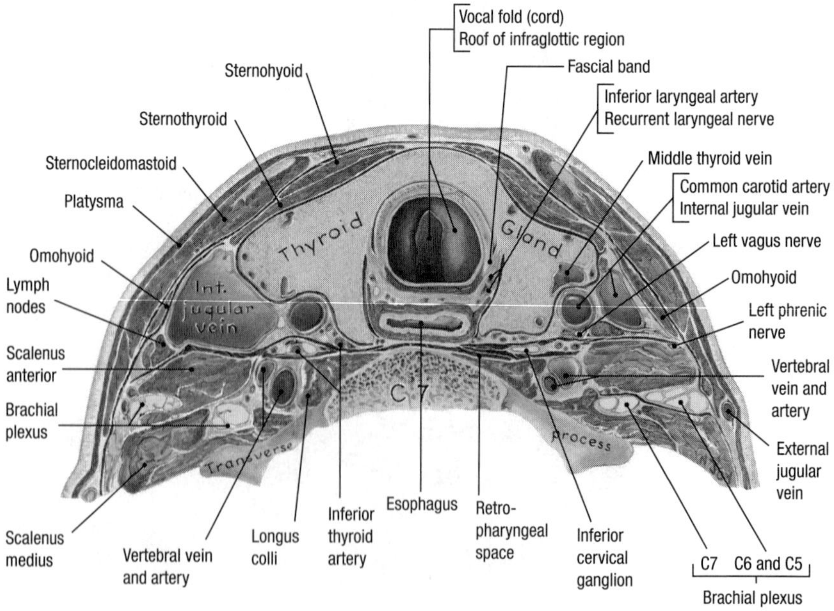

Figure 10. Transverse section of neck through thyroid gland.

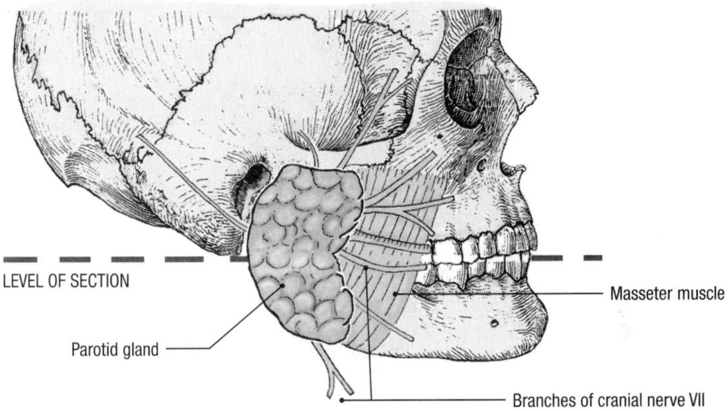

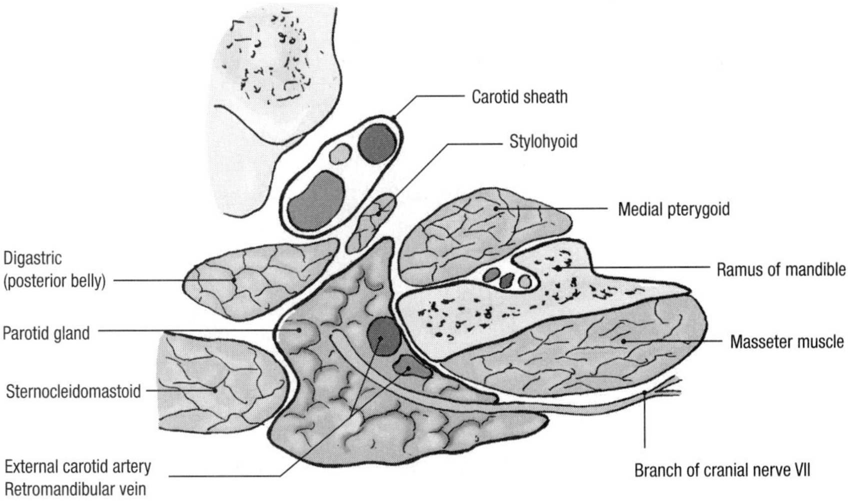

Figure 11. The parotid gland and its topographic relations. Orientation in lateral view and level section for the lower part of the illustration (top). Transverse section demonstrates the relations of the gland to surrounding and traversing structures (bottom).

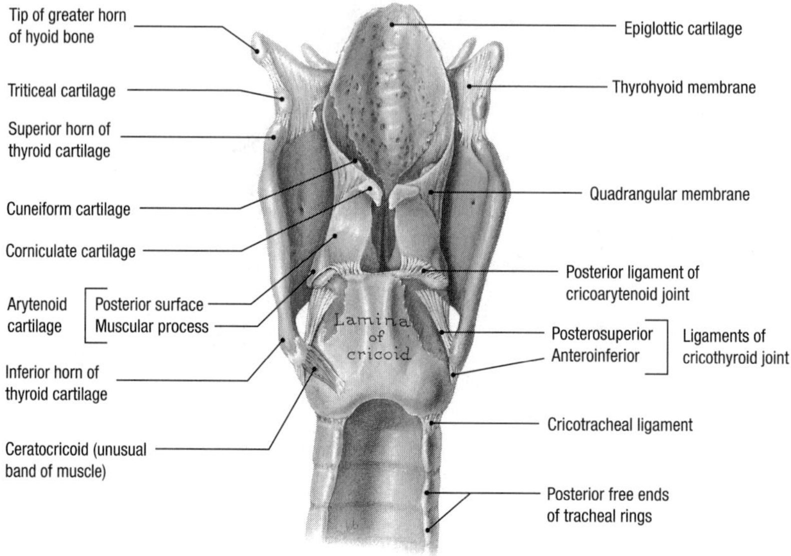

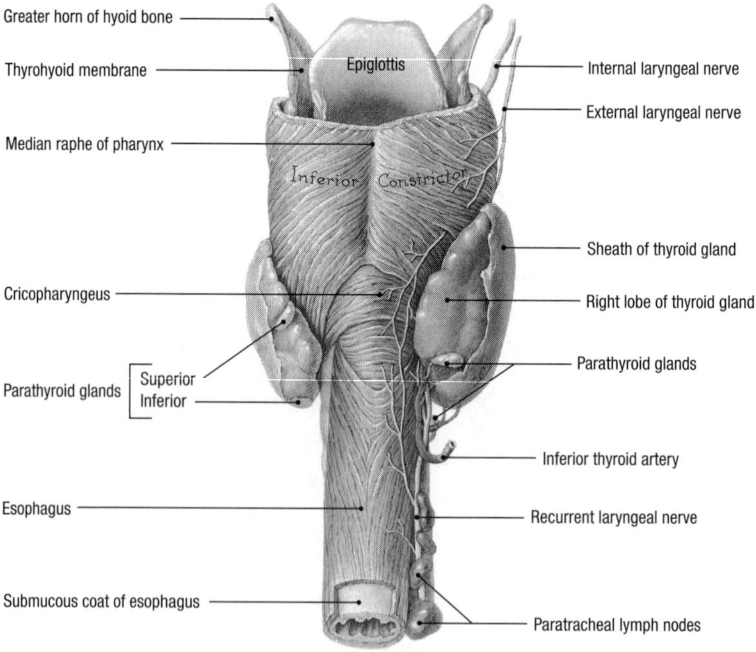

Figure 12. Skeleton of larynx, posterior view (top). Thyroid gland and laryngeal nerves, posterior view (bottom).

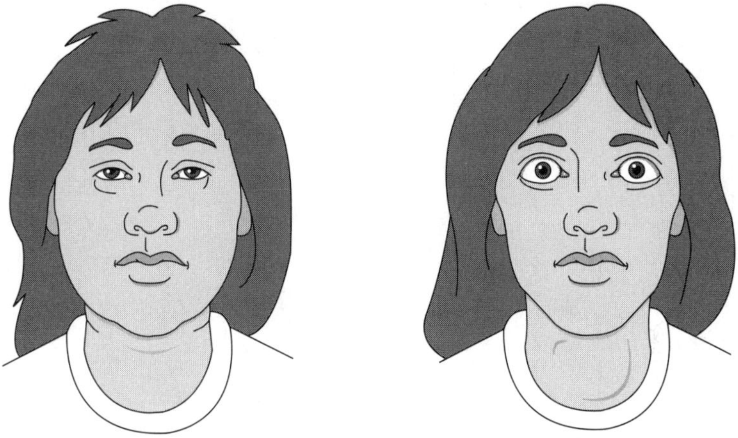

Figure 13. Hypothyroidism (left). Hyperthyroidism (right).

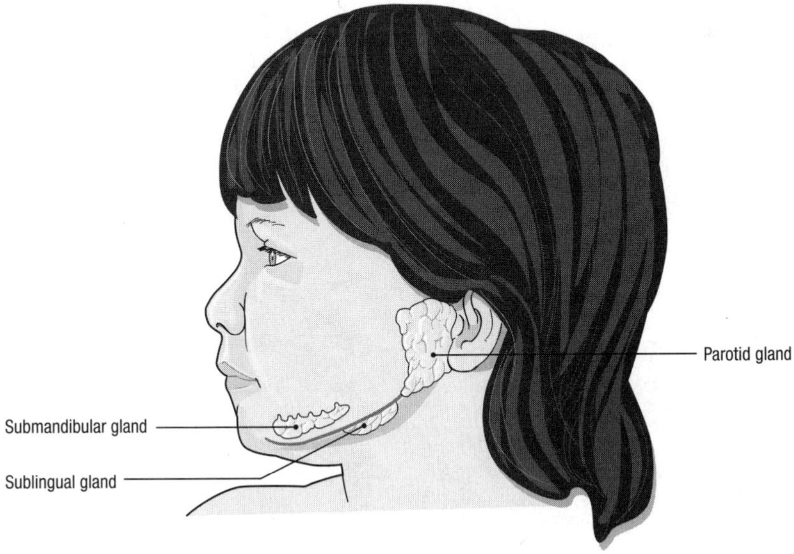

Figure 14. Lateral view of child showing location of the salivary glands.

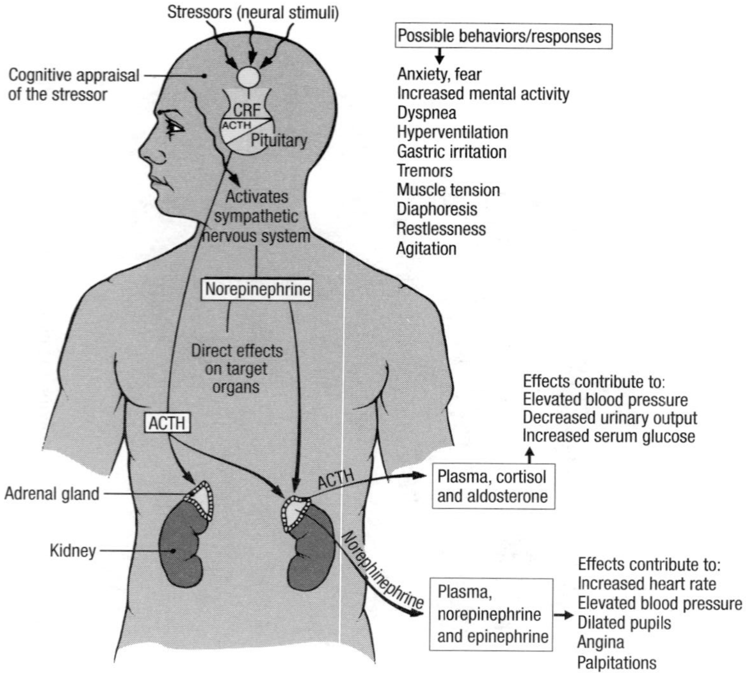

Figure 15. Stress response. Corticotropin releasing factor (CRF). Adrenocorticotropic hormone (ACTH). This image, created by Larry Ward for *Stedman's Medical Dictionary, 27th Edition,* Baltimore, Lippincott Williams & Wilkins, 2000, p. 1708, appears here with permission and courtesy of Lippincott Williams & Wilkins.

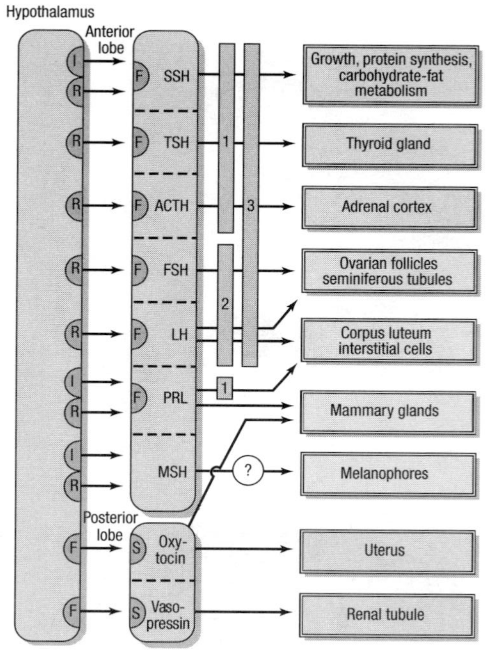

Figure 16. Hypophyseal hormones: (I) inhibiting hormones, (R) releasing hormones, (F) formation, (S) storage, (1) metabolic hormones, (2) gonadotropins, (3) glandotropic hormones. This image, created by Mary Anna Barratt-Dimes for *Stedman's Medical Dictionary, 27th Edition,* Baltimore, Lippincott Williams & Wilkins, 2000, p. 831, appears here with permission and courtesy of Lippincott Williams & Wilkins.

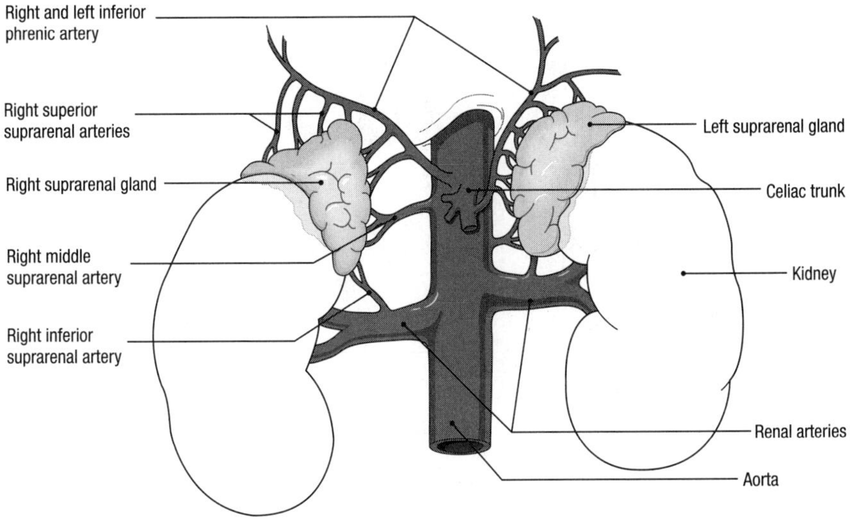

Figure 17. Arterial supply to adrenal glands and kidneys.

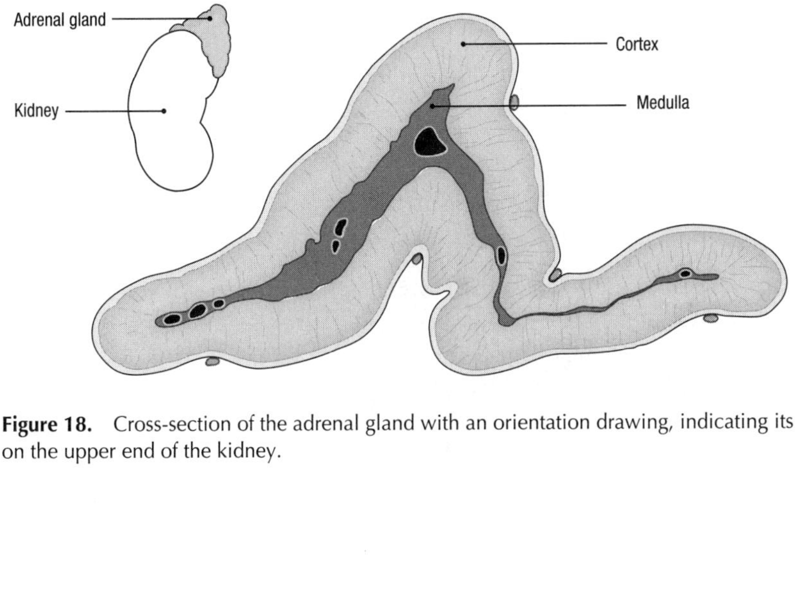

Figure 18. Cross-section of the adrenal gland with an orientation drawing, indicating its location on the upper end of the kidney.

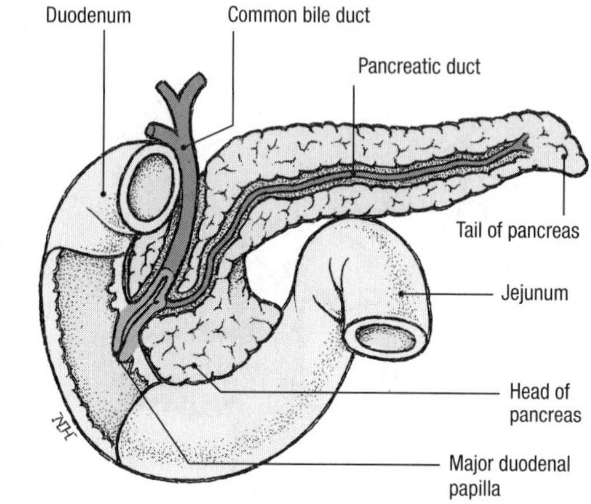

Figure 19. Pancreas (and part of duodenum).

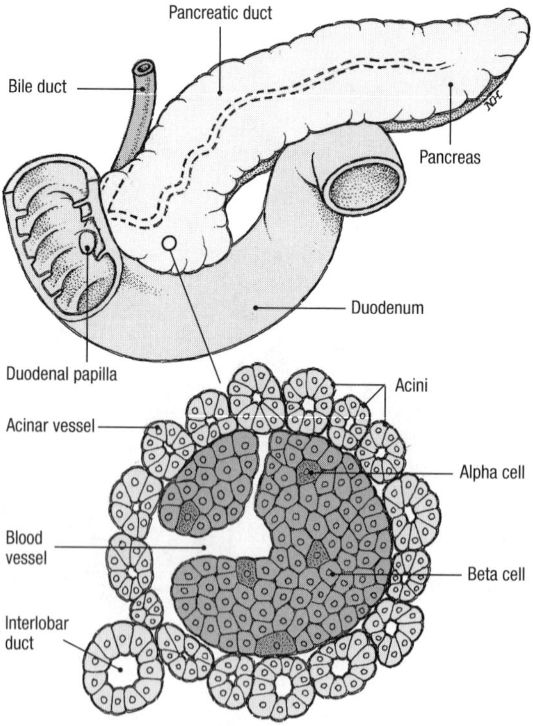

Figure 20. Islets of Langerhans.

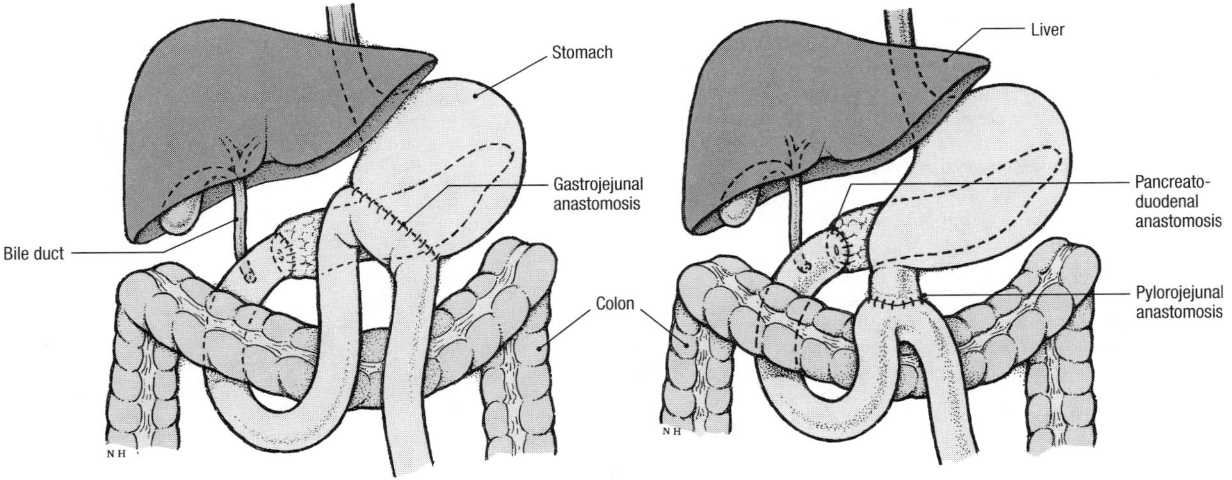

Figure 21. Pancreatoduodenectomy. Excision of all or part of the pancreas together with the duodenum and usually the distal stomach. Whipple operation (left). Pylorus-saving Whipple procedure (right).

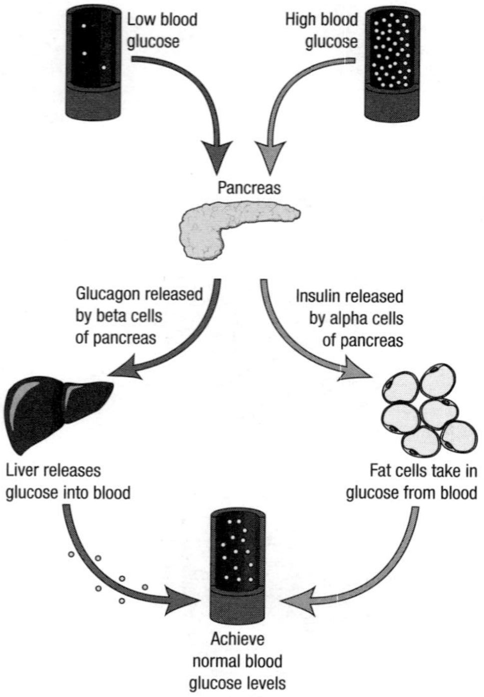

Figure 22. Blood sugar regulation.

Insulin (metabolic effects)			
Metabolic change	**Effect**	**Mechanism**	**Main organ**
1. Glucose transport	+	Unknown	Muscles, fatty tissue
2. Amino acid transport	+	Unknown	Muscles, fatty tissue
3. Potassium transport	+	Unknown; sometimes in connection with glucose transport	Liver, muscles
4. Glucose oxidation	+	Increased glucose transport into cells	Muscles, fatty tissue
5. Glycogen synthesis	+	Increased glucose transport into cells: activation of glycogen synthetase through dephosphorylation of the enzyme	Muscles, liver
6. Fatty acid synthesis	+	As in 4; plus reduction of acyl-CoA, increased acetyl-CoA from glucose resulting from activation of pyruvate dehydrogenase, release of acetyl-CoA-carboxylase	Fatty tissue, liver
7. Lipid synthesis	+	As in 4; plus production of α-glycerophosphate from glucose	Fatty tissue, liver, muscles
8. Protein synthesis	+	Activation of ribosomes (translation of messenger RNA)	Muscles, fibroblasts
9. Lipolysis	–	Antagonistic to lipolytic hormones; inhibition of adenylate cyclase	Fatty tissue, liver
10. Ketogenesis	–	Inhibition of fatty acid production through anti-lipolysis (see 9)	Liver
11. Gluconeogenesis and glycogenolysis	–	Inhibition of glucagon-stimulated glucose release; inhibition of adenylate cyclase	Liver
12. Proteolysis	–	Unknown; inhibition of urea production in the liver, through reduced production of amino acids	Liver, muscle

Figure 23. Insulin (metabolic effects). This table, created by Susan Caldwell for *Stedman's Medical Dictionary, 27th Edition,* Baltimore, Lippincott Williams & Wilkins, 2000, p. 908, appears here with permission and courtesy of Lippincott Williams & Wilkins.

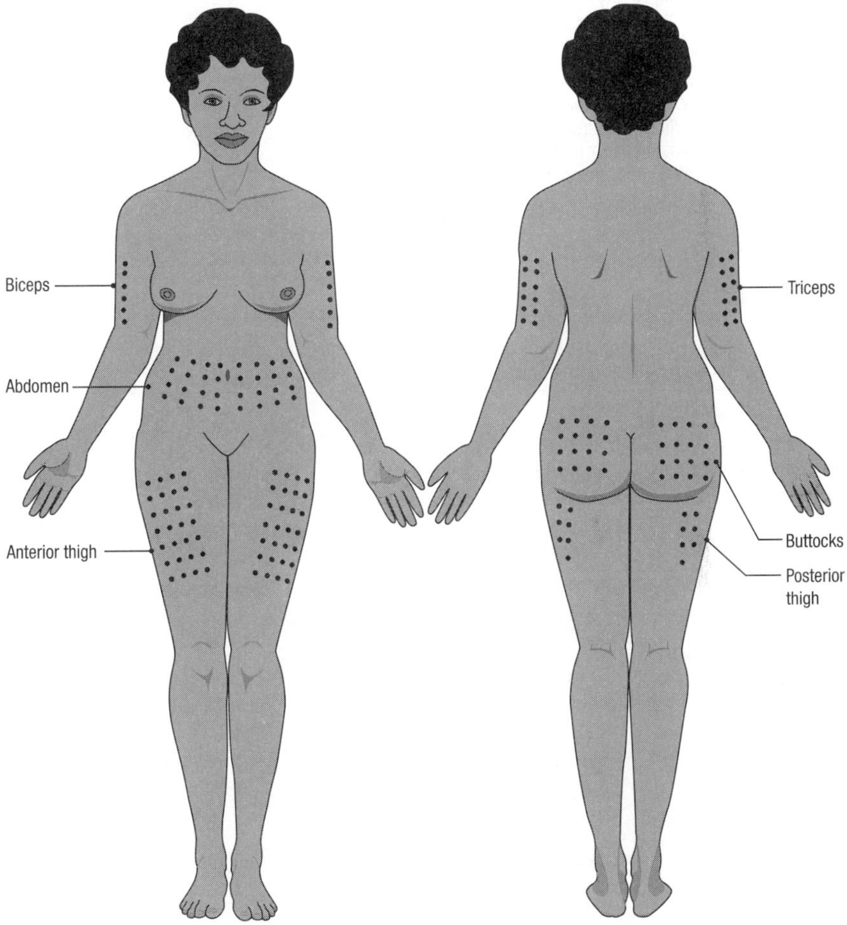

Figure 24. Anterior (left) and posterior (right) views of adult female showing multiple sites for insulin injection.

Diabetes mellitus (DM): Etiologic classification
I. Primary diabetes mellitus (types 1 and 2)
II. Secondary diabetes A. Pancreatic diabetes: – After total or partial pancreatectomy – With extensive destruction of pancreas – Through tumor or wound – Pancreatitis; hemochromatosis
B. Extrapancreatic/endocrine diabetes – With hypersomatotropism (acromegaly) – With hyperadrenalism (Cushing syndrome; Conn syndrome; pheochromocytoma) – With hyperthyroidism – With glucagonoma
C. Drug-induced diabetes – (Somatotropin; ACTH; adrenocorticoid [steroid diabetes]; thyroid hormone) – Thiazides
III. Rare, exceptional forms of diabetes e.g., Lipoatrophic diabetes (Lawrence); myatonic diabetes (Prader-Labhart-Willi); disturbance of insulin receptors; DM with certain genetic syndromes

Figure 25. Diabetes mellitus (DM): Etiologic classification. This table, created by Susan Caldwell for *Stedman's Medical Dictionary, 27th Edition,* Baltimore, Lippincott Williams & Wilkins, 2000, p. 490, appears here with permission and courtesy of Lippincott Williams & Wilkins.

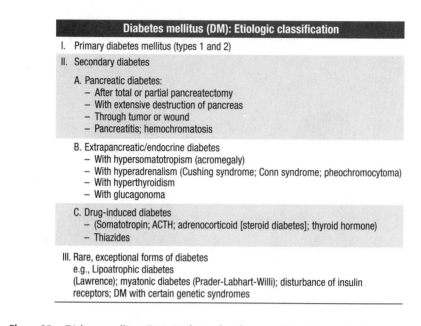

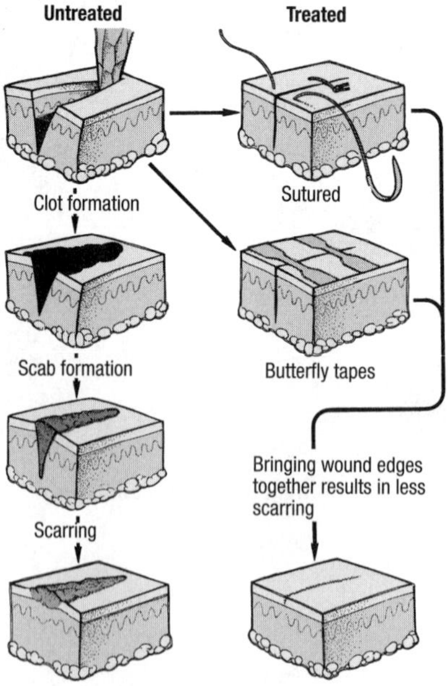

Figure 26. Wound healing.

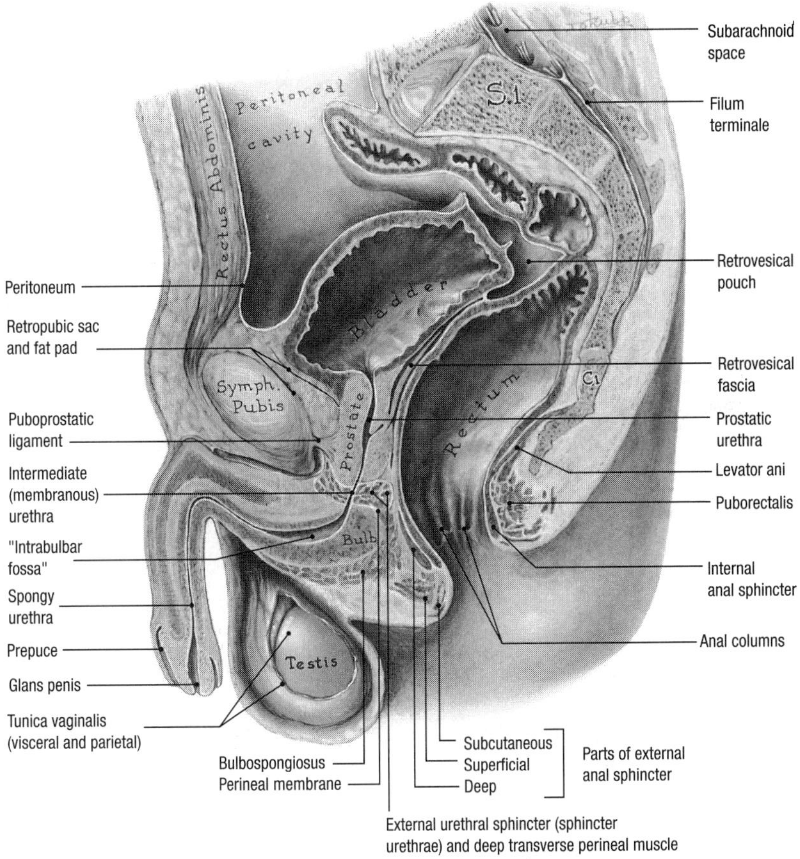

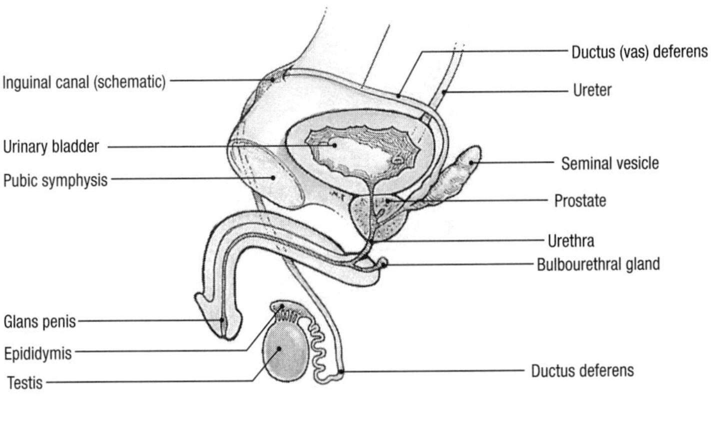

Figure 27. Male pelvis. Median section (top). Overview of urogenital system, median section (bottom).

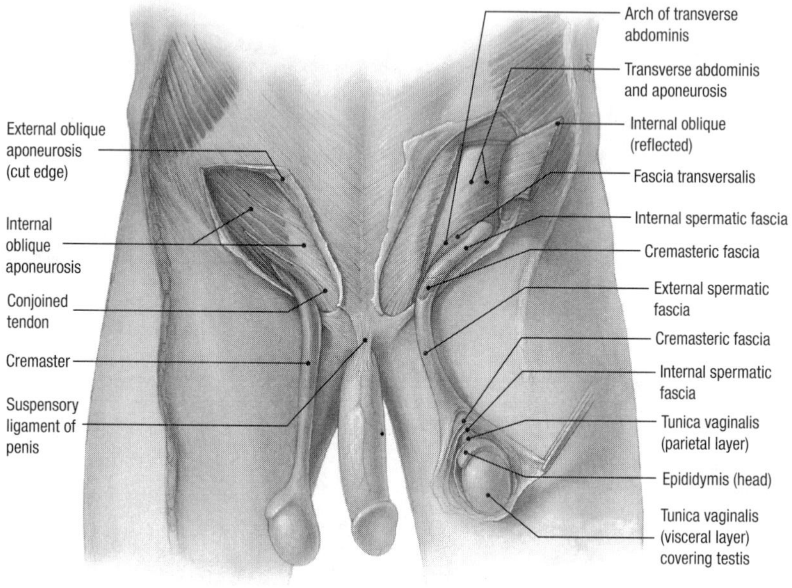

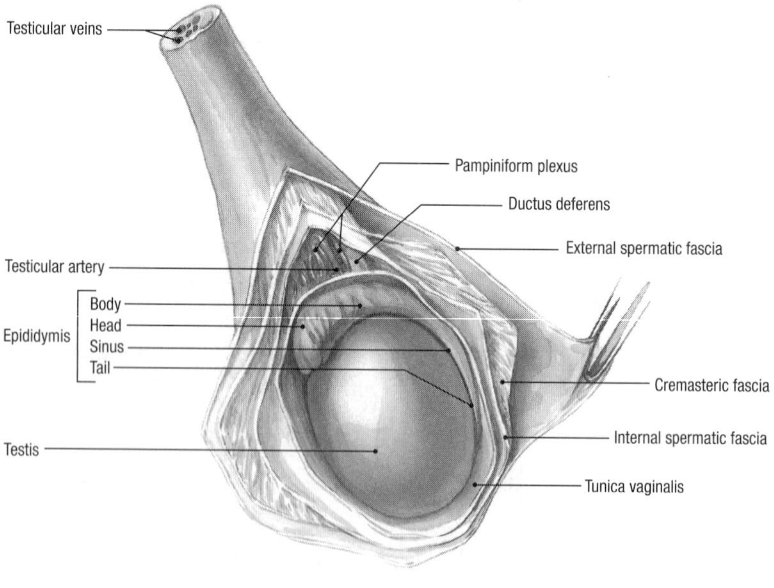

Figure 28. Coverings of spermatic cord and testis. Anterior view (top). Sequential dissection of coverings of testis, anterior view (bottom).

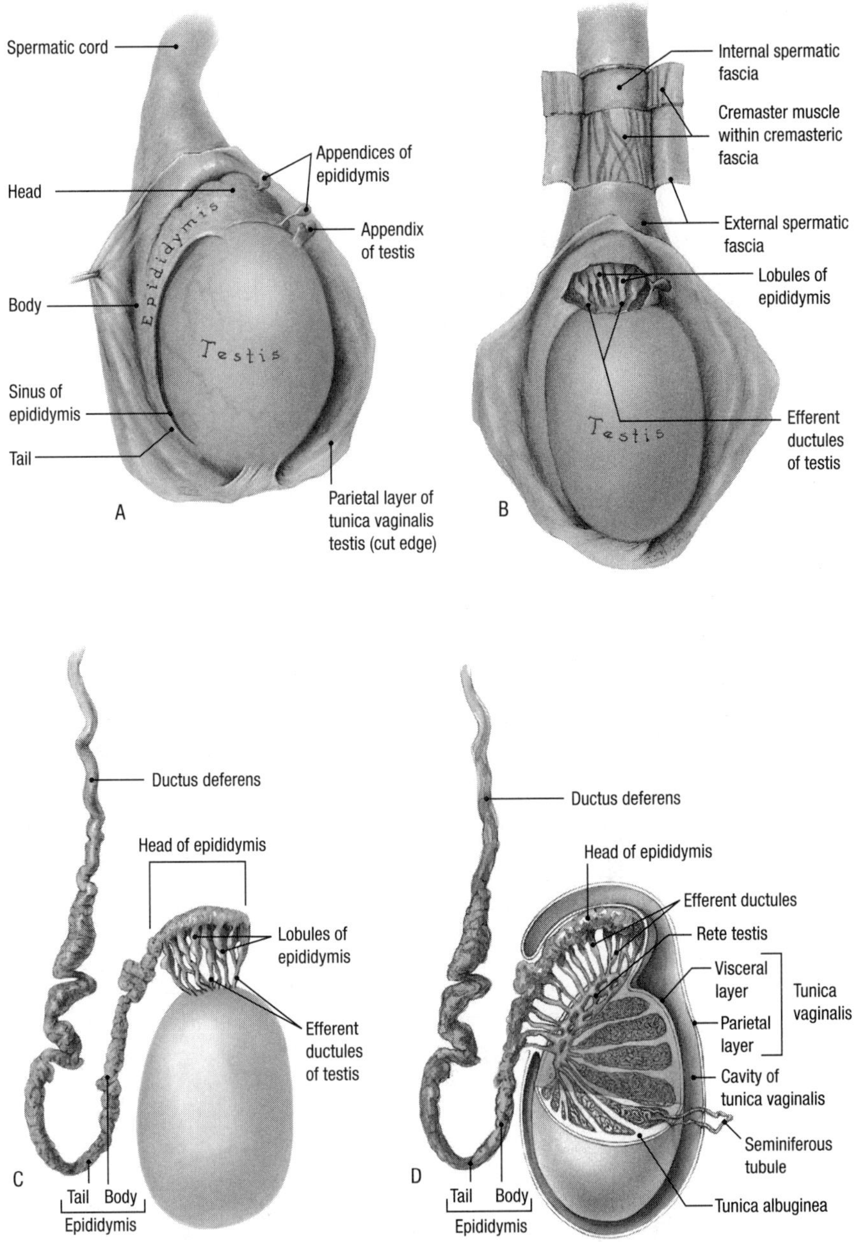

Figure 29. Testis and spermatic cord. (A) Testis, lateral view. (B) Coverings of the spermatic cord, lateral view. (C) Epididymis, lateral view. (D) Structure of the epididymis and testis, schematic vertical section.

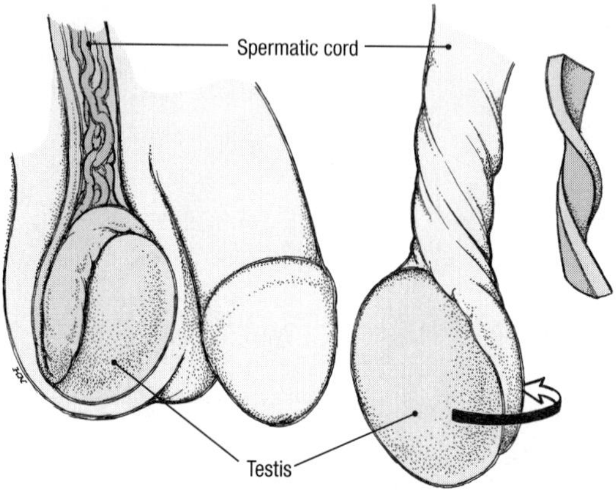

Figure 30. Torsion of the spermatic cord.

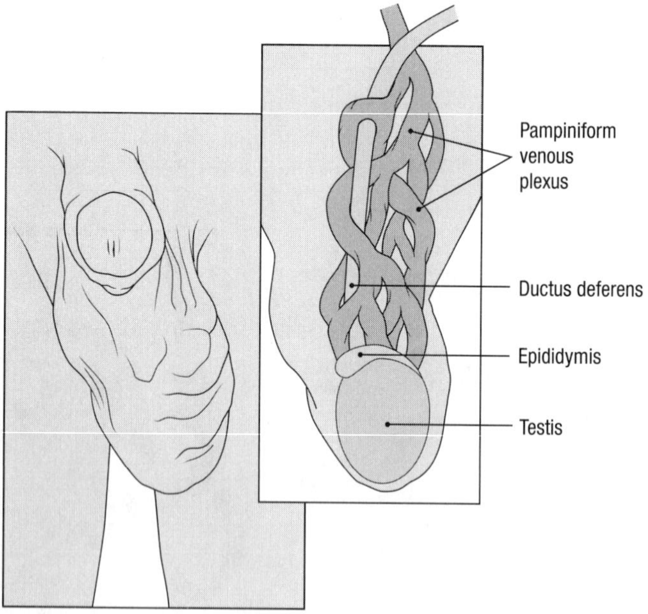

Figure 31. Varicocele. Image of male genitalia showing anatomical abnormality of left scrotum ("bag of worms" appearance). Insert shows internal anatomy of scrotum with abnormal dilation of the cremaster and pampiniform venous plexuses surrounding the spermatic cord.

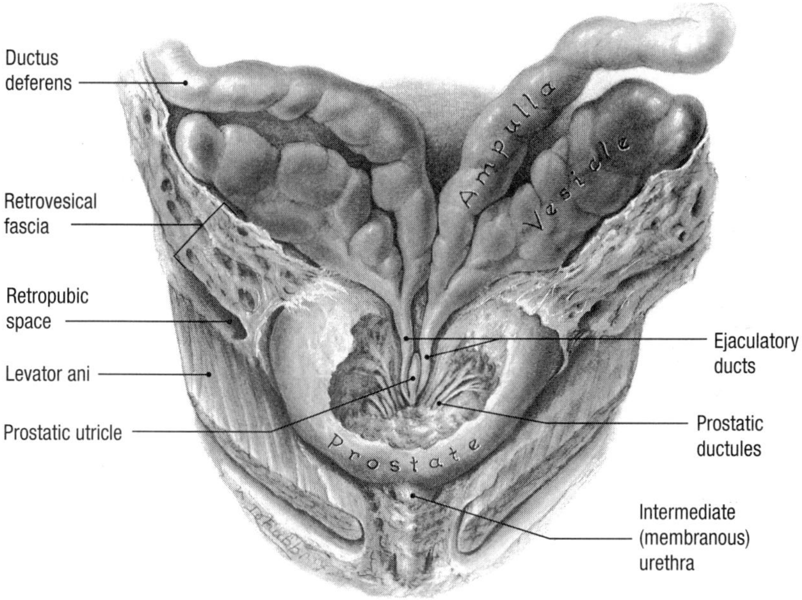

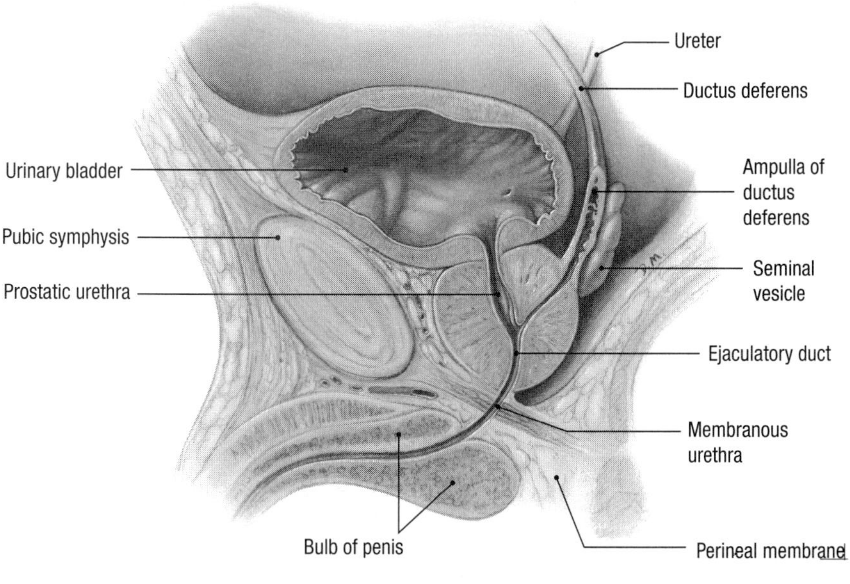

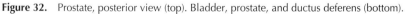

Figure 32. Prostate, posterior view (top). Bladder, prostate, and ductus deferens (bottom).

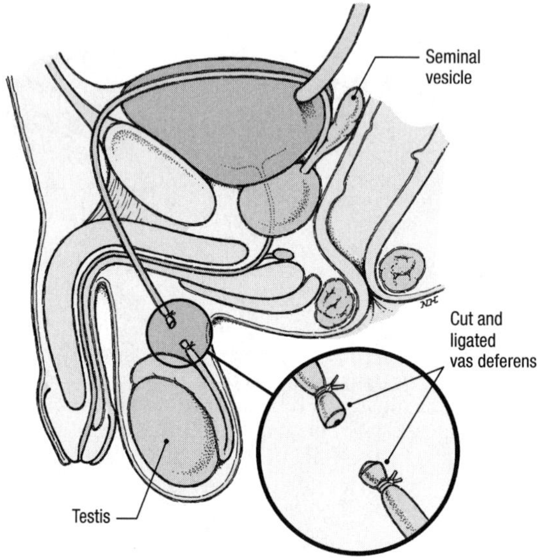

Figure 33. Vasectomy.

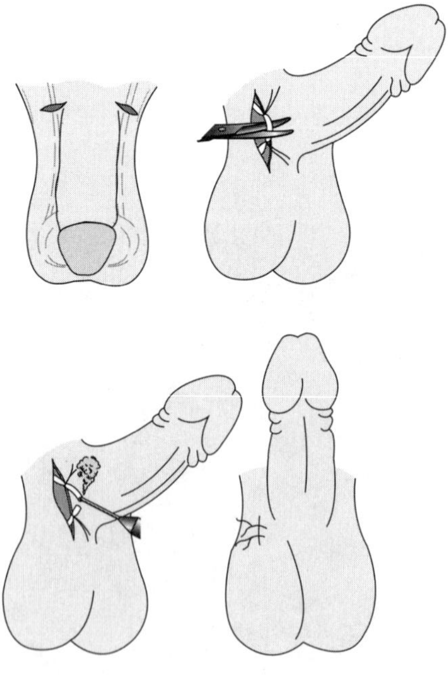

Figure 34. Vasectomy. External view of male genitalia showing vasectomy procedure. Site of incisions and location of vas deferens indicated (top left). Vas deferens pulled outside of body and cut with surgical scissors (top right). Cauterization of vas deferens (bottom left). Skin suture (bottom right).

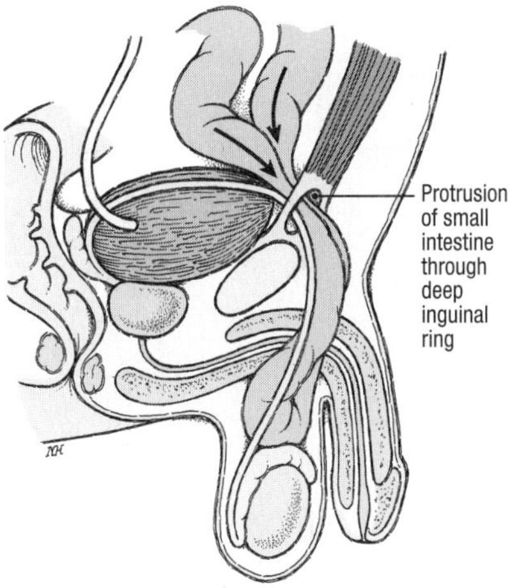

Figure 35. Indirect inguinal hernia.

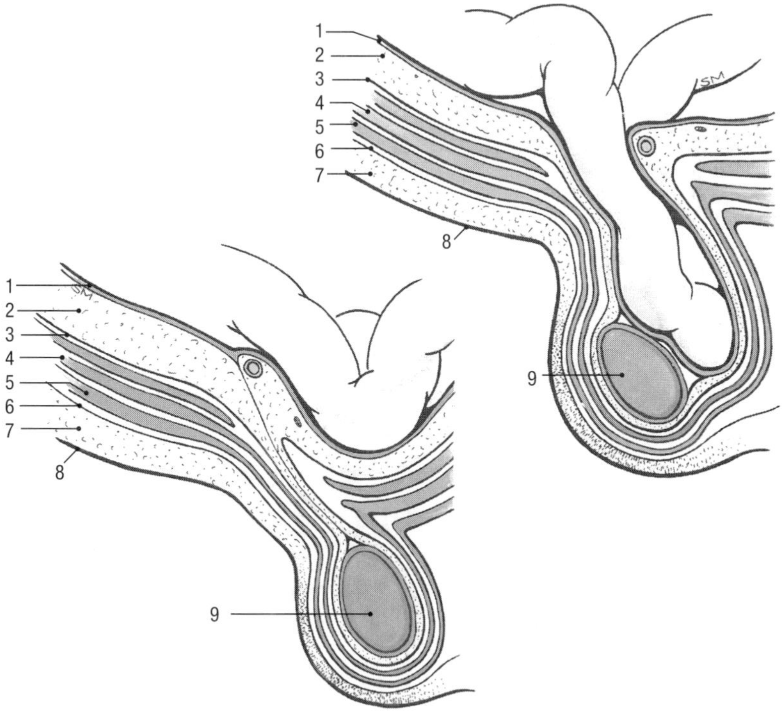

Figure 36. Indirect inguinal hernia (right). Direct inguinal hernia (left). (1) Peritoneum, (2), extraperitoneal fat, (3) fascia transversalis, (4) transversus abdominis, (5) internal oblique, (6) external oblique aponeurosis, (7) subcutaneous fat, (8) skin, (9) testis descending.

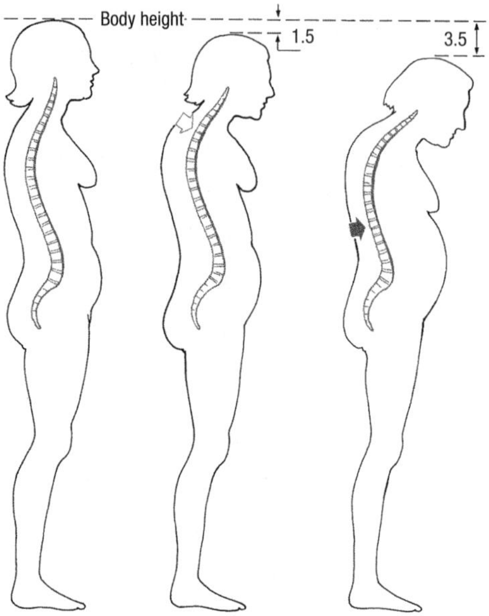

Figure 37. Osteoporosis and aging. Spinal column within outline of woman at 10 years postmenopause (left). Changes (loss of height) at 15 years postmenopause (center). Loss at 25 years postmenopause (right).

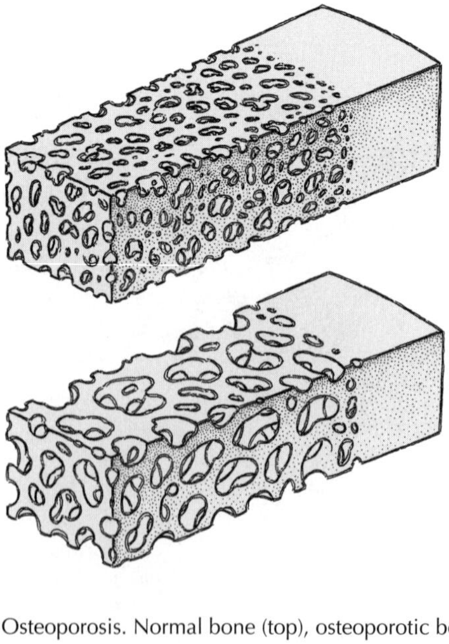

Figure 38. Osteoporosis. Normal bone (top), osteoporotic bone (bottom).

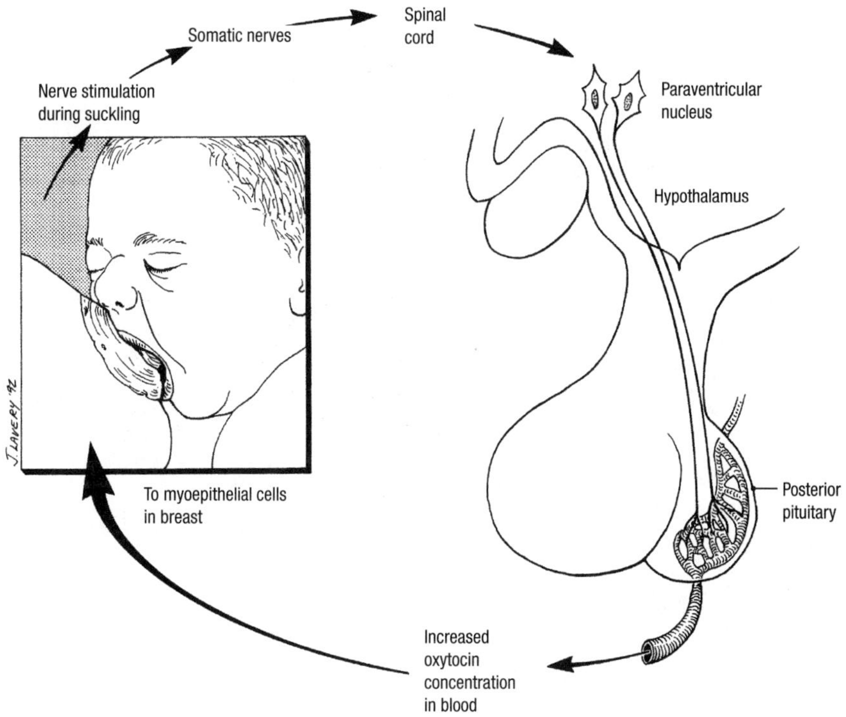

Figure 39. Breast lactation. Somatosensory pathways for the suckling-induced reduced reflex release of oxytocin.

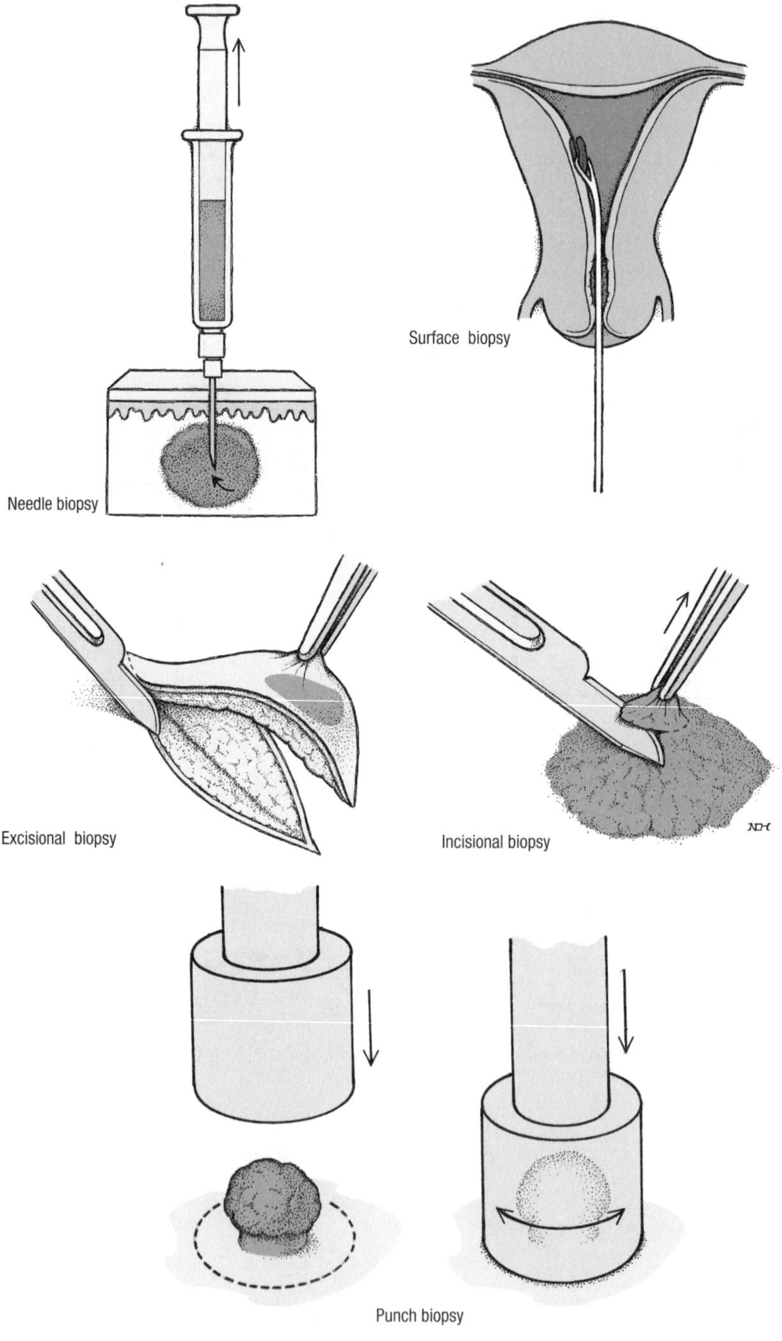

Figure 40. Biopsy techniques.

Appendix 2

Normal Lab Values

Tests	Conventional Units	SI Units
acetone		
serum		
qualitative	negative	negative
quantitative	0.3–2.0 mg/dL	0.05–0.34 mmol/L
urine		
qualitative	negative	negative
adrenocorticotropin (ACTH), plasma		
8 a.m.	<120 pg/mL	<26 pmol/L
midnight (supine)	<10 pg/mL	<2.2 pmol/L
aldosterone		
serum		
supine	3–16 ng/dL	0.08–0.44 nmol/L
standing	7–30 ng/dL	0.19–0.83 nmol/L
urine	3–19 μg/24 h	8–51 nmol/24 h
androstenedione, serum		
male	75–205 ng/dL	2.6–7.2 nmol/L
female	85–275 ng/dL	3.0–9.6 nmol/L
anion gap		
(Na–(Cl + HCO_3))	7–16 mEq/L	7–16 mmol/L
((Na + K)–(Cl + HCO_3))	10–20 mEq/L	10–20 mmol/L
calcium, serum	8.6–10.0 mg/dL	2.15–2.50 mmol/L
calcium, ionized, serum	4.64–5.28 mg/dL	1.16–1.32 mmol/L
calcium, urine		
low-calcium diet	50–150 mg/24 h	1.25–3.75 mmol/24 h
usual diet; trough	100–300 mg/24 h	2.50–7.50 mmol/24 h
cortisol, serum		
plasma		
8 a.m.	5–23 μg/dL	138–635 nmol/L
4 p.m.	3–16 μg/dL	83–441 nmol/L
10 p.m.	<50% of 8 a.m. value	<0.5% of 8 a.m. value
free, urine	<50 μg/24 h	<138 mmol/24 h
creatine kinase (CK), serum		
male	15–105 U/L (30°C)	0.26–1.79 μkat/L (30°C)
female	10–80 U/L (30°C)	0.17–1.36 μkat/L (30°C)
cyclic AMP		
plasma		
male	4.6–8.6 ng/mL	14–26 nmol/L
female	4.3–7.6 ng/mL	13–23 nmol/L
urine, 24 h	0.3–3.6 mg/d or 0.29–2.1 mg/g creatinine	100–723 μmol/d or 100–723 μmol/mol creatinine

continued

Tests	Conventional Units	SI Units
C-peptide, serum	0.78–1.89 ng/mL	0.26–0.62 nmol/L
dehydroepiandrosterone (DHEA), serum		
male	180–1250 ng/dL	6.2–43.3 nmol/L
female	130–980 ng/dL	4.5–34.0 nmol/L
dehydroepiandrosterone sulfate (DHEAS), serum or plasma		
male	59–452 μg/mL	1.6–12.2 μmol/L
female		
premenopausal	12–379 μg/mL	0.8–10.2 μmol/L
postmenopausal	30–260 μg/mL	0.8–7.1 μmol/L
free thyroxine index (FTI), serum	4.2–13	4.2–13
glucose (fasting)		
blood	65–95 mg/dL	3.5–5.3 mmol/L
plasma or serum	74–106 mg/dL	4.1–5.9 mmol/L
glucose, 2 h postprandial, serum	<120 mg/dL	<6.7 mmol/L
glucose, urine		
quantitative	<500 mg/24 h	<2.8 mmol/24 h
qualitative	negative	negative
glycated hemoglobin (hemoglobin A1c), whole blood	4.2%–5.9%	0.042–0.059
growth hormone, serum		
male	<5 ng/mL	<5 μg/L
female	<10 ng/mL	<10 μg/L
17-hydroxycorticosteroids urine		
male	3–10 mg/24 h	8.3–27.6 μmol/24 h (as cortisol)
female	2–8 mg/24 h	5.5–22 μmol/24 h (as cortisol)
insulin, plasma (fasting)	2–25 μU/mL	13–174 pmol/L
17-ketosteroids, urine		
male	10–25 mg/24 h	38–87 μmol/24 h
female	6–14 mg/24 h (decreases with age)	21–52 μmol/24 h (decreases with age)

continued

Tests	Conventional Units	SI Units
L-lactate		
plasma (NaF)		
venous	4.5–19.8 mg/dL	0.5–2.2 mmol/L
arterial	4.5–14.4 mg/dL	0.5–1.6 mmol/L
whole blood, at bedrest		
venous	8.1–15.3 mg/dL	0.9–1.7 mmol/L
arterial	<11.3 mg/dL	<1.3 mmol/L
urine, 24 h	496–1982 mg/d	5.5–22 mmol/d
CSF	10–22 mg/dL	1.1–2.4 mmol/L
lactate dehydrogenase (LDH) total (L→P), 37°C, serum		
adult	100–190 U/L	1.7–3.2 μkat/L
>60 y	110–210 U/L	1.9–3.6 μkat/L
lactate dehydrogenase (LDH) CSF	10% of serum value	0.10 fraction of serum value
magnesium		
serum	1.3–2.1 mEq/L 1.6–2.6 mg/dL	0.65–1.07 mmol/L 16–26 mg/L
urine	6.0–10.0 mEq/24 h	3.0–5.0 mmol/24 h
osmolality		
serum	275–295 mOsm/kg serum water	275–295 mmol/kg serum water
urine	50–1200 mOsm/kg serum water	50–1200 mmol/kg serum water
ratio, urine/serum	1.0–3.0, 3.0–4.7 after 12 h fluid restriction	1.0–3.0, 3.0–4.7 after 12 h fluid restriction
pH		
blood, arterial	7.35–7.45	7.35–7.45
urine	4.6–8.0	4.6–8.0
phosphatase, alkaline, total, serum	38–126 U/L (37°C)	0.65–2.14 μkat/L
phosphate, inorganic, serum	2.7–4.5 mg/dL	0.87–1.45 mmol/L
phosphorus, urine	0.4–1.3 g/24 h	12.9–42 mmol/24 h
potassium		
plasma		
male	3.5–4.5 mmol/L	3.5–4.5 mmol/L
female	3.4–4.4 mmol/L	3.4–4.4 mmol/L
serum		
premature		
cord	5.0–10.2 mmol/L	5.0–10.2 mmol/L
48 h	3.0–6.0 mmol/L	3.0–6.0 mmol/L
newborn, cord	5.6–12.0 mmol/L	5.6–12.0 mmol/L
adult	3.5–5.1 mmol/L	3.5–5.1 mmol/L
urine, 24 h	25–125 mmol/d	25–125 mmol/d
CSF	70% of plasma level or 2.5–3.2 mmol/L	0.70 of plasma level

continued

Tests	Conventional Units	SI Units
prolactin, serum		
male	2.5–15.0 ng/mL	2.5–15.0 μg/L
female	2.5–19.0 ng/mL	2.5–19.0 μg/L
protein, serum		
total	6.4–8.3 g/dL	64–83 g/L
testosterone, serum		
male	280–1100 ng/dL	0.52–38.17 nmol/L
female	15–70 ng/dL	0.52–2.43 nmol/L
pregnancy	3–4 × normal	3–4 × normal
postmenopausal	8–35 ng/dL	0.28–1.22 nmol/L
thyroid-stimulating hormone (TSH), serum	0.4–4.2 μU/mL	0.4–4.2 mU/L
thyroxine (T_4), serum	5–12 μg/dL (higher in pregnant women)	65–155 nmol/L (higher in pregnant women)
thyroxine, free, serum	0.8–2.7 ng/dL	10.3–35 pmol/L
thyroxine-binding globulin (TBG), serum	1.2–3.0 mg/dL	12–30 mg/L
triglycerides, serum, fasting		
desirable	<250 mg/dL	<2.83 mmol/L
borderline high	250–500 mg/dL	2.83–5.67 mmol/L
hypertriglyceridemic	>500 mg/dL	>5.65 mmol/L
triiodothyronine, total (T_3), serum	100–200 ng/dL	1.54–3.8 nmol/L
urea nitrogen, serum	6–20 mg/dL	2.1–7.1 mmol Urea/L
urea nitrogen/creatinine ratio, serum	12:1 to 20:1	48–80 urea/creatinine mole ratio
zinc, serum	70–120 μg/dL	10.7–18.4 μmol/L

Appendix 3

Endocrine Glands and Associated Products

Gland	Primary Products Secreted
adrenal	aldosterone, androstenedione, cortisol, dehydroepiandrosterone (DHEA), dehydroepiandrosterone sulfate (DHEAS), epinephrine, norepinephrine
hypothalamus	antidiuretic hormone (ADH), corticotropin-releasing hormone (CRH), dopamine, gonadotropin-releasing hormone (GnRH), growth hormone-releasing hormone (GHRH), somatostatin, thyrotropin-releasing hormone (TRH)
ovary	androstenedione, estradiol (E2), inhibin, testosterone
pancreas	glucagon, insulin, pancreatic polypeptide, somatostatin
parathyroid	parathyroid hormone (PTH)
pineal	melatonin
pituitary	adrenocorticotrophic hormone (ACTH), follicle-stimulating hormone (FSH), growth hormone, luteinizing hormone (LH), prolactin (PRL), thyroid-stimulating hormone (TSH)
testis	anti-müllerian hormone (AMH), estradiol, inhibin, müllerian inhibitory hormone (MIH), testosterone
thyroid	calcitonin, thyroxine (T4), triiodothyronine (T3)

Appendix 4

Classification of Diabetes

Type	Characteristics
type 1 diabetes mellitus also called insulin-dependent diabetes mellitus (IDDM) or juvenile-onset diabetes	• onset predominantly in youth, but can occur at any age • requires insulin to sustain life
type 2 diabetes mellitus also called noninsulin-dependent diabetes mellitus (NIDDM)	• cause thought to be strongly genetic • does not require insulin to sustain life • has subgroups of obese and nonobese • onset predominantly after age 40, but can occur at any age
gestational diabetes	• glucose intolerance that frequently has onset or recognition during pregnancy
class A gestational diabetes	• transient diabetes that reverts to normal after delivery
class B gestational diabetes	• duration less than 10 years • has been controlled by diet, but patient may become insulin-dependent during the pregnancy • may not need insulin after delivery • onset after age 20
class C gestational diabetes	• onset between ages of 10 and 19 • patient has been insulin-dependent and will need increased doses during pregnancy, but will return to prepregnancy dose after delivery
class D gestational diabetes	• duration more than 20 years • hypertension, diabetic retinopathy, and peripheral vascular disease are present • onset at less than age 10
class E gestational diabetes	• calcification of pelvic vessels is present
class F gestational diabetes	• diabetic nephropathy is present

Appendix 5

Wound Care Products

Bandages, Dressings (Including Foams and Gels)

ABD dressing
AcryDerm dressing
Adaptic gauze dressing
Alginate dressing
Algosteril alginate dressing
Allevyn foam dressing
Aquacel Hydrofiber wound dressing
Aquagel lubricating gel
Aquaphor gauze dressing
Aquasorb dressing
Baza cream
Bioclusive transparent dressing
BioPatch foam dressing
Blisterfilm transparent film dressing
CarboFlex odor control dressing
CarraSmart foam
ClearSite dressing
Coban bandage
Curafoam hydrophilic foam wound dressing
Curagel hydrogel wound dressing
Curasol gel wound dressing
Curasorb calcium alginate dressing
Cutinova foam dressing
Dermagran hydrophilic dressing
Dermagram zinc-saline wet dressing
DermaMend foam dressing
DermAssist glycerin hydrogel wound dressing
DuoDerm hydrocolloid dressing
DuoDerm hydroactive gel
Elasto-Gel occlusive dressing
Exu-Dry wound dressing
Flexderm hydrogel dressing
Flexzan foam dressing
Furacin dressing
Hyalofill dressing
Hydrogel sheet dressing
HyFIL wound gel
IntraSite gel hydrogel wound dressing
Iodoflex gel pad dressing
Iodosorb gel
Kaltostat wound packing dressing
Kerlix dressing
LoProfile foam dressing
Lyofoam polyurethane foam dressing
Medpore dressing
Mepitel nonadhesive silicone dressing
Microdon dressing
MultiPad nonadherent wound dressing
Nu Gauze dressing
Nu-Gel clear hydrogel wound dressing
NutraFil zinc hydrogel
OpSite occlusive dressing
Owen gauze
Polyderm foam dressing
Polymem dressing
PolyWic wound filler
Primapore dressing
ProCyte transparent film dressing
Reston foam dressing
2nd Skin dressing
Sof-Kling conforming bandage
Sofsorb wound dressing
Soft Cloth adhesive wound dressing
SoloSite wound gel
Sorbsan wound dressing
Tegaderm dressing
Tegagel hydrogel wound filler
Tegapore dressing
Telfa dressing
Telfa Clear dressing
TenderSorb Wet-Pruf ABD pad
ThinSite dressing
Tielle hydropolymer dressing
Transorbent dressing
Ventex dressing
Vigilon gel dressing

Webril dressing
Xeroform dressing

Cleansers

Allclenz wound cleanser
Biolex wound cleanser
Cara-Klenz wound cleanser
Chloresium solution
Clinical Care solution
ClinsWound wound cleanser
Curaklense wound cleanser
Debrisan wound cleaning paste
Dermagran wound cleanser
DermaMend
DiaB Klenz cleanser
Elta Dermal wound cleanser
Gentell foam cleanser
Gentell wound cleanser
Hyperion wound cleanser
Iamin wound cleanser
Lobana saline wound cleanser
MPM antimicrobial wound and skin cleanser
Optipore wound cleansing sponge
Puri-Clens wound deodorizer/cleanser
Restore wound cleanser
SAF-Clens wound cleanser
Sea-Clens wound cleanser
SeptiCare wound cleanser
Shur-Clens wound cleanser
Skintegrity wound cleanser
Techni-Care surgical scrub

Compression Dressings/Devices

Ace wrap
Aircast boot
Aircast EdemaFlow system
Circaid Thera-Boot
Coban elastic dressing
Elastikon tape
Elastoplast dressing
Foot Waffle air cushion
PlexiPulse pneumatic compression device
Profore four layer bandaging system
Setopress high compression bandage
SurePress compression bandage
Tubipad bandage
Unna boot
UnnaFlex bandage

Debriding Agents

Accuzyme debriding ointment
Panafil ointment
Pulsavac wound debridement system
Santyl ointment

Ointments, Creams, Lotions, Solutions

Vitamin A and D ointment
Amerigel ointment
Aquaphor ointment
Bactroban ointment
Biafine
Cloderm cream
Dermagran ointment
Diabicream
Domeboro astringent
Eucerin cream
Lac-Hydrin cream
Lamisil cream
Mitrazol cream
Mycolog cream
Neosporin ointment
Panafil ointment
Polysporin ointment
Santyl ointment
Silvadene cream
Ureacin lotion

Powders (antibacterial, antifungal, adhesive)

Furacin powder
Mitrazol powder
Multidex powder
nystatin powder
Stomahesive powder

Appendix 6

Sample Reports and Dictation

ABDOMINAL AND PELVIC CT WITH AND WITHOUT CONTRAST

DIAGNOSIS: Adrenal tumor versus ovarian tumor.

REPORT: Unenhanced axial images through the liver and kidneys followed by routine abdomen and pelvic CT with IV oral and rectal contrast was performed. The liver, spleen, both adrenal glands, both kidneys, and the vascular structures are all within normal limits except for two tiny, calcified splenic granuloma and mild, diffuse, fatty infiltration throughout the liver. There is no significant pelvic or abdominal lymphadenopathy. There are several loops of small bowel in the lower abdomen that appear to be adherent to the anterior abdominal wall, suggesting adhesions. The uterus is not identified, most likely from previous hysterectomy. Pelvic structures are, otherwise, unremarkable. There is a tiny, calcified granuloma in the posterior left lung base. Lung bases are, otherwise, clear.

IMPRESSION

1. Old granulomatous disease involving the spleen and left lower lobe.
2. Possible small bowel adhesions to the anterior abdominal wall but correlation with the patient's surgical history is recommended.
3. Probable previous hysterectomy.

ENDOCRINOLOGY OFFICE CONSULTATION

HISTORY: This is a 59-year-old woman who has been in good health. She had an incident where a thyroid nodule was discovered after referral to a general surgeon for a breast lump. At that time, thyroid ultrasound and fine-needle aspiration of a rather sizable cyst of the right lobe of the thyroid, as well as aspiration of a nodule on the left side were carried out. The findings suggested hemorrhage, and the patient was seen in followup six months later, and since that time she has noted no hoarseness, dysphagia, local tenderness, or other focal symptoms. She also has no symptoms suggestive of thyroid dysfunction, and her baseline thyroid function studies last September were noted to be normal. She does admit to loud snoring and some sleep difficulty with occasional fatigue the following day. This has been commented upon by her husband as being particularly coarse and loud in nature.

MEDICATIONS: She is on no medications except for Estraderm twice weekly.

FAMILY HISTORY: She does have a history of thyroid goiter in mother and grandmother.

PHYSICAL EXAMINATION: This is a healthy-appearing woman. Blood pressure is 130/74. Height is 5 feet 4 inches. Weight is 155 pounds. Integument is normal. She is well tanned. Eyes reveal no ophthalmopathy. Examination of the neck reveals a 2-cm nodular area in the lower part of the neck, which moves with swallowing. Otherwise, there is no enlargement of the thyroid. No lymphadenopathy or other abnormality. Chest is clear. She has no chest wall tenderness. Cardiac exam reveals a slow, regular rate and rhythm. Reflexes are normal.

LABORATORY DATA: Review of the ultrasound shows several cysts, one of which is sizable and compatible with a hemorrhagic cyst, as well as the suggestion of two demarcated adenomas, one of which was aspirated last October. The left-sided nodule did show follicular cells, although it is not stated whether there are adequate numbers, that is, six separate cells present.

IMPRESSION: Probable nodular hyperplasia with rather well-demarcated thyroid nodules, not palpable on clinical exam, and hemorrhagic thyroid cyst which has not changed in the last six months.

PLAN: A free T4 and TSH were obtained, and it was recommended that a re-exam and ultrasound be done in approximately six months.

ENDOCRINOLOGY OFFICE NOTE: DIABETES AND METABOLIC PROBLEMS

HISTORY: This woman is seen for evaluation and subsequent followup for her diabetes and metabolic problems. She has had diabetes for at least the last 20 years and has a rather complex history. But, in summary, her major problems at this time relate to her severe diabetic neuropathy, blindness due to diabetic retinopathy, autonomic neuropathy with orthostatic hypotension, gastroparesis, and what may apparently be a multiinfarct syndrome. She also has a history of hypertension, congestive heart failure, hypoplastic or aplastic anemia requiring intermittent transfusions, seizure disorder, and osteoporosis with multiple small fractures in the lower extremities. She had been on insulin for quite some time and has been on Calcimar in the past, but this was discontinued because of nausea. She has been taking 1000 mg calcium per day.

MEDICATIONS: Treatment of her diabetic neuropathy involves the use of analgesics, including Propacet, which she takes at bedtime. She is also on eyedrops, including Betagan, Antivert 25 mg tablets q.i.d., Trental, Ecotrin, Loprox cream for toenails on the left foot, Procardia XL 60 mg daily, milk of magnesia, Midrin for headaches, Phenergan suppositories p.r.n., selenium, and Synalar for her scalp condition, Entex, docusate, and Tegretol, which she is taking 400 mg at 8 a.m., 200 mg at noon, and 400 mg at bedtime. A recent Tegretol level was obtained. She is currently taking Novolin 70/30, 20 units in the morning, and Novolin N, 10 units in the afternoon, with extra Regular insulin, 2 units for a blood sugar of 201–250, 4 units for a 251–300 blood sugar, 6 units for a 301–350 blood sugar, 8 units for a 351–400 blood sugar, and 10 units for a blood sugar of 401–450. She is also taking Persantine 50 mg q.i.d., amitriptyline 50 mg at bedtime, and Reglan 10 mg q.i.d.

ALLERGIES: Penicillin, sulfa, Rocephin, and Dilantin.

PAST MEDICAL HISTORY: Her past medical history includes bacterial endocarditis in 1987.

Today, her husband is concerned with her chewing motions of the jaw, and blood sugars have been reasonably good of late on her current dose of insulin.

PHYSICAL EXAMINATION: This woman is legally blind. Eyes are not examined. Thyroid is not enlarged. She has a left carotid bruit. Her cardiac exam reveals a harsh grade 2/6 to 3/6 systolic ejection murmur, particularly heard best at the base. The extremities reveal no edema. She has no ischemic changes and has diminished sensation to pinprick on the distal right leg and on the entire left leg. She has absent ankle jerks and some onychomycosis, but no ulcerations.

IMPRESSION

1. Type 2b diabetes mellitus.
   A. Peripheral polyneuropathy.
   B. Autonomic neuropathy manifested by orthostatic hypotension and gastroparesis.
2. Hypertensive and probable arteriosclerotic heart disease with congestive heart failure, compensated.
3. Hypertension.
4. Seizure disorder.
5. Hypoplastic anemia.
6. Osteoporosis.

PLAN: Her primary care physician will continue to monitor blood counts and Tegretol level. I will monitor her blood sugars and any further recommendations for her diabetic neuropathy as it becomes necessary. For her osteoporosis, a bone density was obtained with the possibility of starting her on cyclic Didronel therapy, depending on her baseline studies.

Followup Letter to Referring Physician: Review of Thyroid Disease

Dear Dr. ________,

The patient was seen by me for review of thyroid disease. She has a history of Graves disease which was treated with PTU in January of 1991, and then treated with I-131 therapy in July of 1991. Several weeks following I-131 treatment she was begun on Synthroid replacement, which was increased to maximum dose of 0.15 mg and most recently on 0.125 mg. She has been troubled by palpitations and diarrhea and tremors in the past, which are all significantly improved. She does have some residual tremor. She continues to have irregular periods. She has not had significant local thyroid symptoms. She has mild exophthalmus but no significant impairment of vision. She does experience some moodiness.

Her exam shows height of 5 feet 3–1/4 inches, weight of 128 pounds, pulse 88, blood pressure 140/88. Eye exam shows mild prominence at 92 mm span of 15 mm bilaterally with intact extraocular movements. Thyroid gland is small. Heart shows an intermittent click consistent with mitral valve prolapse. She has a mild tremor. Deep tendon reflexes are normal and remainder of the exam is unremarkable. Thyroid studies are enclosed and show mild elevation of TSH to 8.7, suggesting a need for increased thyroid replacement. I have, therefore, asked her to increase Synthroid to 0.125 mg on Tuesday, Thursday, Saturday, and Sunday, and 0.15 mg on Monday, Wednesday, and Friday. In the past, thyroid studies were elevated with suppressed TSH on a dose of 0.15 mg daily. I have asked her to have these rechecked in six months by you. I would be happy to discuss with you or to see her again for any further thyroid management. Please call me if you need to discuss this with me.

Yours sincerely,

Iodine 123 Uptake and Scan Report

Report: A total of 234.9 mCi of I-123 was orally given to the patient in capsule form. The four-hour thyroid uptake is calculated to be 15.8% (normal is 4%–10%), while the 24-hour uptake is calculated to be 27.1% (normal being 13%–45%).

Posterior and both anterior oblique images of the thyroid gland show the left lobe to be moderately diffusely enlarged with only minimal activity seen within the right thyroid, which is much smaller in size. No focal areas of increased or decreased radiotracer accumulation are seen within either lobe.

IMPRESSION

1. Elevated four-hour uptake but normal 24-hour I-123 thyroid uptake.
2. Moderately diffusely enlarged left lobe of the thyroid gland with the vast majority of the activity within the left lobe but no focal abnormalities present in either lobe of the thyroid gland.

OFFICE VISIT FOR FOLLOWUP OF SCHEDULED TREATMENT FOR HYPERTHYROIDISM AND HYPERANDROGENISM

The patient comes back for a followup visit.

Hyperthyroidism: The patient had her thyroid tests repeated. TSH remains suppressed below 0.04. Free T4 and total T4 remain in the upper limit of normal. Her antimicrosomal antibodies are negative. Thyroid scan and uptake show predominantly active uptake in the left lobe. These findings make the diagnosis of multinodular toxic goiter more likely than Graves disease. The thyroid antibodies are negative as well.

I think that at this point treatment with radioactive iodine would be the best option anyway. I talked about other available options like antithyroid medications and surgery. The patient is more inclined to go with radioactive iodine treatment and understands that she will need to receive lifelong replacement with Synthroid.

Hyperandrogenism: The patient's testosterone is elevated at 71. Sex hormone binding globulin is mid-normal range at 49. Free testosterone is in mid-normal range. Prolactin is normal. This is very puzzling in light of her total hysterectomy and oophorectomy. To confirm that, we obtained operative report from the hospital where she had her surgery. It looks like both ovaries were removed completely. The source of excessive androgens remains unclear to me. The patient does not look cushingoid.

We will obtain some additional tests including ACTH, 17-hydroxyprogesterone, a.m. cortisol, and DHEAS. Differential diagnosis would be between Cushing disease (unlikely), late-onset congential adrenal hyperplasia, and androgen-producing tumor of adrenals or ovaries. Some hilar cells might have been left behind during oophorectomy.

I discussed with the patient that probably the next step would be CT of adrenals and pelvis. For now, we will start Propecia to slow down the hair loss. We also talked about the possibility of telogen effluvium once she is restored to euthyroidism. This should be completely reversible.

Radioactive Iodine Therapy

Exam: NM I-131 therapy hyperthyroid.

Clinical Data: History of Graves disease.

History: This is a 46-year-old female with suppressed TSH and elevated T3 with complaints of tiredness, difficulty sleeping, and increased sweating.

An I-123 uptake and scan demonstrated a four-hour uptake of 15.8% (normal being 4%–10%) and 24-hour uptake at 27.1% (normal being 13%–45%).

Procedure: A single capsule with 21.3 mCi of I-131 was provided for oral ingestion after explaining risk/benefit of radioactive iodine therapy.

Impression: Radioactive iodine therapy provided for hyperthyroidism.

Thyroid Cancer Surgery Discharge Summary

Discharge Diagnosis: Follicular thyroid cancer.

Hospital Course: The patient came into the same-day surgery department on Friday, four days prior to this dictation. She underwent an uneventful left thyroid lobectomy, and intraoperatively her frozen section diagnosis was follicular adenoma. She did well postoperatively and was subsequently prepared for discharge. However, the pathology demonstrated that she had a moderately well-differentiated follicular cancer. A completion thyroidectomy was then planned, and she was returned to the operating room. The contralateral lobe was then removed. Parathyroid glands were well identified as were the recurrent laryngeal nerves bilaterally, and the procedure was well tolerated.

Postoperatively, her calcium level was 7.9, with a preoperative calcium of 8.5. She had no Chvostek or Trousseau sign on postoperative examination and felt no irritability. She had some very mild hoarseness after the second operation but good phonation and was able to cough well. She was instructed on postoperative wound care, and it was discussed with her that she should have radioiodine ablation in several weeks when she becomes hypothyroid.

Plans are to discharge her home on oral Vicodin for pain and have her return to the office later in the week. Additional plans for outpatient ablation will be forthcoming.

THYROID LOBECTOMY AND TOTAL THYROIDECTOMY

PREOPERATIVE DIAGNOSIS: Left thyroid mass, possible malignancy of the thyroid gland.

POSTOPERATIVE DIAGNOSIS: Carcinoma of the left thyroid lobe, possible Hürthle cell, possible papillary. Final diagnosis pending.

OPERATION: Left thyroid lobectomy followed by total thyroidectomy.

ANESTHESIA: General endotracheal.

BRIEF HISTORY: The patient noted a large lump in the left side of the neck. On evaluation by the primary physician, it was felt this was a solid lesion. It was cold on thyroid scanning. The patient was euthyroid. It was felt the patient needed surgical excision of this large mass by thyroid lobectomy, followed by subtotal or total thyroidectomy if carcinoma was identified.

PROCEDURE: With the patient under satisfactory general anesthesia, the neck was prepped and draped in a sterile fashion.

A curvilinear incision was made along the skin lines above the sternal notch. The skin, subcutaneous tissue, and platysma were incised. Large subplatysmal flaps were created superiorly to the level of the thyroid notch and inferiorly to the level of the sternal notch. The strap muscles were split along the midline and retracted laterally. The large left thyroid lobe was dissected from its loose attachments laterally. The superior pole was taken down with ligatures of 2–0 silk and Hemoclips as needed. Mobilizing the lobe inferiorly similarly, the inferior pedicles were taken down with ligatures as well. Rotating the gland medially after this was done allowed visualization of the course of the recurrent laryngeal nerve. No parathyroid tissue was identified on the gland, as the dissection was kept directly on the thyroid gland surface. Hemoclips were used for hemostasis and control of any small tributaries. Following retraction of the entire gland off the trachea, the isthmus was divided with hemostatic ligatures of 2–0 silk.

The isthmus was sent for pathologic examination. The pathologist identified carcinoma in the gland with features suggestive of Hürthle cell carcinoma or papillary. With this information, it was elected to proceed with a total thyroidectomy.

A similar dissection was carried out on the right side with the superior pedicle being controlled first with ligatures of 2–0 silk and Hemoclips. Laterally and inferiorly the loose attachments were taken down. The inferior pedicle was subsequently divided in a similar manner as the superior pedicle. Rotating the gland medially and identifying the course of the recurrent laryngeal nerve, a superior parathyroid gland was found, dissected off the thyroid gland, and left intact. (No parathyroid tissue had been identified thus far, and the specimen was removed.)

Hemostasis was again achieved with Hemoclips. A small tributary that was entered in the gland during the dissection was kept on top of the thyroid gland all the way through. Again, the peritracheal attachments were taken down with ligatures of 2–0 silk. The isthmus was also removed separately.

Both sides of the neck were checked for hemostasis, thoroughly lavaged, and pressure reevaluated. No evidence of bleeding or oozing was noted.

The wound was closed with the strap muscles then closed with 3–0 Vicryl. The platysmal flaps were closed with 3–0 Vicryl as well. The skin was closed with 4–0 Prolene subcuticular suture.

The patient tolerated the procedure well. The subcutaneous tissues and skin were infiltrated with local anesthetic. The patient was taken to the recovery room in satisfactory condition. The patient had good vocal cord function in the recovery room. A calcium level was to be drawn later in a few hours to evaluate for any hypocalcemia.

THYROID SONOGRAM

STUDY: The left gland measures 4.4 x 3.0 x 2.7 cm. The right gland measures 4.4 x 2.2 x 1.6 cm. The right gland is very heterogeneous, and there are multiple small hypoechoic nodules present. Within the left gland there is a large, 3.6-cm, solid mass. Recommend correlating with nuclear medicine study.

IMPRESSION: Heterogenous right gland. Solid, 3.6-cm mass seen within the left gland. Recommend correlation with nuclear medicine study.

Appendix 7

Common Terms by Procedure

Abdominal and Pelvic CT With and Without Contrast

abdomen computed tomography (CT)
abdominal lymphadenopathy
adrenal tumor
axial image
granulomatous disease
ovarian tumor
pelvic computed tomography (CT)
rectal contrast
splenic granuloma
unenhanced axial image

Endocrinology Office Consultation

demarcated adenoma
dysphagia
Estraderm
follicular cell
goiter
hemorrhagic thyroid cyst
hoarseness
lymphadenopathy
nodular hyperplasia
nodule
ophthalmopathy
thyroid function study
thyroid nodule
thyroid ultrasound

Endocrinology Office Note: Diabetes and Metabolic Problems

amitriptyline
Antivert
aplastic anemia
arteriosclerotic heart disease
autonomic neuropathy
bacterial endocarditis
Betagan
blindness
Calcimar
diabetes
diabetic neuropathy
diabetic retinopathy
Didronel therapy
docusate
Ecotrin
Entex
gastroparesis
hypertension
hypoplastic anemia
insulin
Loprox
metabolic problem
multiinfarct syndrome
Novolin 70/30
Novolin N
onychomycosis
orthostatic hypotension
osteoporosis
peripheral polyneuropathy
Persantine
Phenergan
Procardia XL
Propacet
Reglan
Regular insulin
seizure disorder
Synalar
Systolic ejection murmur
Tegretol
Trental

Followup Letter to Referring Physician: Review of Thyroid Disease

diarrhea
exophthalmus
Graves disease

I-131 therapy
palpitations
partial thromboplastin (PTU)
PTU
Synthroid replacement
thyroid disease
thyroid-stimulating hormone (TSH)
tremor
TSH

Iodine 123 Uptake and Scan Report

anterior oblique image
I-123 thyroid uptake
mCi
microcuries (mCi)
radiotracer accumulation
thyroid uptake

Office Visit for Followup of Scheduled Treatment for Hyperthyroidism and Hyperandrogenism

ACTH
active uptake
adrenocorticotropic hormone (ACTH)
androgen
androgen-producing tumor
antimicrosomal antibody
antithyroid medication
congenital adrenal hyperplasia
cortisol
Cushing disease
cushingoid
dehydroepiandosterone sulfate (DHEAS)
DHEAS
effluvium
euthyroidism
free T4
free testosterone
Graves disease
hilar cell
17-hydroxyprogesterone
hyperandrogenism
hyperthyroidism
multinodular toxic goiter
prolactin
Propecia
radioactive iodine
sex hormone binding globulin
Synthroid
telogen
testosterone
thyroid antibody
thyroid scan
thyroid-stimulating hormone (TSH)
thyroid test
thyroid uptake
total T4
TSH

Radioactive Iodine Therapy

elevated T3
Graves disease
hyperthyroidism
I-123 uptake and scan
I-131
radioactive iodine therapy
suppressed thyroid-stimulating hormone (TSH)

Thyroid Cancer Surgery Discharge Summary

Chvostek sign
completion thyroidectomy
contralateral lobe
follicular adenoma
follicular thyroid cancer
hypothyroid
parathyroid gland
phonation
radioiodine ablation
recurrent laryngeal nerve
thyroid lobectomy
Trousseau sign

Vicodin
well-differentiated follicular cancer

Thyroid Lobectomy and Total Thyroidectomy

curvilinear incision
euthyroid
Hemoclip
hemostasis
Hürthle cell carcinoma
hypocalcemia
inferior pedicle
isthmus
lavaged
ligature
papillary carcinoma
parathyroid gland
parathyroid tissue
peritracheal attachment
platysma
4–0 Prolene
recurrent laryngeal nerve
2–0 silk
solid lesion
sternal notch
strap muscle
subcutaneous tissue
subcuticular suture
subplatysmal flap
subtotal thyroidectomy
superior pole
thyroid lobe
thyroid lobectomy
thyroid mass
thyroid notch
thyroid scanning
total thyroidectomy
tributary
3–0 Vicryl

Thyroid Sonogram

heterogeneous right gland
hypoechoic nodule
nuclear medicine study

Appendix 8

Drugs by Indication

ACIDOSIS (METABOLIC)

Alkalinizing Agent
- Polycitra®-K
- potassium citrate and citric acid
- sodium acetate
- sodium bicarbonate
- sodium lactate
- THAM®
- THAM-E®
- tromethamine

Electrolyte Supplement, Oral
- Enemol™ (Can)
- Fleet® Phospho®-Soda [OTC]
- sodium phosphates

ACROMEGALY

Ergot Alkaloid and Derivative
- Apo® Bromocriptine (Can)
- bromocriptine
- Parlodel®
- pergolide
- Permax®

Somatostatin Analog
- octreotide
- Sandostatin®
- Sandostatin LAR®

ADDISON DISEASE (SEE ADRENOCORTICAL FUNCTION ABNORMALITIES)

ADENOSINE DEAMINASE DEFICIENCY

Enzyme
- Adagen™
- pegademase (bovine)

ADRENAL HYPERPLASIA (SEE ADRENOCORTICAL FUNCTION ABNORMALITIES)

ADRENOCORTICAL FUNCTION ABNORMALITIES

Adrenal Corticosteroid
- Acthar®
- Adlone® Injection
- A-hydroCort® Injection
- Amcort® Injection
- A-methaPred® Injection
- Apo®-Prednisone (Can)
- Aristocort® Forte Injection
- Aristocort® Intralesional Injection
- Aristocort® Oral
- Aristospan® Intra-articular Injection
- Aristospan® Intralesional Injection
- Atolone® Oral
- betamethasone (systemic)
- Celestone® Oral
- Celestone® Phosphate Injection
- Celestone® Soluspan®
- Cel-U-Jec® Injection
- Cortef® Oral
- corticotropin
- cortisone acetate
- Cortone® Acetate
- Decadron® Injection
- Decadron®-LA
- Decadron® Oral
- Decaject®
- Decaject-LA®
- Delta-Cortef® Oral
- Deltasone®
- depMedalone® Injection
- Depoject® Injection

Depo-Medrol® Injection
Depopred® Injection
dexamethasone (systemic)
Dexasone®
Dexasone® L.A.
Dexone®
Dexone® LA
D-Med® Injection
Duralone® Injection
Haldrone®
Hexadrol®
H.P. Acthar® Gel
hydrocortisone (systemic)
Hydrocortone® Acetate Injection
Hydrocortone® Oral
Hydrocortone® Phosphate Injection
Jaa-Prednisone® (Can)
Kenacort® Oral
Kenaject® Injection
Kenalog® Injection
Key-Pred® Injection
Key-Pred-SP® Injection
Liquid Pred®
Medralone® Injection
Medrol® Oral
Medrol® Veriderm® Cream (Can)
methylprednisolone
Meticorten®
M-Prednisol® Injection
Novo-Prednisolone® (Can)
Novo-Prednisone® (Can)
Orasone®
paramethasone acetate
Pediapred® Oral
Predicort-50®
Prednicen-M®
prednisolone (systemic)
Prednisol® TBA Injection
prednisone
Prelone® Oral
Selestoject® (Can)
Solu-Cortef® Injection
Solu-Medrol® Injection
Solurex L.A.®
Stemex®
Tac™-3 Injection
Tac™-40 Injection
Triam-A® Injection
triamcinolone (systemic)
Triam Forte® Injection
Triamonide® Injection
Tri-Kort® Injection
Trilog® Injection
Trilone® Injection
Trisoject® Injection
Winpred (Can)

Adrenal Corticosteroid (Mineralocorticoid)
Florinef® Acetate
fludrocortisone

ALDOSTERONISM

Diuretic, Potassium Sparing
Aldactone®
Novo-Spiroton® (Can)
spironolactone

ALOPECIA

Antiandrogen
finasteride
Proscar®

Progestin
hydroxyprogesterone caproate
Hylutin®
Hyprogest® 250

Topical Skin Product
Apo®-Gain (Can)
Gen-Minoxidil (Can)
minoxidil
Minoxigaine™ (Can)
Rogaine® Topical

AMENORRHEA

Antihistamine
cyproheptadine
Periactin®

Ergot Alkaloid and Derivative

bromocriptine
Parlodel®
Gonadotropin
Factrel®
gonadorelin
Lutrepulse®
Progestin
Amen® Oral
Aygestin®
Crinone™
Curretab® Oral
Cycrin® Oral
Depo-Provera® Injection
hydroxyprogesterone caproate
Hylutin®
Hyprogest® 250
medroxyprogesterone acetate
Micronor®
norethindrone
NOR-QD®
Progestasert®
progesterone
Provera® Oral

ANGIOEDEMA (HEREDITARY)

Anabolic Steroid
stanozolol
Winstrol®
Androgen
Cyclomen® (Can)
danazol
Danocrine®

BALDNESS (SEE ALOPECIA)

BARTTER SYNDROME

Nonsteroidal Antiinflammatory Drug (NSAID)
Aches-N-Pain® [OTC]
Actiprofen® (Can)
Advil® [OTC]
Apo®-Ibuprofen (Can)
Apo®-Indomethacin (Can)
Children's Advil® Suspension
Children's Motrin® Suspension [OTC]
Excedrin® IB [OTC]
Genpril® [OTC]
Haltran® [OTC]
Ibuprin® [OTC]
ibuprofen
Ibuprohm® [OTC]
Ibu-Tab®
Indocin® I.V. Injection
Indocin® Oral
Indocin® SR Oral
Indocollyre® (Can)
indomethacin
Indotec (Can)
Junior Strength Motrin® [OTC]
Medipren® [OTC]
Menadol® [OTC]
Midol® IB [OTC]
Motrin®
Motrin® IB [OTC]
Novo-Methacin® (Can)
Novo-Profen® (Can)
Nu-Ibuprofen® (Can)
Nu-Indo® (Can)
Nuprin® [OTC]
Pamprin IB® [OTC]
Pedia-Profen™
Pro-Indo® (Can)
Saleto-200® [OTC]
Saleto-400®
Trendar® [OTC]
Uni-Pro® [OTC]

BREAST ENGORGEMENT (POSTPARTUM)

Androgen
fluoxymesterone
Halotestin®
Estrogen and Androgen Combination
Andro/Fem®

Deladumone®
depAndrogyn®
Depo-Testadiol®
Depotestogen®
Duo-Cyp®
Duratestrin®
estradiol and testosterone
Valertest No.1®

Estrogen Derivative
Alora® Transdermal
Cenestin™
C.E.S.™ (Can)
chlorotrianisene
Climara® Transdermal
Congest (Can)
depGynogen® Injection
Depo®-Estradiol Injection
Depogen® Injection
Dioval® Injection
Esclim® Transdermal
Estrace® Oral
Estraderm® Transdermal
estradiol
Estra-L® Injection
Estring®
Estro-Cyp® Injection
estrogens, conjugated, A (synthetic)
estrogens, conjugated (equine)
Gynogen L.A.® Injection
Premarin®
TACE®
Vivelle™ Transdermal

CACHEXIA

Antihistamine
cyproheptadine
Periactin®
PMS-Cyproheptadine (Can)

Progestin
Megace®
megestrol acetate

CARCINOMA

Androgen
Anabolin®
Androderm® Transdermal System
Android®
Andro-L.A.® Injection
Androlone®
Androlone®-D
Andropository® Injection
bicalutamide
Casodex®
Deca-Durabolin®
Delatest® Injection
Delatestryl® Injection
depAndro® Injection
Depotest® Injection
Depo®-Testosterone Injection
Duratest® Injection
Durathate® Injection
Everone® Injection
fluoxymesterone
Halotestin®
Histerone® Injection
Hybolin™ Decanoate
Hybolin™ Improved Injection
methyltestosterone
nandrolone
Neo-Durabolic
Oreton® Methyl
Tesamone® Injection
Teslac®
Testoderm® Transdermal System
testolactone
Testopel® Pellet
testosterone
Testred®
Virilon®

Antiandrogen
Androcur® (Can)
Androcur® Depot (Can)
cyproterone Canada only
Euflex® (Can)

Eulexin®
flutamide
Antineoplastic Agent, Hormone (Antiestrogen)
Femara™
letrozole
Estrogen and Androgen Combination
Estratest®
Estratest® H.S.
estrogens and methyltestosterone
Premarin® With Methyltestosterone
Estrogen Derivative
chlorotrianisene
diethylstilbestrol
estradiol
estrogens, conjugated (equine)
estrone
polyestradiol
Premarin®
Stilphostrol®
TACE®
Gonadotropin Releasing Hormone Analog
goserelin
Zoladex® Implant
Progestin
Amen® Oral
Androcur® (Can)
Androcur® Depot (Can)
Crinone™
Curretab® Oral
Cycrin® Oral
cyproterone (Can)
Depo-Provera® Injection
hydroxyprogesterone caproate
Hylutin®
Hyprogest® 250
medroxyprogesterone acetate
PMS-Progesterone (Can)
Progestasert®
progesterone
Progesterone Oil (Can)
Provera® Oral
Somatostatin Analog
octreotide
Sandostatin®
Sandostatin LAR®
Thyroid Product
Armour® Thyroid
Cytomel® Oral
Eltroxin®
Levo-T™
Levothroid®
levothyroxine
Levoxyl®
liothyronine
liotrix
PMS-Levothyroxine Sodium (Can)
S-P-T
Synthroid®
Thyrar®
thyroid
Thyroid Strong®
Thyrolar®
Triostat™ Injection

CONGENITAL SUCRASE-ISOMALTASE DEFICIENCY

Enzyme
sacrosidase
Sucraid™

CRYPTORCHIDISM

Gonadotropin
A.P.L.®
Chorex®
chorionic gonadotropin
Choron®
Corgonject®
Follutein®
Glukor®
Gonic®
Pregnyl®
Profasi® HP

CUSHING SYNDROME (SEE ADRENOCORTICAL FUNCTION ABNORMALITIES)

CUSHING SYNDROME (DIAGNOSTIC)

Diagnostic Agent
- metyrapone

CYSTIC FIBROSIS

Enzyme
- dornase alfa
- Pulmozyme®
- ZNP® Bar [OTC]
- phenelzine
- Prozac®
- Remeron®
- sertraline
- Zoloft™

DIABETES INSIPIDUS

Antidiuretic Hormone Analog
- Diapid® Nasal Spray
- lypressin

Hormone, Posterior Pituitary
- Pitressin®
- Pressyn® (Can)
- vasopressin

Vasopressin Analog, Synthetic
- DDAVP®
- desmopressin acetate
- Octostim® (Can)
- Stimate®

DIABETES MELLITUS, INSULIN-DEPENDENT (IDDM)

Antidiabetic Agent, Parenteral
- Humalog®
- Humulin® 50/50
- Humulin® 70/30
- Humulin® L
- Humulin® N
- Humulin® R
- Humulin® U
- Iletin® (Can)
- Iletin® II Pork (Can)
- Insulin Lente® L
- insulin preparations
- Lente®
- Lente® Iletin® I
- Lente® Iletin® II
- Novolin® 70/30
- Novolin® ge (Can)
- Novolin® L
- Novolin® N
- Novolin-Pen® II, -3 (Can)
- Novolin® R
- NPH Iletin® I
- NPH Insulin
- NPH-N
- Pork NPH
- Pork Regular Iletin® II
- Regular [Concentrated] Iletin® II U-500
- Regular Iletin® I
- Regular Insulin
- Regular Purified Pork Insulin
- Velosulin®

DIABETES MELLITUS, NON-INSULIN-DEPENDENT (NIDDM)

Antidiabetic Agent
- Actos™
- Diamicron® (Can)
- gliclazide (Can)
- pioglitazone

Antidiabetic Agent, Oral
- acarbose
- acetohexamide
- Albert® Glyburide (Can)
- Amaryl®
- Apo-Chlorpropamide® (Can)

- Apo-Glyburide® (Can)
- Apo-Tolbutamide® (Can)
- chlorpropamide
- Diabeta®
- Diabinese®
- Dymelor®
- Euglucon® (Can)
- Gen-Glybe (Can)
- glimepiride
- glipizide
- Glucophage®
- Glucotrol®
- Glucotrol® XL
- glyburide
- Glynase™ PresTab™
- Glyset®
- metformin
- Micronase®
- miglitol
- Mobenol® (Can)
- Novo-Butamide® (Can)
- Novo-Glyburide (Can)
- Novo-Metformin (Can)
- Novo-Propamide® (Can)
- Nu-Glyburide (Can)
- Orinase® Diagnostic Injection
- Orinase® Oral
- Precose®
- tolazamide
- tolbutamide
- Tolinase®

Antidiabetic Agent, Parenteral

- Humalog®
- Humulin® 50/50
- Humulin® 70/30
- Humulin® L
- Humulin® N
- Humulin® R
- Humulin® U
- Iletin® (Can)
- Iletin® II Pork (Can)
- Insulin Lente® L
- insulin preparations
- Lente®
- Lente® Iletin® I
- Lente® Iletin® II
- Novolin® 70/30
- Novolin® ge (Can)
- Novolin® L
- Novolin® N
- Novolin-Pen® II, -3 (Can)
- Novolin® R
- NPH Iletin® I
- NPH Insulin
- NPH-N
- Pork NPH
- Pork Regular Iletin® II
- Regular [Concentrated] Iletin® II U-500
- Regular Iletin® I
- Regular Insulin
- Regular Purified Pork Insulin
- Velosulin®

Hypoglycemic Agent, Oral

- Avandia®
- Diamicron® (Can)
- gliclazide (Can)
- Prandin™
- repaglinide
- rosiglitazone

Sulfonylurea Agent

- Diamicron® (Can)
- gliclazide (Can)

Thiazolidinedione Derivative

- Actos™
- Avandia®
- pioglitazone
- Rezulin®
- rosiglitazone
- troglitazone

DWARFISM

Growth Hormone

- Genotropin®
- human growth hormone
- Humatrope®

Norditropin®
Nutropin®
Nutropin® AQ
Protropin®
Saizen®
Serostim®

DYSMENORRHEA

Nonsteroidal Antiinflammatory Drug (NSAID)
Aches-N-Pain® [OTC]
Actron® [OTC]
Advil® [OTC]
Aleve® [OTC]
Anaprox®
Ansaid® Oral
Cataflam® Oral
Children's Advil® Suspension
Children's Motrin® Suspension [OTC]
diclofenac
diflunisal
Dolobid®
Excedrin® IB [OTC]
Feldene®
flurbiprofen
Genpril® [OTC]
Haltran® [OTC]
Ibuprin® [OTC]
ibuprofen
Ibuprohm® [OTC]
Ibu-Tab®
Junior Strength Motrin® [OTC]
ketoprofen
Medipren® [OTC]
mefenamic acid
Menadol® [OTC]
Midol® IB [OTC]
Motrin®
Motrin® IB [OTC]
Naprosyn®
naproxen
Nuprin® [OTC]
Orudis®
Orudis® KT [OTC]
Oruvail®
Pamprin IB® [OTC]
Pedia-Profen™
piroxicam
Saleto-200® [OTC]
Saleto-400®
Trendar® [OTC]
Uni-Pro® [OTC]
Voltaren® Oral
Voltaren®-XR Oral
Selective Cyclooxygenase-2 Inhibitor
rofecoxib
Vioxx®
Urispas®

GALACTORRHEA

Antihistamine
cyproheptadine
Periactin®
Ergot Alkaloid and Derivative
bromocriptine
Parlodel®

GOITER

Thyroid Product
Armour® Thyroid
Cytomel® Oral
Eltroxin®
Levo-T™
Levothroid®
levothyroxine
Levoxyl®
liothyronine
liotrix
PMS-Levothyroxine Sodium (Can)
S-P-T
Synthroid®
Thyrar®
thyroid
Thyroid Strong®

Thyrolar®
Triostat™ Injection

GROWTH HORMONE (DIAGNOSTIC)

Diagnostic Agent
Geref®
sermorelin acetate

GROWTH HORMONE DEFICIENCY

Diagnostic Agent
Dopar®
Larodopa®
levodopa
Growth Hormone
Genotropin®
human growth hormone
Humatrope®
Norditropin®
Nutropin®
Nutropin® AQ
Protropin®
Saizen®
Serostim®

HAIR LOSS (SEE ALOPECIA)

HARTNUP DISEASE

Vitamin, Water Soluble
niacinamide
Gastrointestinal Agent, Gastric or Duodenal Ulcer Treatment
ranitidine bismuth citrate
Tritec®
Gastrointestinal Agent, Miscellaneous
Bismatrol® [OTC]
bismuth subsalicylate
Pepto-Bismol® [OTC]
Macrolide (Antibiotic)
Biaxin™
clarithromycin
Penicillin
amoxicillin
Amoxil®
Trimox®
Wymox®
Tetracycline Derivative
Nor-tet® Oral
Panmycin® Oral
Robitet® Oral
Sumycin® Oral
Tetracap® Oral
tetracycline

HORMONAL IMBALANCE (FEMALE)

Progestin
Amen® Oral
Aygestin®
Crinone™
Curretab® Oral
Cycrin® Oral
Depo-Provera® Injection
hydroxyprogesterone caproate
Hylutin®
Hyprogest® 250
medroxyprogesterone acetate
Micronor®
norethindrone
NOR-QD®
PMS-Progesterone (Can)
Progestasert®
progesterone
Progesterone Oil (Can)
Provera® Oral

HYPERMENORRHEA (TREATMENT)

Contraceptive, Oral
Alesse™
Brevicon®
Demulen®
Desogen®
Estrostep® 21

Estrostep® Fe
ethinyl estradiol and desogestrel
ethinyl estradiol and ethynodiol diacetate
ethinyl estradiol and levonorgestrel
ethinyl estradiol and norethindrone
ethinyl estradiol and norgestimate
ethinyl estradiol and norgestrel
Genora® 0.5/35
Genora® 1/35
Genora® 1/50
Jenest-28™
Levlen®
Levlite®
Levora®
Loestrin®
Lo/Ovral®
mestranol and norethindrone
Modicon™
N.E.E.® 1/35
Nelova™ 0.5/35E
Nelova® 1/50M
Nelova™ 10/11
Nordette®
Norethin™ 1/35E
Norethin 1/50M
Norinyl® 1+35
Norinyl® 1+50
Ortho-Cept®
Ortho-Cyclen®
Ortho-Novum® 1/35
Ortho-Novum® 1/50
Ortho-Novum® 7/7/7
Ortho-Novum® 10/11
Ortho Tri-Cyclen®
Ovcon® 35
Ovcon® 50
Ovral®
Preven™
Tri-Levlen®
Tri-Norinyl®
Triphasil®
Zovia®

Contraceptive, Progestin Only
- norgestrel
- Ovrette®

HYPERPARATHYROIDISM

Vitamin D Analog
- doxercalciferol
- Hectorol®
- paricalcitol
- Zemplar™

HYPERTHYROIDISM

Antithyroid Agent
- methimazole
- Pima®
- potassium iodide
- propylthiouracil
- Propyl-Thyracil® (Can)
- SSKI®
- Tapazole®
- Thyro-Block®

Beta-Adrenergic Blocker
- Apo®-Propranolol (Can)
- Betachron®
- Detensol® (Can)
- Inderal®
- Inderal® LA
- Nu-Propranolol® (Can)
- propranolol

HYPOALDOSTERONISM

Diuretic, Potassium Sparing
- amiloride
- Midamor®

HYPOGLYCEMIA

Antihypoglycemic Agent
- B-D Glucose® [OTC]
- diazoxide
- glucagon
- glucose, instant
- Glutose® [OTC]
- Insta-Glucose® [OTC]
- Proglycem® Oral

HYPOGONADISM

Androgen
- Androderm® Transdermal System
- Android®
- Andro-L.A.® Injection
- Andropository® Injection
- Delatest® Injection
- Delatestryl® Injection
- depAndro® Injection
- Depotest® Injection
- Depo®-Testosterone Injection
- Duratest® Injection
- Durathate® Injection
- Everone® Injection
- Histerone® Injection
- methyltestosterone
- Oreton® Methyl
- Tesamone® Injection
- Testoderm® Transdermal System
- Testopel® Pellet
- testosterone
- Testred®
- Virilon®

Diagnostic Agent
- Factrel®
- gonadorelin
- Lutrepulse®

Estrogen Derivative
- Alora® Transdermal
- Aquest®
- Cenestin™
- C.E.S.™ (Can)
- chlorotrianisene
- Climara® Transdermal
- Congest (Can)
- depGynogen® Injection
- Depo®-Estradiol Injection
- Depogen® Injection
- diethylstilbestrol
- Dioval® Injection
- Esclim® Transdermal
- Estinyl®
- Estrace® Oral
- Estraderm® Transdermal
- estradiol
- Estra-L® Injection
- Estratab®
- Estring®
- Estro-Cyp® Injection
- estrogens, conjugated, A (synthetic)
- estrogens, conjugated (equine)
- estrogens, esterified
- estrone
- estropipate
- ethinyl estradiol
- Femogen® (Can)
- Gynogen L.A.® Injection
- Honvol® (Can)
- Kestrone®
- Menest®
- Neo-Estrone® (Can)
- Oestrillin® (Can)
- Ogen® Oral
- Ogen® Vaginal
- Ortho-Est® Oral
- Premarin®
- Stilphostrol®
- TACE®
- Vivelle™ Transdermal

HYPOPARATHYROIDISM

Diagnostic Agent
- Parathar™
- teriparatide

Vitamin D Analog
- Calciferol™
- Calcijex™
- calcitriol
- DHT™
- dihydrotachysterol
- Drisdol®
- ergocalciferol
- Hytakerol®
- Ostoforte® (Can)
- Radiostol® (Can)
- Rocaltrol®

HYPOTHYROIDISM

Thyroid Product
- Armour® Thyroid
- Cytomel® Oral
- Eltroxin®
- Levo-T™
- Levothroid®
- levothyroxine
- Levoxyl®
- liothyronine
- liotrix
- PMS-Levothyroxine Sodium (Can)
- S-P-T
- Synthroid®
- Thyrar®
- thyroid
- Thyroid Strong®
- Thyrolar®
- Triostat™ Injection
- salicylic acid and propylene glycol

IMPOTENCY

Androgen
- Android®
- methyltestosterone
- Oreton® Methyl
- Testred®
- Virilon®

Miscellaneous Product
- Aphrodyne™
- Dayto Himbin®
- Yocon®
- yohimbine
- Yohimex™

Vasodilator
- ethaverine

INFERTILITY

Antigonadotropic Agent
- Antagon™
- ganirelix

Ovulation Stimulator
- Follistim®
- follitropin alpha
- follitropin beta
- Gonal-F®

INFERTILITY (FEMALE)

Ergot Alkaloid and Derivative
- bromocriptine
- Parlodel®

Gonadotropin
- A.P.L.®
- Chorex®
- chorionic gonadotropin
- Choron®
- Corgonject®
- Follutein®
- Glukor®
- Gonic®
- Humegon™
- menotropins
- Pergonal®
- Pregnyl®
- Profasi® HP
- Repronex™

Ovulation Stimulator
- Clomid®
- clomiphene
- Milophene®
- Serophene®

Progestin
- Crinone™
- Progestasert®
- progesterone
- Progesterone Oil (Can)

INFERTILITY (MALE)

Gonadotropin
- A.P.L.®
- Chorex®
- chorionic gonadotropin
- Choron®
- Corgonject®
- Follutein®
- Glukor®
- Gonic®
- Humegon™

menotropins
Pergonal®
Pregnyl®
Profasi® HP
Repronex™

KETOSIS (SEE ACIDOSIS—METABOLIC)

LACTATION (SUPPRESSION)

Ergot Alkaloid and Derivative
Apo® Bromocriptine (Can)
bromocriptine
Parlodel®

MALNUTRITION

Electrolyte Supplement, Oral
zinc sulfate
Nutritional Supplement
cysteine
glucose polymers
Moducal® [OTC]
Polycose® [OTC]
Sumacal® [OTC]
Trace Element
Chroma-Pak®
Iodopen®
Molypen®
M.T.E.-4®
M.T.E.-5®
M.T.E.-6®
MulTE-PAK-4®
MulTE-PAK-5®
Neotrace-4®
PedTE-PAK-4®
Pedtrace-4®
P.T.E.-4®
P.T.E.-5®
Sele-Pak®
Selepen®
Trace-4®
trace metals
Zinca-Pak®
zinc chloride
Vitamin
Adeflor®
ADEKs® Pediatric Drops
Becotin® Pulvules®
Cefol® Filmtab®
Chromagen® OB [OTC]
Eldercaps® [OTC]
Icaps® (Can)
LKV-Drops® [OTC]
Multi Vit® Drops [OTC]
M.V.C.® 9 + 3
M.V.I.®-12
M.V.I.® Concentrate
M.V.I.® Pediatric
Natabec® [OTC]
Natabec® FA [OTC]
Natabec® Rx
Natalins® [OTC]
Natalins® Rx
NeoVadrin® [OTC]
Niferex®-PN
Poly-Vi-Flor®
Poly-Vi-Sol® [OTC]
Pramet® FA
Pramilet® FA
Prenavite® [OTC]
Secran®
Stresstabs® 600 Advanced Formula Tablets [OTC]
Stuartnatal® 1 + 1
Stuart Prenatal® [OTC]
Therabid® [OTC]
Theragran® [OTC]
Theragran® Hematinic®
Theragran® Liquid [OTC]
Theragran-M® [OTC]
Tri-Vi-Flor®
Tri-Vi-Sol® [OTC]
Unicap® [OTC]
Vicon Forte®
Vicon® Plus [OTC]

- Vi-Daylin® [OTC]
- Vi-Daylin/F®
- vitamin, multiple (injectable)
- vitamin, multiple (oral)
- vitamin, multiple (pediatric)
- vitamin, multiple (prenatal)

Vitamin, Fat Soluble

- Amino-Opti-E® [OTC]
- Aquasol A®
- Aquasol E® [OTC]
- Del-Vi-A®
- E-Complex-600® [OTC]
- E-Vitamin® [OTC]
- Palmitate-A® 5000 [OTC]
- vitamin A
- vitamin E
- Vita-Plus® E Softgels® [OTC]
- Vitec® [OTC]

Vitamin, Water Soluble

- Apatate® [OTC]
- Betalin®S
- Gevrabon® [OTC]
- Lederplex® [OTC]
- Lipovite® [OTC]
- Mega B® [OTC]
- Megaton™ [OTC]
- Mucoplex® [OTC]
- NeoVadrin® B Complex [OTC]
- Nestrex®
- Orexin® [OTC]
- pyridoxine
- Surbex® [OTC]
- thiamine
- vitamin B complex

MARFAN SYNDROME

Rauwolfia Alkaloid

- reserpine
- Serpalan®

MENOPAUSE

Ergot Alkaloid and Derivative

- belladonna, phenobarbital, and ergotamine tartrate
- Bellergal-S®
- Bel-Phen-Ergot S®
- Phenerbel-S®

Estrogen and Androgen Combination

- Andro/Fem®
- Deladumone®
- depAndrogyn®
- Depo-Testadiol®
- Depotestogen®
- Duo-Cyp®
- Duratestrin®
- estradiol and testosterone
- Valertest No. 1®

Estrogen and Progestin Combination

- Activelle™
- estradiol and norethindrone
- estrogens and medroxyprogesterone
- Premphase™
- Prempro™

Estrogen Derivative

- Alora® Transdermal
- Cenestin™
- chlorotrianisene
- Climara® Transdermal
- depGynogen® Injection
- Depo®-Estradiol Injection
- Depogen® Injection
- diethylstilbestrol
- Dioval® Injection
- Esclim® Transdermal
- Estinyl®
- Estrace® Oral
- Estraderm® Transdermal
- estradiol
- Estra-L® Injection
- Estratab®
- Estring®
- Estro-Cyp® Injection
- estrogens, conjugated, A (synthetic)
- estrogens, conjugated (equine)
- estrogens, esterified
- ethinyl estradiol
- Gynogen L.A.® Injection

Menest®
Premarin®
Stilphostrol®
TACE®
Vivelle™ Transdermal

MENORRHAGIA

Androgen
danazol
Danocrine®

METABOLIC BONE DISEASE

Vitamin D Analog
calcifediol
Calderol®

OBESITY

Adrenergic Agonist Agent
Acutrim® 16 Hours [OTC]
Acutrim® II, Maximum Strength [OTC]
Acutrim® Late Day [OTC]
Control® [OTC]
Dexatrim® Pre-Meal [OTC]
Maximum Strength Dex-A-Diet® [OTC]
Maximum Strength Dexatrim® [OTC]
Phenoxine® [OTC]
Phenyldrine® [OTC]
phenylpropanolamine
Unitrol® [OTC]
Amphetamine
Adderall®
amphetamine
Desoxyn®
Dexedrine®
dextroamphetamine
dextroamphetamine and amphetamine
methamphetamine
Anorexiant
benzphetamine
Bontril PDM®
Bontril® Slow-Release
Didrex®
diethylpropion
Dital®
Dyrexan-OD®
Mazanor®
mazindol
Melfiat-105® Unicelles®
Meridia™
phendimetrazine
Plegine®
Prelu-2®
Rexigen Forte®
Sanorex®
sibutramine
Tenuate®
Tenuate® Dospan®

OSTEOPOROSIS

Bisphosphonate Derivative
alendronate
Aredia™
Didronel®
etidronate disodium
Fosamax®
pamidronate
Electrolyte Supplement, Oral
calcium glubionate
calcium lactate
calcium phosphate, dibasic
Neo-Calglucon® [OTC]
Posture® [OTC]
Estrogen and Progestin Combination
estrogens and medroxyprogesterone
Premphase™
Prempro™
Estrogen Derivative
Alora® Transdermal
Cenestin™
chlorotrianisene
Climara® Transdermal
Congest (Can)
depGynogen® Injection
Depo®-Estradiol Injection

Depogen® Injection
diethylstilbestrol
Dioval® Injection
Esclim® Transdermal
Estinyl®
Estrace® Oral
Estraderm® Transdermal
estradiol
Estra-L® Injection
Estratab®
Estring®
Estro-Cyp® Injection
estrogens, conjugated, A (synthetic)
estrogens, conjugated (equine)
estrogens, esterified
ethinyl estradiol
Gynogen L.A.® Injection
Menest®
Premarin®
Stilphostrol®
TACE®
Vivelle™ Transdermal

Mineral, Oral
fluoride

Polypeptide Hormone
Calcimar®
calcitonin
Cibacalcin®
Miacalcin®
Miacalcin® Nasal Spray
Osteocalcin®
Salmonine®

Selective Estrogen Receptor Modulator (SERM)
Evista®
raloxifene

OVARIAN FAILURE

Estrogen and Progestin Combination
estrogens and medroxyprogesterone
Premphase™
Prempro™

Estrogen Derivative
Alora® Transdermal
Aquest®
Cenestin™
Climara® Transdermal
depGynogen® Injection
Depo®-Estradiol Injection
Depogen® Injection
Dioval® Injection
Esclim® Transdermal
Estrace® Oral
Estraderm® Transdermal
estradiol
Estra-L® Injection
Estratab®
Estring®
Estro-Cyp® Injection
estrogens, conjugated, A (synthetic)
estrogens, conjugated (equine)
estrogens, esterified
estrone
estropipate
Gynogen L.A.® Injection
Kestrone®
Menest®
Ogen® Oral
Ogen® Vaginal
Ortho-Est® Oral
Premarin®
Vivelle™ Transdermal

OVULATION

Ovulation Stimulator
Clomid®
clomiphene
Milophene®
Serophene®

OVULATION INDUCTION

Gonadotropin
A.P.L.®
Chorex®
chorionic gonadotropin
Choron®
Corgonject®
Follutein®

Glukor®
Gonic®
Humegon™
menotropins
Pergonal®
Pregnyl®
Profasi® HP
Repronex™
Ovulation Stimulator
Fertinex®
Metrodin®
urofollitropin

PAIN (DIABETIC NEUROPATHY NEURALGIA)

Analgesic, Topical
capsaicin
Capsin® [OTC]
Capzasin-P® [OTC]
Dolorac™ [OTC]
No Pain-HP® [OTC]
R-Gel® [OTC]
Zostrix® [OTC]
Zostrix®-HP [OTC]

PANCREATIC EXOCRINE INSUFFICIENCY (DIAGNOSTIC)

Diagnostic Agent
secretin
Secretin-Ferring Powder

PANCREATIC EXOCRINE INSUFFICIENCY

Enzyme
Cotazym®
Cotazym-S®
Creon®
Creon® 10
Creon® 20
Digepepsin®
Digess®8000 (Can)
Donnazyme®
Hi-Vegi-Lip®
Ilozyme®
Ku-Zyme® HP
Pancrease®
Pancrease® MT
pancreatin
Pancrecarb®
pancrelipase
Protilase®
Ultrase® MT
Viokase®
Zymase®

PITUITARY FUNCTION TEST (GROWTH HORMONE)

Diagnostic Agent
arginine
R-Gene®

PSEUDOHYPOPARATHYROIDISM

Vitamin D Analog
Calciferol™
Calcijex™
calcitriol
DHT™
dihydrotachysterol
Drisdol®
ergocalciferol
Hytakerol®
Ostoforte® (Can)
Radiostol® (Can)
Rocaltrol®

PUBERTY (DELAYED)

Androgen
Androderm® Transdermal System
Android®
Andro-L.A.® Injection

Andropository® Injection
Delatest® Injection
Delatestryl® Injection
depAndro® Injection
Depotest® Injection
Depo®-Testosterone Injection
Duratest® Injection
Durathate® Injection
Everone® Injection
fluoxymesterone
Halotestin®
Histerone® Injection
methyltestosterone
Oreton® Methyl
Tesamone® Injection
Testoderm® Transdermal System
Testopel® Pellet
testosterone
Testred®
Virilon®

Diagnostic Agent
Factrel®
gonadorelin
Lutrepulse®

PUBERTY (PRECOCIOUS)

Gonadotropin Releasing Hormone Analog
histrelin
Supprelin™

Hormone, Posterior Pituitary
nafarelin
Synarel®

Luteinizing Hormone-Releasing Hormone Analog
leuprolide acetate
Lupron®
Lupron Depot®
Lupron Depot-3® Month
Lupron Depot-4® Month
Lupron Depot-Ped®

SALIVATION (EXCESSIVE)

Anticholinergic Agent
Anaspaz®
A-Spas® S/L
atropine
Cantil®
Cystospaz®
Cystospaz-M®
Donnamar®
ED-SPAZ®
Gastrosed™
glycopyrrolate
hyoscyamine
I-Tropine®
Levbid®
Levsin®
Levsinex®
Levsin/SL®
mepenzolate
Robinul®
Robinul® Forte
scopolamine

SERUM THYROGLOBULIN (TG) TESTING

Diagnostic Agent
Thyrogen®
thyrotropin alpha

SWEATING

Alpha-Adrenergic Blocking Agent
Dibenzyline®
phenoxybenzamine

SYNCOPE

Adrenergic Agonist Agent
Adrenalin® Chloride
epinephrine
isoproterenol
Isuprel®

Respiratory Stimulant
- ammonia spirit, aromatic
- Aromatic Ammonia
  - Aspirols®

SYNDROME OF INAPPROPRIATE SECRETION OF ANTIDIURETIC HORMONE (SIADH)

Tetracycline Derivative
- Declomycin®
- demeclocycline

THYROID FUNCTION (DIAGNOSTIC)

Diagnostic Agent
- Combantrin® (Can)
- protirelin
- Relefact® TRH
- Thypinone®
- Thyrel® TRH
- thyrotropin
- Thytropar®

THYROIDITIS

Thyroid Product
- Armour® Thyroid
- Cytomel® Oral
- Eltroxin®
- Levo-T™
- Levothroid®
- levothyroxine
- Levoxyl®
- liothyronine
- liotrix
- PMS-Levothyroxine Sodium (Can)
- S-P-T
- Synthroid®
- Thyrar®
- thyroid
- Thyroid Strong®
- Thyrolar®
- Triostat™ Injection

THYROTOXIC CRISIS

Antithyroid Agent
- methimazole
- Pima®
- potassium iodide
- propylthiouracil
- Propyl-Thyracil® (Can)
- SSKI®
- Tapazole®
- Thyro-Block®

TURNER SYNDROME

Androgen
- Oxandrin®
- oxandrolone

ULCER, DIABETIC FOOT OR LEG

Topical Skin Product
- becaplermin
- Regranex®

WILSON DISEASE

Chelating Agent
- Syprine®
- trientine

VASOACTIVE INTESTINAL PEPTIDE-SECRETING TUMOR (VIP)

Somatostatin Analog
- octreotide
- Sandostatin®
- Sandostatin LAR®

ZOLLINGER-ELLISON SYNDROME (DIAGNOSTIC)

Diagnostic Agent
- secretin
- Secretin-Ferring Powder

ZOLLINGER-ELLISON SYNDROME

Antacid
- calcium carbonate and simethicone
- magaldrate
- magaldrate and simethicone
- magnesium hydroxide
- magnesium oxide
- Maox®
- Phillips'® Milk of Magnesia [OTC]
- Riopan® [OTC]
- Riopan Plus® [OTC]
- Titralac® Plus Liquid [OTC]

Antineoplastic Agent
- streptozocin
- Zanosar®

Diagnostic Agent
- pentagastrin
- Peptavlon®

Gastric Acid Secretion Inhibitor
- Aciphex™
- lansoprazole
- omeprazole
- Prevacid®
- Prilosec™
- rabeprazole

Histamine H2 Antagonist
- cimetidine
- famotidine
- Pepcid®
- Pepcid RPD®
- ranitidine hydrochloride
- Tagamet®
- Tagamet-HB® [OTC]
- Zantac®
- Zantac® 75 [OTC]

Prostaglandin
- Cytotec®
- misoprostol

NOTES

NOTES

NOTES

NOTES

NOTES

NOTES

NOTES

NOTES

NOTES